JOE FRIEL'S HIGH-PERFORMANCE CYCLIST

This book is dedicated to the hundreds of athletes
I've trained during my coaching career.

JOE FRIEL'S HIGH-PERFORMANCE CYCLIST

THE COMPLETE TRAINING MANUAL

BLOOMSBURY SPORT
LONDON · OXFORD · NEW YORK · NEW DELHI · SYDNEY

BLOOMSBURY SPORT
Bloomsbury Publishing Plc
50 Bedford Square, London, WC1B 3DP, UK
Bloomsbury Publishing Ireland Limited
29 Earlsfort Terrace, Dublin 2, Ireland

BLOOMSBURY, BLOOMSBURY SPORT and the Diana logo are trademarks of Bloomsbury Publishing Plc

First published in Great Britain 2025

Copyright © Joe Friel, 2025

Joe Friel has asserted his right under the Copyright, Designs and Patents Act, 1988, to be identified as Author of this work

For legal purposes the Acknowledgments on p. 255 constitute an extension of this copyright page

All rights reserved. No part of this publication may be: i) reproduced or transmitted in any form, electronic or mechanical, including photocopying, recording or by means of any information storage or retrieval system without prior permission in writing from the publishers; or ii) used or reproduced in any way for the training, development or operation of artificial intelligence (AI) technologies, including generative AI technologies. The rights holders expressly reserve this publication from the text and data mining exception as per Article 4(3) of the Digital Single Market Directive (EU) 2019/790

Bloomsbury Publishing Plc does not have any control over, or responsibility for, any third-party websites referred to or in this book. All internet addresses given in this book were correct at the time of going to press. The author and publisher regret any inconvenience caused if addresses have changed or sites have ceased to exist, but can accept no responsibility for any such changes

Every reasonable effort has been made to trace copyright holders of material reproduced in this book, but if any have been inadvertently overlooked the publishers would be glad to hear from them.

A catalogue record for this book is available from the British Library

Library of Congress Cataloguing-in-Publication data has been applied for

ISBN: PB: 978-1-3994-1850-8; eBook: 978-1-3994-1854-6; ePDF: 978-1-3994-1853-9

2 4 6 8 10 9 7 5 3 1

Typeset in Helvetica Neue

Design by Emil Dacanay and Sian Rance for D.R. Ink

Interior images by Getty Images, with the exception of pp. 32/3 and 111/2 by Shutterstock

Printed and bound in China by C&C Offset Printing Co., Ltd.

To find out more about our authors and books visit www.bloomsbury.com and sign up for our newsletters. For product safety related questions contact productsafety@bloomsbury.com

Note: While every effort has been made to ensure that the content of this book is as technically accurate and as sound as possible, neither the author nor the publishers can accept responsibility for any injury or loss sustained as a result of the use of this material.

CONTENTS

- **PROLOGUE** — 6
- **1. GETTING STARTED** — 12
- **2. TRAINING BASICS** — 32
- **3. EXERTION** — 56
- **4. PLANNING** — 82
- **5. TRAINING DETAILS** — 110
- **6. STRESS AND REST** — 144
- **7. MINDSET** — 168
- **8. COMMON QUESTIONS** — 186
- **9. RACE DAY** — 210
- **EPILOGUE** — 232

APPENDIX — 240
GLOSSARY — 249
ACKNOWLEDGMENTS — 255
REFERENCES — 256
ABOUT THE AUTHOR — 269
INDEX — 270

PROLOGUE

Exactly what "high performance" means in cycling is surprisingly hard to nail down. It's a term usually meant for those who race at the highest levels in cycling sports—grand tours, monuments, Olympics, world championships, and such. But that's not who this book is meant for. So, I'd like to refocus that term. Rather than being a catchphrase only for riders at the elite levels of racing, let's instead think of it as the level of performance that will help you achieve *your* goals this season. It's *your* achievements that you and I are concerned about, not how the latest winner of France's *maillot jaune* goes about training. If you set a high race goal—high for you—and perform at a level that achieves it, then you are a high-performance athlete in my book.

It really doesn't make any difference what anyone else might do. It's just about how you perform relative to your lofty goal on race day. For you to accomplish this at *your* highest level, you and I must come up with a unique and personalized way of training. We'll do that, but it will be no small task.

As you work your way through my book, I will prompt you to make decisions about your goal, the training methods you will use, equipment choices, your support team, and many other matters. You may eventually decide the task is just too great and so you will go back to what you've done in the past. If that was successful, and you truly were a high-performance rider, I have no problem with such a decision. Everyone is unique. But if you've not achieved what you sense you are capable of then I'd strongly suggest hanging in there with me through the entire book. I think I can help you.

There are endless ways to prepare for competition. And I've been studying them for decades. While I've got a fairly good idea of how to train, I don't know anything about you. You're exceptional as an athlete in many ways, but you'll have to pay close attention to the training details in the following chapters to

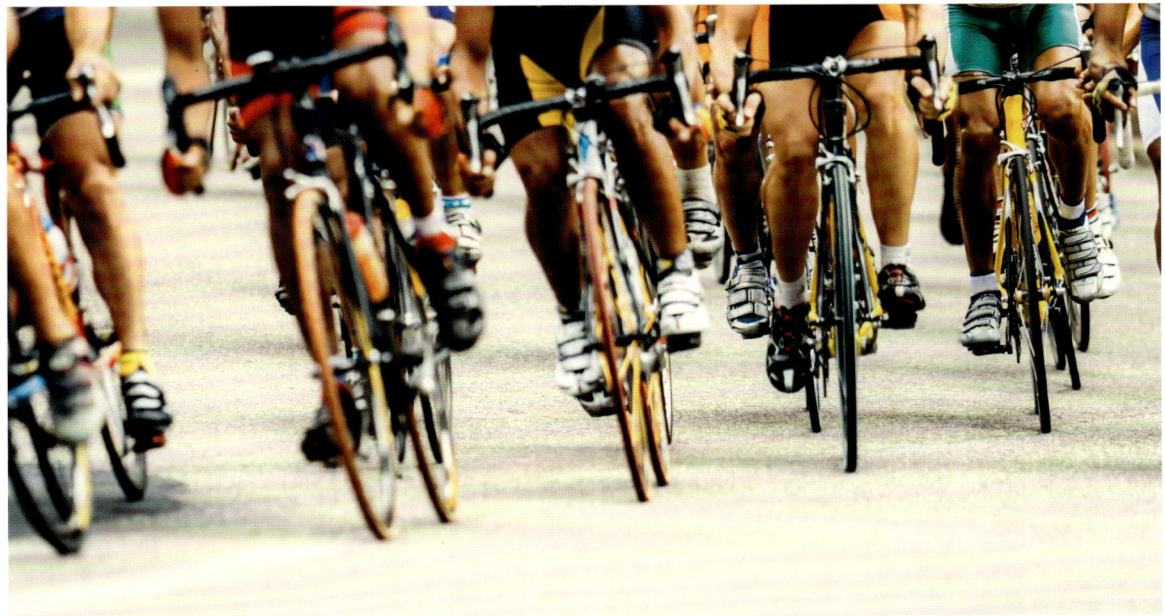

determine the best way for *you* to train given your uniqueness. How do you respond to frequent workouts? How often do you need a day off? When should your extended rest and recovery (R&R) breaks be? Do you get through long rides without difficulty or do a few hours in the saddle take a serious toll on you? How about training intensity? If you do a set of high-intensity intervals, does that workout wipe you out for the next few days or do you bounce back quickly? What's the best diet for you leading up to the race? How quickly do you respond to training? Those are all good questions, but that's a lot for you to ponder. Unfortunately, there's a lot more. I'm just skimming the surface here. Training for high-performance racing is certainly not simple.

Here's another way of thinking about a high-performance season. If you search "high performance" online, you'll soon come across comments about beating an opponent. That's a problematic concept. Of course, your goal could mean a position on the podium, which indeed does imply that you beat other riders that day, but performance is strictly about you and your goal, not about anyone else in the race. Or, on the other end of the spectrum, it could mean you finish the event and that could be a great accomplishment given where you may be as a rider right now. High performance for us going forward means accomplishing *your* challenging event goal and building on that in future seasons. It is not about who you beat.

As athletes, we need to move away from measuring our success by whether we "beat others." That's a narrow and somewhat egotistical way of measuring achievement in sport. While it's okay to gauge your race performances on how well you did relative to your competition, basing your success entirely on who you beat is a bit misguided. Such a result often comes down to who showed up that day and what kind of shape they were in.

There are more important outcomes we can measure. Performance in sport is more about what you accomplish relative to yourself. If at the end of the season you are performing at a higher level than previously, that's a success. If you are getting faster under similar conditions, then you are improving regardless of what anyone else has achieved.

Being a high-performance cyclist is challenging, but it really isn't complicated. It's mostly about having a dream and pursuing it persistently and patiently. I'll come back to this topic frequently in the following chapters. I'll talk about how to believe in yourself—like you never have before. And how riding your bike must have a purpose that you fully accept and pursue every day of every week of every month. You can't let up. That doesn't mean you can't have fun on your bike and enjoy life along the way. You can. And I'm sure you will. But when it's time to do a serious ride, you need to get focused. I'll also tell you how to do that.

I'll make a confession upfront: I don't have a guaranteed formula for your high-performance cycling success. There is no secret, perfect way of training. Each athlete is unique in many ways. It's my job as your coach in this book to help you figure out what that way is—with your help, of course. There are, however, certain principles that have proven to be effective across the board in pursuing high performance, which we'll pay close attention to. Without digging too deeply into the science behind these principles, I'll briefly explain what they are about. Some may surprise you.

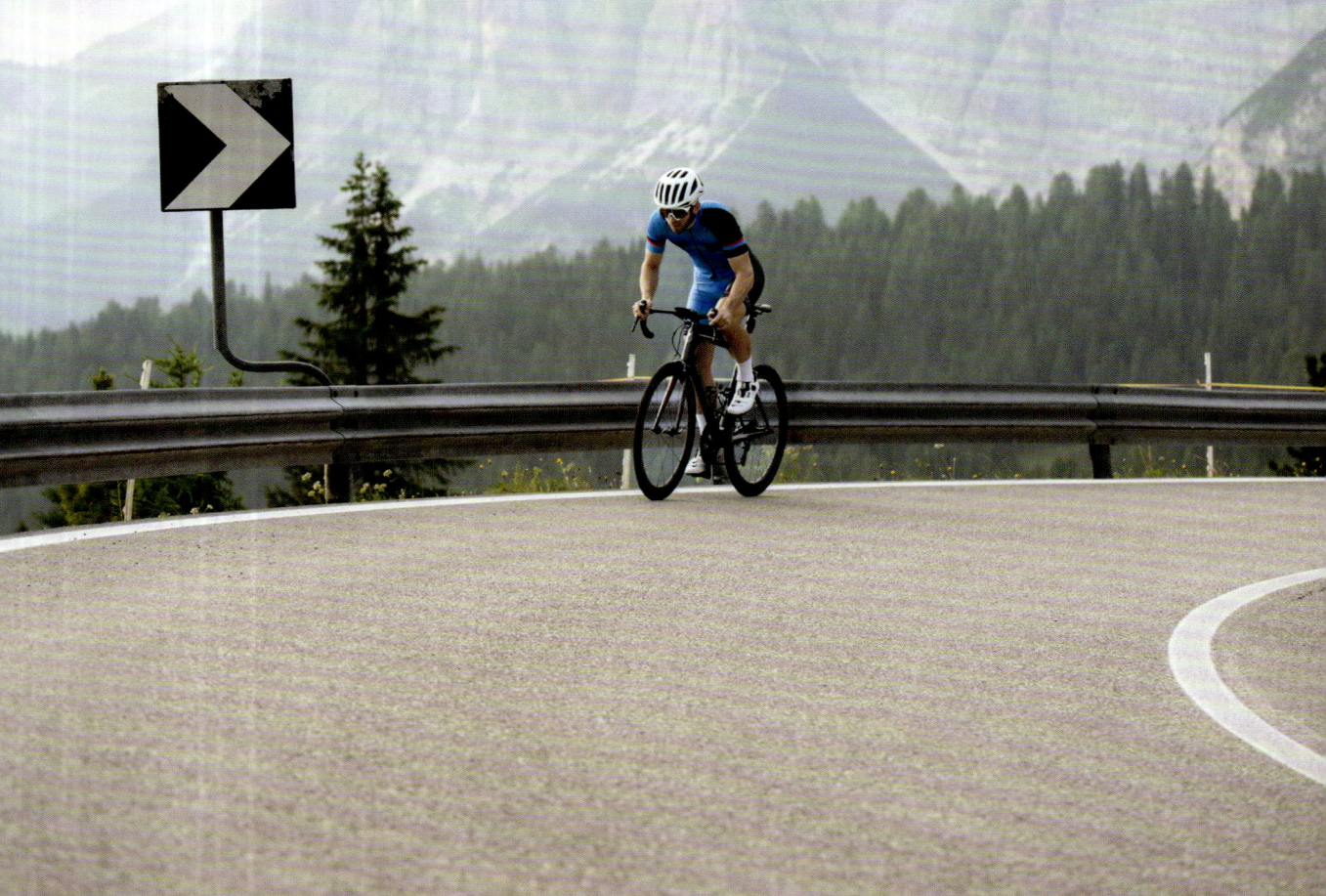

PROLOGUE

Being a high-performance cyclist is challenging, but it really isn't complicated. It's mostly about having a dream and pursuing it persistently and patiently.

The first principle of training is *individuality*. This just means that you are an individual with unique genes, talents, needs, lifestyle, habits, and lots more. We must always keep that in mind as we search for what is right for *your* training. Just because a pro or even a training partner does something that is very effective for them, that doesn't mean it's what you should do.

The second principle is *specificity*. You must train for your goal event, not something else. And the closer you get to that event, the more your training must become like the race. We will, however, start the season by doing things that aren't specific. For example, you'll do some cross-training in the very early season and lift weights. Those aren't "like" your race at all. But as the season progresses, we'll gradually cut back on the non-specific stuff and increase your focus on the bike. You'll need to trust me here. I know how effective the non-bike training can be very early in the year. It'll pay off. Of course, that doesn't mean you won't ride the bike at all. You most certainly will. Just not a lot at first. And we'll start making a gradual change in your training several weeks out from your first high-priority race. In the last few weeks before your race you will be training to match the expected demands of the race. Specificity is something we will gradually apply in your workouts as the season advances until you come to race day fully primed and ready to go.

Next is the principle of *progression*. What does that mean? We will start with a level of training which you know is manageable. Then over the course of the season, we will gradually increase the load. That doesn't mean I'm going to overwhelm you later with a bunch of workouts that leave you wasted. Instead, we will strive to keep the progression at a rate your body can easily adapt to. *Adaptation* is the key to progression. This will lead to you gradually becoming more fit and race-ready. This is critical for high performance.

Finally, the principle of *reversibility* simply says that if you stop training or significantly reduce the training load for a long time you will lose fitness. That's no surprise, I'm sure. But there's a caveat here. We will most certainly have to reduce your training load in the last few weeks before your most important race. I know that probably sounds like a problem given this principle. But there is a powerful reason and we'll do it in such a way that the impact on your fitness is minimal. I know, it probably sounds counterproductive to cut back on training approaching the race. But we must do it for you to come into *form* (I'll explain that later), which will bring you to a peak of fitness and race readiness. The purpose of coming into form is to get rid of fatigue while keeping fitness as high as you can, albeit with a very small amount lost. Because of this you'll feel great on race day and be ready for a truly

You'll have to keep a very close eye on your progress and make changes as you see the need. I'll help you make decisions. It will be challenging but a fun journey!

high-performance race. I know losing any fitness before a race sounds scary. Hang in there with me. It works.

Bottom line is that I don't know what exactly you'll have to do in training throughout the season yet, but I have a good idea of how you'll get started and what generally will happen along the way. You'll have to keep a very close eye on your progress and make changes as you see the need. I'll help you make decisions. It will be challenging but a fun journey!

Let me tell you about this book. There are nine chapters. Each starts with a featured athlete I've coached whose story represents the chapter's key topic. The athlete's story is intended to give you a realistic and in-depth look at how the athlete and I succeeded (or failed) to implement the concepts of that chapter. Each chapter also includes a brief explanation by a leading expert in the field on one of the key topics mentioned there. This may help you understand a complex topic by describing, from a different perspective than mine, how it is applied in training and racing. Along the way in each chapter, I'll provide "Key Takeaways" to summarize important topics. This is to help reinforce what you've just read and may also be used to quickly refresh your memory on the main points of a chapter when you come back to the book after an extended break from reading.

Chapter 1 is about getting started, laying the groundwork for your upcoming season. Here I'll describe how to set up your "team," determine your season's goals, and the equipment you will need to train for a high-performance season.

In Chapter 2 I'll tell you about "breakthrough" training and the fundamentals of a high-performance season. The most important points here have to do with the determiners of your race-day fitness—aerobic capacity, stamina, and sprint power. You'll read about these throughout the book. Read very carefully when you come to these topics. They are critical to your performance.

Chapter 3 does a deep dive into the most complex and misunderstood subject of training and racing—intensity. Here I'll tell you how to set your training zones, how to gauge fitness progress, and the use of heart rate and power to measure workout and race efforts. I always strive to keep this topic simple and easy to grasp as you will come to rely on it almost daily for the next few months.

How to plan your training and race season is covered in Chapter 4. We'll look at differing methodologies for training and when to use each one, laying out a training plan for the season, and designing your weekly training routine. This is a very important subject as you will come to rely on this plan to guide you to a high-performance season.

Chapter 5 carries the overview topics from Chapter 4 to a deeper level with an emphasis on preparing to race. Here I'll explain the basic and advanced abilities and how you can use them to prepare for your A-priority event.

Perhaps the most important part of the book is Chapter 6. It has to do with both stress and rest, which are probably the most ignored topics in endurance sports among self-coached athletes. If you read only one chapter, this should be it. Knowing when to go hard and when to back off is critical to success, yet it is often ignored. Understanding that stress and rest must be taken seriously is crucial if you are to succeed as a high-performance cyclist.

Chapter 7 simplifies some of the basic concepts of sport psychology. This is also a topic often disregarded by self-coached athletes. The athlete's training and racing mindset has been shown to be just as important to event outcomes as physical training. The body can achieve at a higher level if the mind allows it to.

I get questions from athletes on an almost daily basis. Chapter 8 addresses some of the most common ones I'm asked on topics such as diet, bodyweight, use of training time, and the consequences of age—both old and young.

Chapter 9 fittingly takes you right up to race day and immediately after. The key points have to do with the most challenging race conditions you can experience, what to do during Race week, race-day details, and managing your post-race review. Don't put off reading this chapter until the week of your race. There is a great deal that must be done in the preceding weeks to be ready for those last few days.

There are a lot of details on the following pages, many of which involve terminology you may not recognize. To help with this I've included a Glossary near the end of the book. Here you can look up words that you may not understand. Also near the end is an Appendix of workouts. These are the most basic types of rides I have cyclists do. At the start of the Appendix I'll suggest a way to design custom workouts.

I often get feedback from readers on how one of my books affected their training and racing, things they don't understand in my book, what they would like to know more about, and a broad range of questions on a wide array of subjects. I'm happy to answer your questions if I can. Should you need to reach me it can be done through my website at JoeFrielTraining.com. Please be patient as I get lots of inquiries. I will respond.

I look forward to helping you achieve your high-performance goal. Let's get started.

Chapter 6 on stress and rest is perhaps the most important part of this book. Knowing when to go hard and when to back off is critical to success.

1.
GETTING STARTED

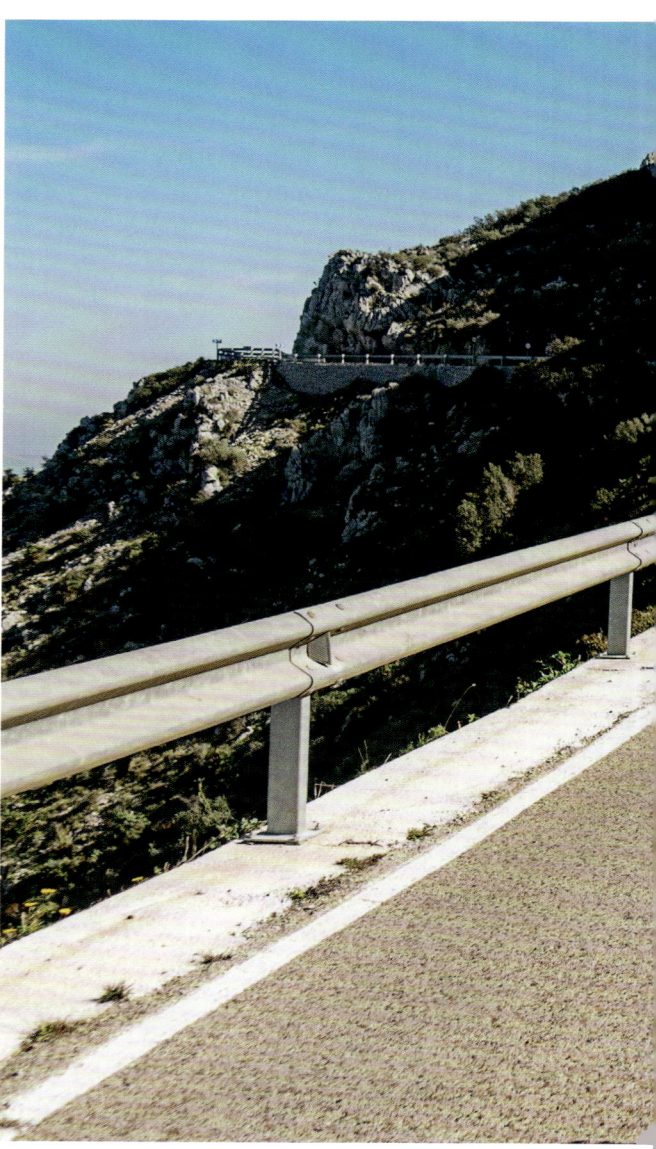

What does it take to perform at a high level, and how do you go about pulling all the details together? I'll touch on things such as how the coach and athlete work together, why you should surround yourself with a high-performance team, defining your goal for the season, how we will go about achieving it, the basics of a workout, and the first steps to be taken in preparing for the coming season.

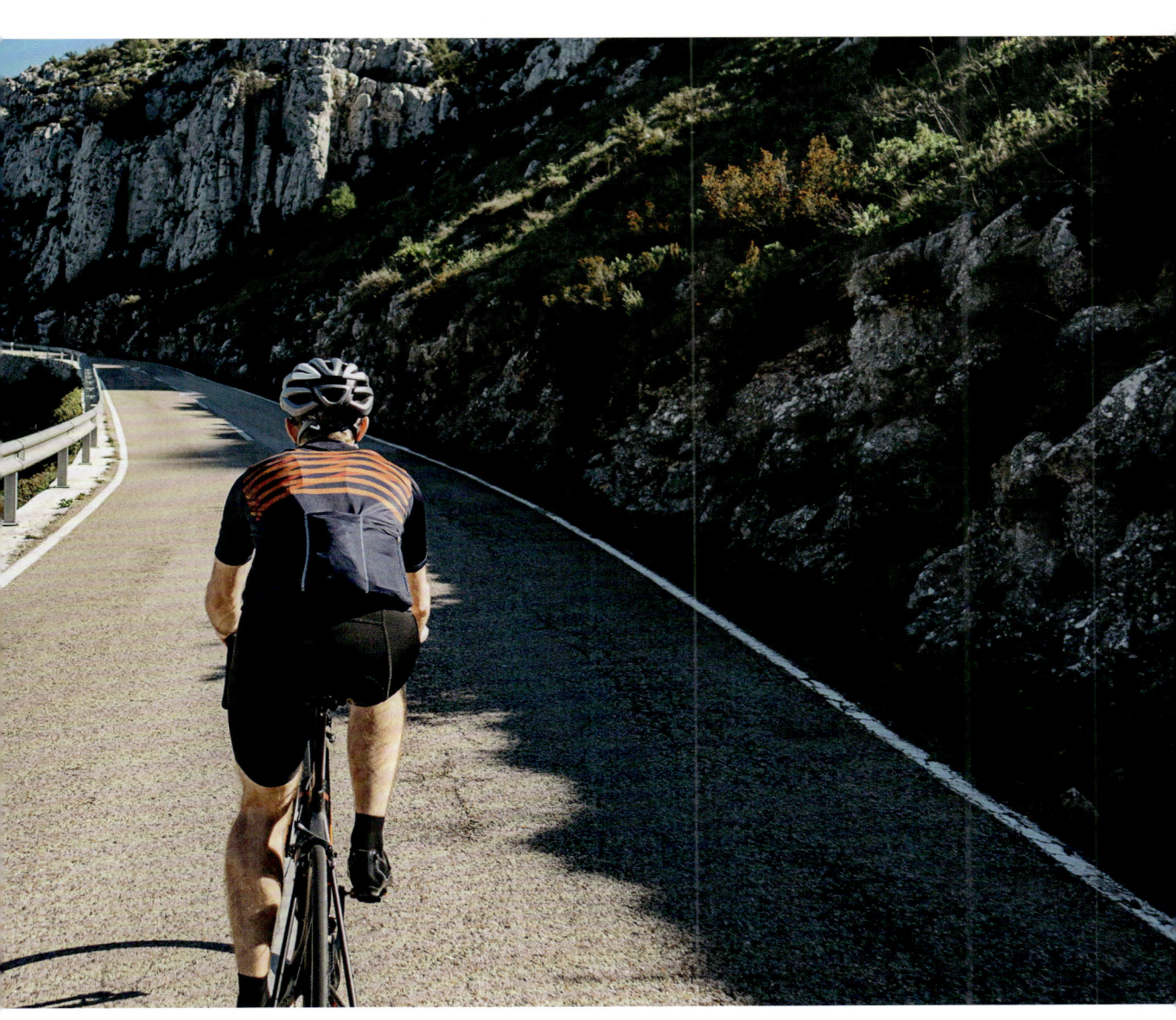

STEVE'S STORY

He sounded like a steam locomotive coming up behind me. The heavy breathing could be heard from 20 meters back. There was no greeting as he went by. Not even a smile. He wasn't holding anything back and had nothing to spare. At five years my senior he demolished my two-minute head start. Not only did he win his category that day, but he also set a new national time trial record for 60+ riders. Regardless of my outcome, however, his success made my day. You could never find a nicer guy—nor one who trained and raced as all-in as Steve did. He was a big guy for a cyclist. That's what made the National Time Trial Championship that summer just right for him. I had started coaching him the previous winter. We had never met before then, but as it turned out, we were aiming at the same race in late summer. His goal, since this would be his first year in the new race category, was to win the USA 20km National Time Trial Championship for his 60+ age category. No small task. He did it. Here's how.

Steve is an example of the kind of athlete I have been fortunate enough to coach over the last 40-some years. He stands out in many ways. He came to me with a truly high-performance goal. And while there was some doubt in his mind if he could pull it off at that first meeting, as I got to know him, the more I came to believe in his chances for success.

When we met, he had been riding for just short of a decade and was well known among central Nebraska riders for his power. But if the course turned uphill, he was off the back. At his size, he wasn't cut out to be a climber. Local, flat time trials were his specialty. He was hard to beat. As soon as he heard that the National Time Trial Championship would be on a flat course in New Mexico he made it a goal to be on the podium in his race category. However, when he sat down with me that winter there was a gnawing doubt in his mind. After all, he had never raced at Nationals and didn't know who the competition might be. This would be his first race outside of Nebraska and his first national championship event.

It was certainly a very high-performance goal so we talked about what it would take. I didn't pull any punches. It was obvious how big the challenge was and how little experience he had to back it up. He would have to be fully dedicated to the goal.

It meant his life for the next several months would have to be laser-focused on one thing—the National Championship.

We talked about what all the aspects of the training would mean: high volume weeks, very challenging interval sessions, serious weightlifting, a strict diet, 100 percent family support, and lots of sleep. Fortunately, he had retired from his career as a mechanical engineer recently. He had the time. He also demonstrated that he had the desire, but I had frequently seen athletes talk big months in advance. Could his enthusiasm make it through the next several months?

As he trained through that year, I came to feel quite positive about the direction we were heading. And I told him that. But I also told him upfront that he needed more racing experience. He needed to find a few time trials to enter that had top performers in his category. He set about doing some research and came up with three races spread over the course of the spring and summer. Two were state time trial championships and the third was a three-day stage race starting with a 20km time trial. Perfect. From this I was able to lay out a framework training plan for his season. And we got started training.

I also suggested that he do some research on previous podium riders in his category, what the time trial courses were like in those years, and their times. He must know what to expect. Winning a national championship isn't easy and he needed to have some idea upfront who the competition might be and how they had performed in past years. Another reason I asked him to do this research is that getting to know something about possible contenders is also a great motivator.

Along the way Steve faced some setbacks—a lingering head cold in late winter, a nasty crash on a group ride in the spring, and a few missed workouts due to family matters. This is all normal stuff for a rider. I didn't see them as being major obstacles as they occurred many weeks out from his goal race. I told him so. We just needed to become more cautious with such matters as we closed in on Nationals.

I didn't mollycoddle him or sugar-coat his chances. One thing I never do is lie to an athlete or exaggerate my expectations. Those will always come back to haunt both me and the rider. It's far better to be truthful, but it also means I must have a flexible plan just in case. Wishing and hoping won't do it. Regardless of all my initial seasonal planning, unanticipated change has always been the norm. I've never had an athlete finish a season without significant alterations to the annual training plan. It was no different with Steve.

Throughout the season he and I talked by phone at least once weekly. And, of course, I reviewed the workout spreadsheets he sent to me daily (this was before my business partners and I started TrainingPeaks). Our conversations always revolved around the same matters: how he was feeling and what he was thinking, how he felt about his recent training, what he thought was necessary going forward, my views on possible changes in our plan, what his lifestyle was like for the coming weeks, and what I saw the workout details to be for the following week. He always asked good questions and remained unflinchingly focused on his high-performance goal. He was the perfect client-athlete in so many ways.

THE COACH-ATHLETE RELATIONSHIP

Steve and I got along great. I believe our relationship had a lot to do with his success. The coach-athlete bond is always at the heart of the athlete's training. You've got to like and trust each other as you will spend a lot of time facing problems and making decisions together. In the same way, you and I must become a team. How you perform in this coming season depends largely on how well we blend. The problem is, I'm going to be a distant coach working from this book and there won't be weekly conversations, but we both want the same outcome—your race-day success. Of course, we haven't yet defined what "success" means. We will come back to that shortly.

YOUR TRAINING PLAN

I will help you lay out a training plan that will eventually lead to success in your race—I hope. There are no guarantees in sport. Your plan will be more than a schedule of workouts. That's the easy part. Going beyond the workouts, the plan will also include several lifestyle-related matters such as your support system, daily nutrition, race-day diet, sleep, R&R, mental focus, likely setbacks, injury avoidance, weight management, workouts, and race day details. With your help in identifying your personal needs, I'll make suggestions for these matters and more as we proceed.

There may well be times when you have concerns about the direction I'm taking you in or you may even disagree with what's in the plan. That's okay and to be expected. It's just a part of the coach-athlete relationship. My methodology when preparing an athlete for competition is to make it a "team" approach. You and I are at the team's core. We will expand the team a bit as I'll explain shortly. If I suggest something in the following chapters and you are sure there is a better way for you to do it, you win. I won't stand in your way. You are central to our purpose and certainly know yourself better than I ever will. I respect your understanding of how you respond to all aspects of training. So, if there appears to be some incongruity, we will do it your way.

SEEKING HELP

If you ever become confused or unsure about something I suggest in the following pages, go to my blog at JoeFrielTraining.com and search for the topic of your concern. There you will find nearly two decades of articles I've written on a broad array of topics. If that doesn't resolve the matter, and it's truly critical to your performance, reach out to me through my website by clicking on "About." It may take me a while to get back to you, but I promise I will answer. I'm here for you.

COACH-ATHLETE RELATIONSHIP:
ANDY KIRKLAND

For me, the most important aspect of developing a good coach-athlete relationship relates to the fact that the knowledge, beliefs, and values of an athlete are different from mine. Furthermore, we, as humans, do not always act logically and rationally in our own best interests and are not always truthful with ourselves. Maladaptive things like exercise addiction, overtraining, eating disorders and the associated Relative Energy Deficit in Sport (REDs) can emerge as a result. Such things are prevalent in high-performance cycling, greater than 30 percent in some instances. Therefore, my job is to help athletes be honest with themselves as well as with me. To do so means "getting inside their heads" to understand what drives athlete behaviors and then taking appropriate action to support more adaptive ones. This is only possible through developing strong coach-athlete relationships.

Of course, sometimes relationships do not work and are not meant to. This usually occurs where there are different expectations and a lack of role clarity. For example, if a rider simply wants me to prescribe workouts and my expectations of my role as a coach are more holistic, then frustration on both sides will occur and cracks in the relationship will appear very quickly. Challenges can also occur in cycling teams or funded programs where coaches and riders are "imposed" on each other in processes that are akin to arranged marriage.

Similarly, when an athlete requests that I coach them, I ask "Why me?" "Why am I the best coach for you, and who else have you contacted?" Unless they can answer such questions, I will ask them to come back to me when they can. Recently, I was contacted by a rider who had won at the highest level. They said they were looking for a coach but were speaking to other coaches, too. Over the next month we shared emails, chatted online, and got to know each other relatively well. I was questioned on what my approaches would be to training prescription, altitude training, and various other performance-related questions. In turn, I asked myself questions relating to how committed I could be to the rider, if I was willing to prioritize them above my own partner, and if I had the skills to support them achieve their goals. My answer was a clear "yes." I respected the fact that they expected me to provide deep justification for all my answers, and I liked them and enjoyed chatting, too. I also answered questions honestly, not simply telling them what I thought they wanted to hear. Ultimately, when the rider told me they had chosen to be coached by someone else and why, I respected them even more. After all, a good coach-athlete relationship should be an intimate and long-lasting one, built on openness, respect, and trust. The coach-athlete relationship is not one to be entered into lightly.

Of course, there is also a business element to coaching for many coaches. They need to develop a sustainable business model, through providing services that cyclists want and value in a cost-effective way. "Want" is different from "need" though. Better coaches balance them both, recognizing that a relationship cannot develop without addressing the want in the short-term, slowly helping athletes understand what they need over time. Less agile coaches may have a method or approach to address the wants of all their riders without adequately addressing needs. This often works in the short-to-medium term and can be an effective business model. The danger is that what is effective in business terms may be less sustainable in performance terms. Rather, a strong, agile, coach-athlete relationship and holistic practices are required to maintain a dynamic state of equilibrium in the long term.

Dr. Andrew Kirkland is a Lecturer in Sport Coaching at the University of Stirling, Scotland. He is a Chartered Scientist, an experienced triathlon coach, and an expert in endurance performance.

YOUR HIGH-PERFORMANCE TEAM

It takes a team to accomplish a truly high-performance goal. Assuming your goal will push you to your limits, we will need all the help we can get. For that, we must include others. The more supportive people we have behind you, the greater your chances of success.

YOUR TEAM'S CORE

The place to start is with those who already support you—your family and friends. They need to know what your goal is and why it's important to you. They must also understand that it's going to stretch you to your limits. Their help and support will be central to your success. Of course, they also have things in their lives that are important to them. Offer to assist them in whatever ways you can. If you are a parent, by doing this you are demonstrating a great way of seeing the world for your kids. It will serve as a huge lesson for them. Mutual support for those close to you goes a long way when everyone is striving together—and bonding—because of it.

YOUR CYCLING TEAM

If you ride for a team, bring them onboard next. Make sure they know what your goal is. A cycling team can do a lot to aid you in race success. They understand what is facing you and will be there for support if you make them aware of your goal. Besides riding with you, they can offer suggestions on your race, especially if you haven't done that event before. Other riders may be aware of the terrain, surfaces, weather, who typically shows up to race, and a host of other minute details. As with your family, you should offer to help your teammates prepare for their high-performance goal races. The more you help each other, the stronger your team becomes.

If you don't have a cycling team, you may have some training partners you frequently ride with. You're probably the best of buddies. Treat them as you would a team. Let them know your goal and ask for their help in achieving it. And, of course, return the favor. The more people who are aware of your goal behind you, the greater your chances of success.

OTHER MEMBERS OF YOUR TEAM

In this book I'm going to provide a few other "team" members as examples. These are the experts I call on when I seek help, whether that's for sport science, health, bike fit, equipment purchase, mechanical fixes, training expertise, sport psychology, data analysis, or nutritional needs. In each chapter one of these experts will offer a brief glance into their field of knowledge with a unique suggestion that may prove beneficial in your training. I'd strongly suggest that you also create such a team of experts where you live. They are the folks you can turn to when you need expert assistance. If you don't have local access to such an expert, follow such people through your social media and reach out to them if stymied. I'm always impressed by how willingly people at the top in their field of study give help to their followers. Just don't overstay your welcome.

Here's the most important requirement for anyone who becomes a member of your high-performance team: they must be happy and positive people who never doubt or mock you or your goal. That approach goes well beyond cycling. Surrounding yourself with sincerely supportive people is an important key to success in any aspect of your life. Avoid people who don't have these fundamental qualities. They will only drag you down.

KEY TAKEAWAYS

- Your race success depends, in large part, on your support team.
- Share your goals with those closest to you—your family and friends.
- Your cycling team or training partners can help you achieve your goal; include them in your support team.
- A team of experts will make your goal much more achievable.
- All your team members must be happy, positive, and successful people who never doubt or mock you or your goal.

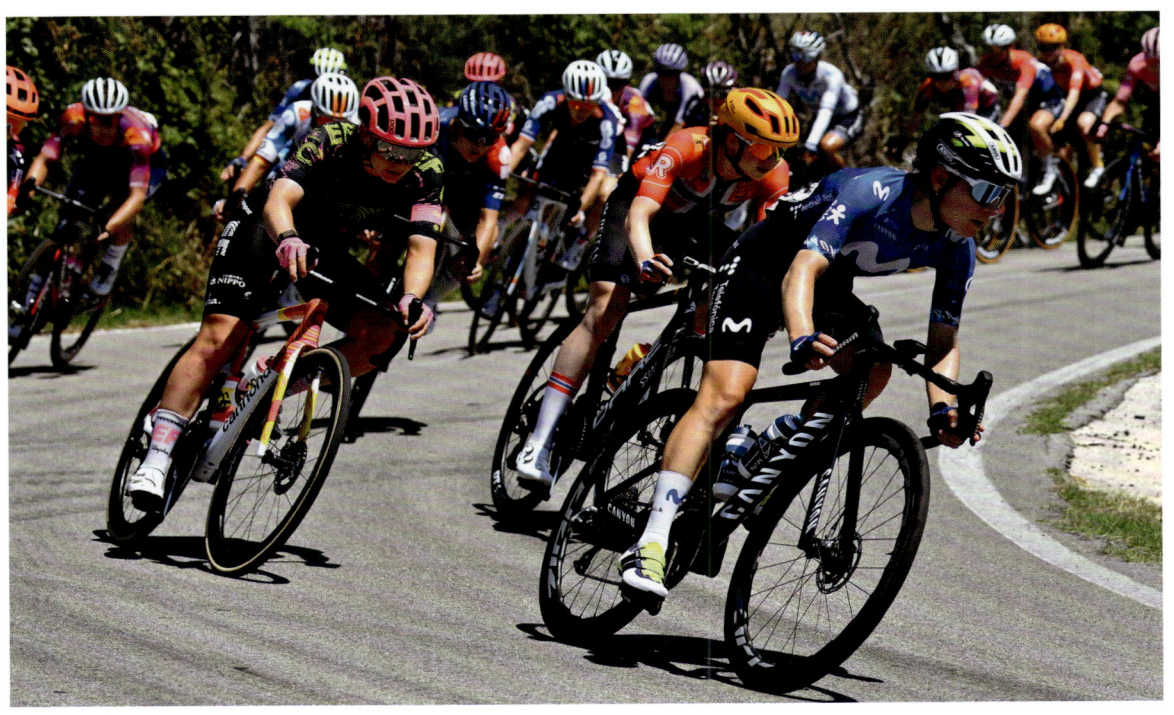

YOUR GOAL

While the principles in this book work with almost any endurance sport, there are many topics here that relate only to cycling. Chances are that you're a cyclist given the book's title, but cycling is also a wide territory. The types of events this book and I can help you with are road races, criteriums, stage races, time trials, gravel races, cross-country mountain bike races, cyclocross, and virtual races. Others that may find my coaching guidelines helpful but not as sport specific are ultra-distance bike races, track cycling, gran fondos, cyclosportives, randonneuring, and century rides. Triathletes and duathletes may also benefit from reading this book but it does not offer guidance with swimming or running (for that I suggest reading my *Triathlete's Training Bible*). If you participate in another endurance sport, you can probably still find ways my training methodology will prove helpful, but there will also be a great deal that is not specific to your sport. (By the way, I've coached a wide array of sports besides cycling, including triathlon, duathlon, running, rowing, and even endurance horse racing. All endurance sports have a lot in common: The motor is the same for each; it's the drivetrain and chassis that differ.)

Remember Steve's goal at the start of this chapter? He wanted the top step of the podium at a national championship. That was clearly a high-performance goal. But as mentioned in the Prologue, your goal doesn't have to be winning. It could be that you want to have a personal best performance in a local race. Or maybe it's simply finishing a very long or otherwise challenging event. Those and similar types of goals are great. If it causes you to stretch your limits to achieve something at the edge of your ability, then it's a high-performance goal.

What are you and I aiming for this coming season? Let me give you some things to think about when it comes to goal races. Some riders have multiple goals for their season. That's okay, but I'd strongly suggest that you have no more than three high-priority race goals within a year. Two is better and one is great, so long as it's a late-season race. Why not more? It has to do with physiology. We'll taper your workouts, especially workout durations, for each high-priority race for two to three weeks prior. And, as I mentioned in the Prologue, tapering means cutting back on your training volume. You'll do fewer hours on the bike each week as you taper, although we'll keep the intensity high (we'll come back to the details in Chapters 4 and 5). Remember the *reversibility principle* in the Prologue? In brief, it says that whenever you reduce the training load, fitness begins to decline. We can get by quite easily with that if there's only one late-season race. If there are two or three, they are best separated by several weeks. Three races spread over the early spring, midsummer, and late fall are probably not going to present a problem. But the closer their timing on the calendar, the greater the risk of losing too much fitness due to the tapering only to wind up having a poor follow-up race. That's why two is better and one is perfect. Steve's focus on only one race in the fall made for a highly focused season.

While we are on this topic of race importance, let's give category names to these most important events. I call them the A-priority races. These are the ones you will taper for. They are the most important in your season—the reason for your training. Then there are the B-priority races. They are important to you but not as much as the A-priority races. For the B races we will reduce your workout volume for only three days prior, and that will be mostly just resting and recovering. There won't be a long taper as with the A races. But because of the pre-race resting, you will go into the race feeling pretty good, just not as good as when you come to a peak after a two-week taper. You may have a half dozen or so B races over the course of a year. Last are the C-priority races. These are treated just as you would treat a hard group ride or other high-intensity workout. And that's just what it is—a workout, which we are calling a "race." There is no tapering or extended resting. You show up at the start line and race, regardless of what you've done in the previous days. There may be a lot of these in your season since each serves as a workout. From now on I will refer to your races as A-priority, B-priority, and C-priority, or as A, B, and C races.

Let's get back to your goal or goals for the season. What are you aiming for? Setting a season goal is very important since you'll be devoting your time and energy to it for several months. To set effective goals, what should you take into consideration? The following is a suggested goal-setting structural tool that is used by many in sport, business, and life in general when setting goals. You may be familiar with it. It's called SMART, which stands for Specific, Measurable, Achievable, Relevant, and Timed. These are the key issues to consider in setting your season goal.

SPECIFIC

There's no doubt that Steve's goal was specific. He wanted to win the US National Time Trial Championship for his race category. To be specific, your goal should include a verb which is action oriented. For Steve the verb was "win." Others may be "finish," "improve," "qualify," "achieve," or some other positive, action-related word that defines what you want the outcome to be. You also need a specific event for your goal as Steve had—the National Time Trial Championship. What is your event?

MEASURABLE

What will your success look like? Can it be measured? Some sports lend themselves to being measured quite nicely, while other sports are a bit more difficult to measure. Running, for example, is quite easily measured and a finish time can be the goal. For Steve the measurable part was to be on the top step of the podium. That's certainly measurable, but is also determined, to some extent, by who shows up on race day. You have no control over that, but don't let that stop you from setting the bar high.

ACHIEVABLE

Knowing yourself quite well, can you reasonably expect to achieve the goal? Is it realistic given your focused preparation? With Steve we really didn't know if it was achievable. But he obviously had a great background in time trialing, albeit local, that we could assume put the goal within his reach. That's why I suggested he do more races with other top-end riders.

Multiple goals must be complementary, not contradictory.

Of course, we never know months in advance if a goal is truly achievable. That's what sport is all about—can I do it?

RELEVANT
This is perhaps the trickiest goal-setting criterion. It comes down to me asking you why this particular goal is so important. Here we're getting into the mental side of goal setting. The goal was relevant for Steve because time trialing was his strength and he wanted to see how he would stack up with riders from all over the country.

TIMED
Your goal must have a timeline—when will it be achieved? Steve's goal was timed by the date of the National Time Trial Championship in late summer of that same year he came to me seeking coaching. What is the date for your A-priority event?

WHAT IS YOUR GOAL?
With all of this in mind, what is your goal? You don't have to answer that question right now, but you will need to eventually. You should be thinking about it. Your goal must meet the guidelines for all five criteria above. The goal should also excite you with the thought of exploring your limits. There should be a lingering question in the back of your mind: *Can I really do that?* The mere thought of trying to achieve such a goal should cause the hair to stand up on the back of your neck or increase your heart rate and breathing. In other words, it should feel really challenging. If it's something you've already done before and it's easy there's no excitement, no wondering. But at the same time, it shouldn't be impossible. Having an unrealistic goal is the same as having no goal at all. If you don't believe it's achievable then it's just a waste of time. Please give it some thought. We'll come back to this in Chapter 4 when we begin to lay out the plan for achieving your goal.

And there's just one more thing on goals. If you have more than one, it's possible for them to be in conflict. That's not good. For example, what if Steve had said in our first meeting that he also had a second goal that season of losing weight so he could climb better at another A-priority road race? How would that have impacted his time trial performance? Well, it would have been a huge mistake and probably would have cost him a national championship and a new record. His weight on a flat course was not a handicap. In fact, it was beneficial. Losing weight would have caused him to also lose some muscle mass. He would be less powerful and therefore slower. Weight on a flat course is of little consequence on a bike. The only significant matter when the course is flat is wind resistance—drag. The difference in drag between a large rider and a small one is so slight as to be inconsequential, assuming both are in an aerodynamic position. My point is that multiple goals must be complementary, not contradictory.

APPROPRIATE GOALS

Let's dig a little bit deeper into this idea of seasonal goals. Several years ago I coached an athlete who got on the podium in all three of his major races by the end of our first season together. It was quite an impressive accomplishment, but in talking with him the day after that last race of the season, it was obvious he wasn't thrilled about it. In fact, he seemed a bit down in the dumps.

Perplexed, I began to dig into what I *thought* his goals were for the just-finished season. *Did I get something wrong?* I soon came to realize that deep down he had wanted to beat a certain athlete that year but never had. Even though the rider I was coaching was considered one of the best in the region, he was upset because he failed to beat one other cyclist. I was dumbfounded. He had never mentioned that specific goal, but the other rider's name had popped up a few times in our weekly conversations. Looking back, I didn't take those comments seriously enough. His goal was stored away some place in his head, and if he had ever shared it with me, I suspect that it would have led to a serious talk.

WHAT IS RACE SUCCESS?

As athletes, we need to move away from measuring our success by whether we "beat others." That's a narrow and somewhat egotistical way of measuring achievement in sport. While it's okay to gauge your race performances on how well you did relative to your competition, basing your success entirely on who you beat is a bit misguided. The outcome comes down to who showed up that day and what kind of shape they were in.

There are more important outcomes we can measure. Performance in sport is more about what you accomplish relative to yourself, not others. If at the end of the season you are performing at a higher level than previously, I see that as success. If you are getting faster under similar conditions, then you are improving regardless of what anyone else in the race does.

COMPETITION

Don't get me wrong, competition with other athletes is okay. It's not, however, the be-all and end-all we make it out to be. We too often assume that if we are *competing* with someone, our goal is to beat that person. While that might be how the word is commonly often used today, that's not what it originally meant. Let's dig a bit deeper into the word *competition*. "Compete" is from the Latin *competere* and means, in one early definition, to "strive together." You are not striving *against* other people. You are striving *together*. Yes, you're pushing each other to your individual limits and one of you is going to come out on top, but you're actually working together. Regardless of the mano-a-mano outcome, you are both becoming better athletes because of your competition. Another way of thinking about this is that without the other competitors you wouldn't be as good as you are. When seen in that light, you owe your competitors a measure of gratitude for what they are doing for you, regardless of how it turns out.

One of the best indicators of a successful athlete, and a good competitor, is how they act when they lose. It's heartwarming to see the "loser" seek out the "winner" after a race to offer congratulations. A post-race smile and handshake exemplify what competition is all about. Compare that with the athlete who frowns, places blame on others for the loss, and avoids contact with the winner. Which do you prefer to see? Which do you prefer to *be*? That will say a lot about who you are both as a person and as an athlete.

KEY TAKEAWAYS

- To be *specific* a goal must include an action verb. What do you want to happen?
- Your goal must state the *measurable* part. How will you know if you are successful?
- A good goal is achievable. Can you do it?
- The goal must be appropriate for you. Is it?
- A timeline must be attached to any goal. When will you achieve your goal?

PREDICTORS OF GOAL SUCCESS

Research and experience tells me that there are predictors of high-performance success for athletes. There are obviously physiological markers, such as how high your aerobic capacity is (more on that later) and a whole lot more in this physical category. I expect that when you set your goal for the season these will be uppermost in your mind. I doubt if you will strive to attain a goal that is well beyond your reach physically. That should be obvious to you. If you are like most athletes, you give less attention to the mental markers.

Then there are historical markers, such as how much experience you have in the sport. The more experience you have in cycling, the greater the chances of your success. You will probably also be better at defining your goals, and you will have a sense of what it will take to reach a high goal.

Your lifestyle can play a role in your success, too. Do you have enough time to prepare for that goal? Is your career physically or mentally demanding? Do you have a lot of psychological stress in your life? We'll return to all these topics in later chapters.

MENTAL PREDICTORS

There are many physical, as opposed to psychological, predictors. Many books have been written on just that subject. But the most important, I believe, is your mental dedication to the goal, as evidenced by five mental predictors that I consider critical to your success, based on my experiences in coaching lots of athletes. The greater your chance of goal success, the more of these mental success predictors you have:

- An unquenchable curiosity for the sport.
- Strong bonds with other cyclists.
- The support of family and friends.
- Riding is seen as enjoyable and fun, not laborious.
- Training is thought of in years, not weeks or months.

I've coached athletes who had high levels of each of these qualities and some who didn't have any. My experience has been that when an athlete has all these mental qualities there is a very high likelihood they will perform at a high level. In the following chapters I will introduce you to some of my athletes who had successful seasons and some who didn't. Steve had all five predictors. That's why, as I came to know him, I felt very confident of his potential for success.

Of course, high level performance is based on much more than these five mental success predictors. As mentioned, the physical side is obviously critical to performance, but I'm afraid that when we think of preparing for a high-performance race, our primary focus is on the physical side. While that is obviously important, there is considerable research demonstrating that the psychological side is just as important. We'll check into your mental readiness to race in Chapter 7.

KEY TAKEAWAYS

- Mental determiners of success are just as important as physical determiners (see Chapter 7).
- Your experience in cycling has a lot to do with your success.
- Your lifestyle must allow you to train without frequent interruptions or undue stress.
- You must be completely dedicated to your goal for success.
- Mindset is often the key determiner of success; believing in yourself is vital.

HOW I CAN HELP WITH YOUR GOAL

I can help you stay focused on your goal and point you in the right direction with your training, but I can't endow you with the five mental success predictors described earlier. That's something that must come from within you. Ultimately, your success is about commitment—simply doing what you said you would do long after the mood you were in when you said it has passed. The bigger your goal, the greater your challenge to stay committed. Keeping the dream alive for weeks, months, and even years demands unwavering dedication and long-term discipline. The athlete who has both commitment and dedication has a highly beneficial quality—passion. But passion takes some time to develop. After setting his national championship goal and beginning to prepare for it, Steve eventually became passionate about succeeding. That's what kept him going when he faced setbacks early in the season. You'll also face setbacks. Some will be physical, such as an illness, but the most challenging will be a loss of passion. I'll remind you of that commitment as you go forward in this book.

Unfortunately, one of the common reasons that the passion fades for athletes is their misbeliefs about how to train. Many self-coached athletes think their workouts must be grueling to the point of daily suffering. They don't understand how to build fitness. They seem to think that every workout should be as hard as they can bear, otherwise it's a waste of time and there is no benefit. Nothing could be further from reality. Easy workouts are also necessary. In fact, there should be far more easy rides than hard ones. We'll come back to this in Chapter 2, and I'll teach you how to train effectively without the excessive suffering. Sure, there will be some, but probably not as much as you expect. While you may not believe me, this is how the best riders in the world train. They don't hammer themselves every day. They maintain a balance between hard and easy with the scales tilting significantly toward the easy side. I'll keep reminding you of this as we progress with your training plan. This is the key not only to your goal commitment, dedication, and passion, but also to your fitness.

Of course, having a goal without a plan for achieving it is of little value. A goal without a plan is nothing more than a wish. In Chapters 4 and 5 I'll lead you step by step through the process of creating an annual training plan. By then we'll need to know your goal since that's our ultimate destination this season and the platform for your plan. If you don't have a goal in mind now, please give this some serious thought. Aim high.

Ultimately, your success is about commitment—simply doing what you said you would do long after the mood you were in when you said it has passed.

WHAT YOU NEED TO GET STARTED

Other than a good bike, there are two things you will need to fully reap the benefits of this book. Those things have to do with the intensity of workouts. I'll explain. There are only two variables we measure in a ride—duration and intensity. Duration is easy. It just takes a watch. Intensity is much more complicated, not only in terms of how we measure it, but also what the intensity numbers mean. I'm going to talk about this with you frequently throughout this book. The main topic will be the importance of how hard the ride *feels* to you. This is the single most important marker of intensity. I'll make that point over and over as you read the following chapters. This, however, doesn't rule out any other ways of measuring intensity. The key in training is to relate the measured intensity to how you are feeling at that moment—your "rating of perceived exertion" (RPE). (I'll come back to this topic in much greater detail in Chapter 3.)

POWER METER AND HEART RATE MONITOR

What will you need? More than 20 years ago I started requiring all my clients to have a heart rate monitor and power meter. Why? Because we will learn a lot about you by having both heart rate and power data. I can almost guarantee you'll become a better rider because of this. I've seen it happen many times, but I also know there is some resistance to having one or both tools. And they are just that—tools. You can get by without a heart rate monitor and power meter, but the product of your work would also be of a lower quality. You'd be missing the finer points of training. I'll introduce those to you in Chapter 3.

The most common argument against using these tools is cost. I understand. They're not cheap. However, you've got a bike that probably cost you a lot of money, and you're probably willing to spend even more to upgrade the wheels and other components. I will guarantee you that the combined use of a heart rate monitor and power meter will make you faster than new wheels. Yes, I know, a power meter is expensive. When I got my first one, some 30 years ago, I recall weighing both sides of this dilemma. Should I spend the money or not? Back then power meters were more than five times as expensive as they are now (without an adjustment for inflation). And the prices keep coming down these days. You may even be able to find a secondhand one when another rider upgrades. Check with your local bike shop as they may know of someone looking to sell a used power meter or start saving your money for a new one. Of course, you will need both, but heart rate monitors are comparatively inexpensive.

The other argument against using a heart rate monitor and power meter is technology. There are lots of people who want to keep cycling basic—a bike and that's it. Nothing else. It reminds me of the early 19th-century Luddites in England who were opposed to the advancement of technology. They were against mechanization in the spinning and weaving industry. Well, guess what? We now have advanced spinning and weaving machines. It's not done by hand anymore. The same thing happened with cycling in the early days. It was

34 years after they were invented before the Tour de France allowed derailleurs. In the early days, riders changed gears when they came to a climb by getting off the bike and reversing the rear wheel, which had a gear on either side. Notice that we don't do that anymore. The world of cycling has moved on, and heart rate monitors and power meters are not going to go away.

Another reason I require both devices is that they provide unbiased information about your training. For example, I'll teach you how to compare power and heart rate to measure your aerobic efficiency—an excellent indicator of improving (or fading) fitness. That's just the tip of the iceberg. There's much more to come in Chapters 3 and 5, when I teach you how to use these tools to find out how you're responding to training, and what you need to work on going forward. There's a lot to be learned on this topic that will help you become a high-performance cyclist.

SAFETY FIRST

Of course, not every rider needs a heart rate monitor and a power meter. Novices, for example, need to be more concerned with workout frequency than with their heart rates or wattage. Just getting out the door regularly is the key to their growth as a rider, but I suspect you're well beyond that stage now. You'll improve by being able to precisely measure how your training and racing are progressing.

Unfortunately, numbers appearing on the handlebars while riding aren't always beneficial. There are some riders who become so fixated on the data flow that they increase the risk of an accident. When I've coached riders like that who were new to heart rate and especially to power, I had them cover their handlebar devices with tape so they couldn't see the numbers. When we really need the data is after the ride. Safety is much more important than data analysis.

KEY TAKEAWAYS

- You need both a heart rate monitor and a power meter to follow my coaching guidelines in this book.
- Heart rate and power both play key roles in achieving high goals, but in different ways.
- Use your heart rate monitor and power meter every time you ride.
- Power meters can be expensive. Ask around at shops for used ones.

GETTING STARTED

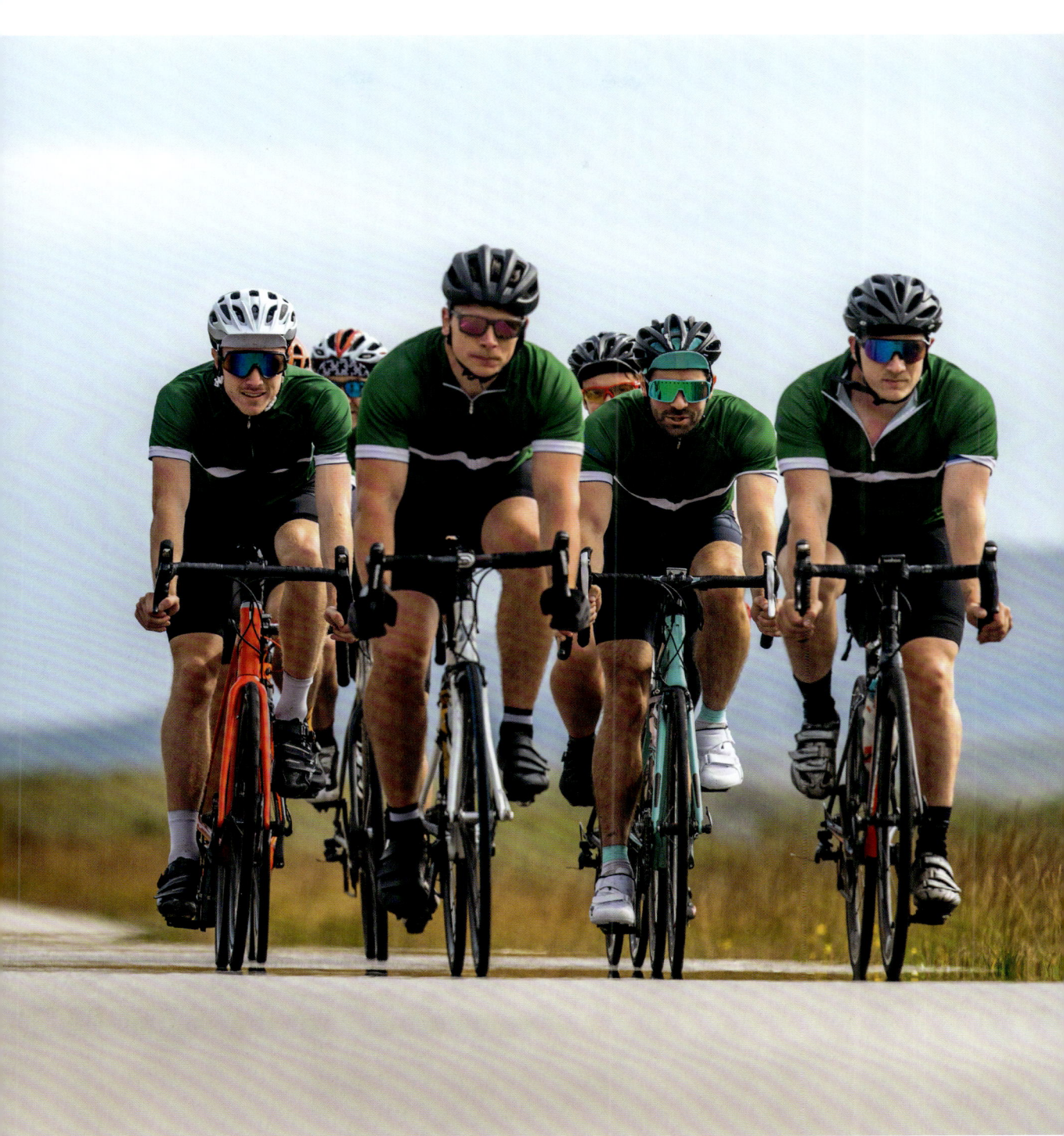

PHYSICAL AND EQUIPMENT ASSESSMENT

In this chapter I'm treating you much as I would any client-athlete I coach. There are certain things that must be done upfront before you do the first workout. These have to do with ensuring that you are physically ready before throwing a leg over the bike for a serious ride. We'll get to that in detail in Chapter 5. For now, let's make sure you are ready to begin.

There are two things I have riders do at the start of every season. Both have to do with injury avoidance and optimal bike positioning for a high-performance season. Even if you are reading this book at a time well beyond the start of your season, I'd still recommend that you follow these guidelines.

SEE A PHYSICAL THERAPIST

Earlier in this chapter I suggested that you create a high-performance team of experts who can help you as matters pop up during the season. One of those expert categories was health and a medical expert I'd suggest enlisting into your team is a physical therapist or a physiotherapist, especially one with experience working with endurance athletes. Make an appointment and explain that you are just starting your season and want to avoid injuries, improve performance, and provide information for your bike fit, which will be the next step in this assessment.

What the physical therapist will do is assess your soft-tissue flexibility, joint mobility, structural balance, and muscular strength, looking for anything that may lead to a breakdown once the hard workouts and racing begin. If something is found, which is highly likely, the physical therapist should provide you with guidance on how to correct the discrepancy with exercises that can be done at home or in a gym. This may also have to do with the type of shoes you wear, your saddle type, handlebar reach, and other possibilities. This information should then be taken to your bike fitter, which is the next expert you should see before starting to train seriously.

NEXT, SEE A FITTER

Make an appointment with a professional bike fitter. Don't ask a training partner, spouse, or friend to check your fit. And don't do it yourself with an indoor trainer and mirror. A good bike fit is incredibly complex and not to be done by amateurs (see Chapter 2). Also, don't assume your fit is fine as is. Just because you've become used to the setup doesn't mean that it's best for your training and racing. If you don't know of a fitter, ask other riders if they would recommend someone. Make sure the fitter you see has considerable experience with your unique cycling sport. Some fitters may do very well with road bikes, but not so well with fitting a time trial bike or a mountain bike. When you go in for the fitting take the physical therapist's findings with you. There may be information about leg length differences, lower back issues, tight hamstrings, or something else that will have a bearing on your fitting.

   I'd strongly recommend that you repeat both steps—seeing a physical therapist and a bike fitter—at the start of every season as things change over time. It's likely that small tweaks are needed annually to make sure you are ready for the upcoming race season.

> **KEY TAKEAWAYS**
> - The starting point for a new season is a physical therapist checking you for physical weaknesses that need correcting.
> - A professional bike fit is essential for success.
> - Do both at the start of every season.

THE REST OF STEVE'S STORY

Steve is a great example of someone who set a high goal and then persistently pursued it. At Nationals I was happy when he passed me, and I was even happier when he stood atop the podium. It could not have happened to a more deserving person.

2. TRAINING BASICS

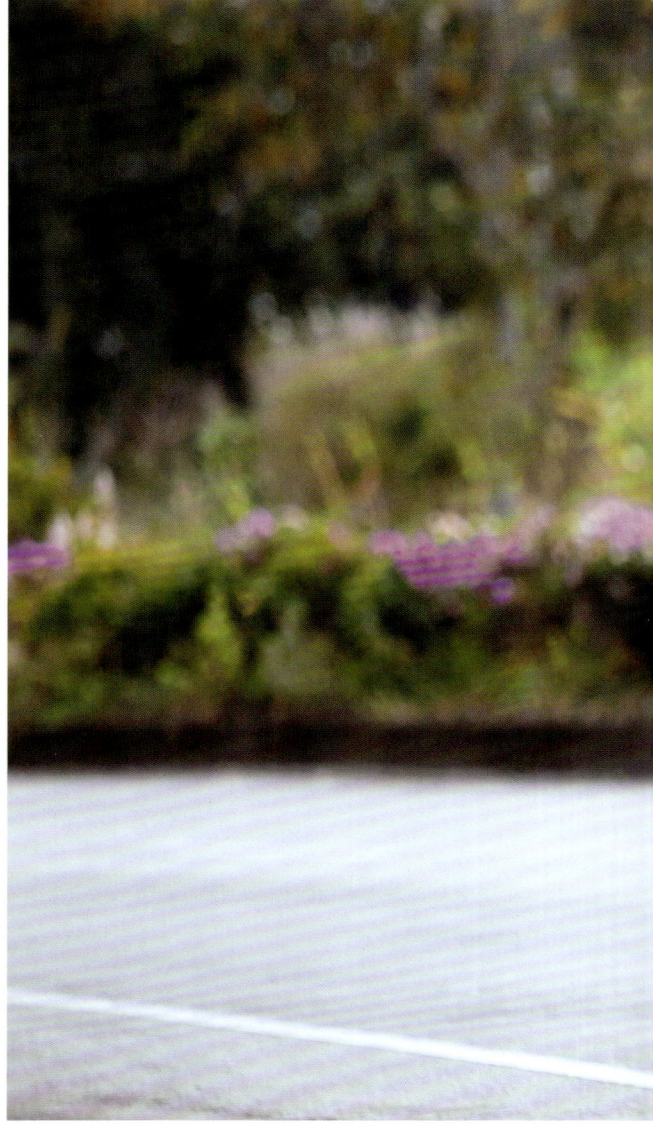

Chapter 2 is all about what it takes to perform at a high level in this sport. First, I'll tell you about several little things in training that can make a big difference when taken together. I'll introduce you to the three key physiological determiners of high performance. We'll come back to these frequently throughout this book so please make sure you understand them before moving on. The benefits of aerobic training are discussed in some detail here. This is something I will repeatedly return to in later chapters, too. As I think you'll come to see, this aspect of training is much more important to performance than most riders understand.

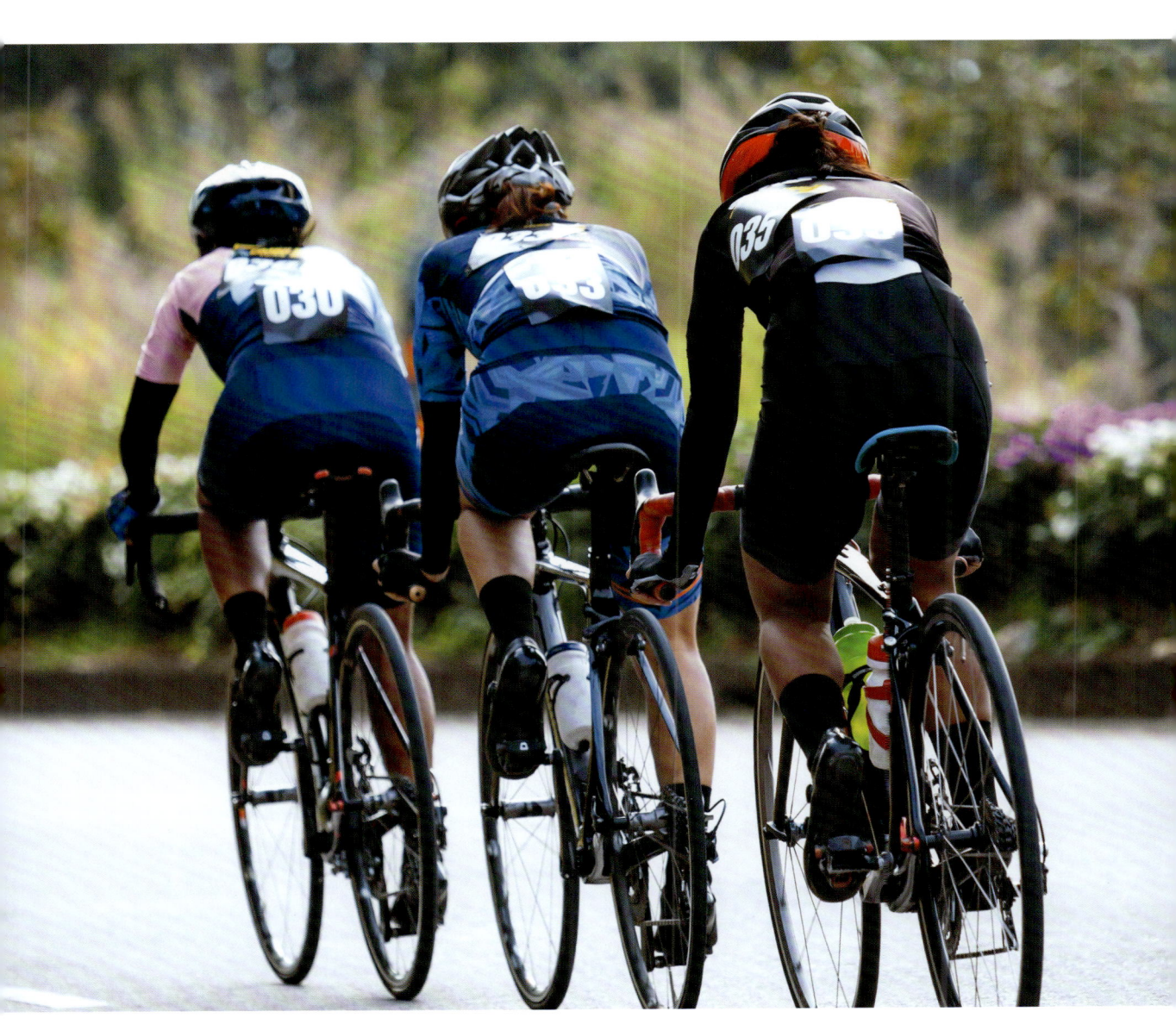

DIRK'S STORY

I was in the garage tinkering with a woodworking project on a warm day in June when my son, who was then 12 years old, rolled up the driveway on his get-around-town bike. Before he even fully stopped, he asked if I would help him take the kickstand off. "How come?" I asked. Still panting from the ride, he told me there was a criterium with a junior race in town in October and he wanted to do it. Little did I know at the time that this was the start of a lifetime passion and, eventually, a career for him. It's become an epic moment in our family.

I recall thinking, "There's no way he's going to stay focused on a race four months in the future." Dirk seemed like a typical pre-teen. I figured he'd soon be back to his regular summer routine: shooting hoops, playing games, and hanging out all day with his neighborhood buddies. His race goal sounded good, but I didn't think his motivation could possibly last that long. "But what the heck, I'll remove the kickstand anyway," I thought.

What happened over the next few months was remarkable. He rode laps around the neighborhood almost daily, mostly alone. There weren't many laps at first, but he always rode hard as if he was racing. As a coach and father, I decided to stay out of what he was doing. I was certainly impressed that he maintained such a high level of motivation at such a young age. My concern was that if I got involved the goal might shift from being his to mine. And besides, I wanted to see if he could pull this off on his own.

He kept riding almost daily for the next several weeks. I had never seen a pre-teen have such a passion for a "fringe" sport before. What had happened to his interest in football, baseball, and basketball? My wife and I were so impressed with his new-born enthusiasm for cycling that we bought him a much nicer machine—a Peugeot race bike. He helped pick it out. That was a big change from the old clunker he had been riding. And it seemed to boost his enthusiasm even higher.

He made it to race day without losing his focus. His mother and I continued to be impressed. That October day was a bit chilly and blustery. We drove him to the race venue—the library near the center of town. Other than a pair of bike shorts and a T-shirt, Dirk didn't really have a traditional kit. Since the weather was a bit cool, he decided to wear a jacket and some basketball warm-up pants over his shorts. The race would be a few laps on the streets around the building. In warming up while the older riders were racing, I could tell he was nervous and hyped up.

At the start line he took a position in the middle of a rather small group of 12-year-olds who also looked quite nervous. If I recall right, they did three laps of the block. He finished last. His baggy basketball pants flapping in the wind didn't help. When he rode over to us, I was afraid he might be so disappointed that it would be the end of cycling for him. I was wrong. He was really pumped up!

That winter he kept on riding whenever the weather in Northern Colorado would allow it. He also started talking about doing more races the following spring and summer. And he did. The last-place finish in his first race was never given a second thought. I continued to stay away from telling him what to do, with one exception. The following school year he told me he didn't want to do any other sports at his junior high school as he had done the previous year. He just wanted to ride his bike, he told me. This is when I decided to get involved. I told him his mom and I were now his sponsors. We bought him a bike and would provide entry fees and transportation to all his races.

If he wanted us to continue sponsoring him, he had to participate in at least one other sport at his school every year. My reasoning was that it simply didn't sound like a good idea for a 13-year-old to become overly focused on one sport. "But," I said, "when you are 16 you can specialize in cycling." He reluctantly agreed.

Three years later, on the day he turned 16, Dirk came to me and said he would only do bike races from now on. No other sports. I, of course, was okay with that. That was our agreement. Next, I hired a young cycling coach to work with him. I told the coach there was only one thing I wanted him to do. That was to make sure that Dirk had fun. And just as important, I wanted him to still be riding his bike in 10 years and enjoying it. Winning was not important. The coach did a great job. Dirk is now in his 50s and still racing—and having fun.

THE BIKE FIT: PARAIC MCGLYNN

Bike fitting is the science of customizing a bicycle to accommodate the unique physical traits of a cyclist. A bike fit is performed on your existing bike or on a special, highly adjustable "fit bike." A bike fitter gathers information about the cyclist's physical makeup, analyzes pedaling and movement patterns, and optimizes the rider's bike contact points to ensure comfort, longevity, and performance. A professional bike fitter transforms a generic bike setup into one that is perfectly suited to the cyclist's needs.

The Initial Bike Fit Process

The fitting process starts with an in-depth interview to understand the cyclist's lifestyle, riding preferences, goals, injury history, and any current discomfort. This initial conversation provides valuable insights that guide the rest of the fitting process. The fitter gathers clues about the cyclist's symptoms, their severity, onset, and the circumstances of any discomfort. Skilled fitters can recognize correlations between these factors and how they influence each step of the bike fitting process.

Foot Evaluation

The physical assessment typically begins with the feet, as they play a crucial role in cycling biomechanics. Fitters evaluate various aspects of the feet, including size, width, volume, arch length, arch height, and forefoot orientation. This helps determine if the cyclist has the correct shoes, foot support (footbed), and pedal and cleat setup.

Muscular, Skeletal, and Stability Evaluation

Next, the fitter assesses the muscles and joints to understand their needs and limitations. This involves three types of assessment.

The cyclist's muscles are the engine. Understanding the strength and flexibility of the key muscle groups allows the fitter to set the riding position. For example, hamstring flexibility will define the limits of saddle height.

The skeletal structure is the infrastructure the muscles depend on to create the force. Bike fitters will perform assessments of body symmetry to determine if there are differences that require accommodation. In rare cases fitters may suggest a referral to a medical professional to help resolve more complex issues.

Core strength determines how the body performs on the bike. The cyclist's ability to be stable enough to deal with the large, more powerful muscles pushing on the pedals is important, especially for riders tackling longer distances or great volumes of training.

On-Bike Assessment

The rider begins by warming up on a stationary trainer or fit bike. Bike fitters will use static or dynamic angle-measurement equipment used to analyze the cyclist's position and determine adjustments.

Static tools include goniometers for determining angles, plumb bobs, and lasers to measure joint angles and joint positions. Static tools require the rider to pause at a specific point in the pedal stroke while maintaining the same form exhibited when pedaling under load. Kinematics measures the motion of specific points and joint angles.

Dynamic angle measurement tools, such as 2D video or 3D analysis, provide more accurate and reproducible measurement of cycling kinematics. These tools allow the fitter to observe and analyze body angles simultaneously and in real-time. This is accomplished by placing markers on the cyclist's joints and using cameras to track their angles and motion.

This data allows for precise adjustments to the bike to ensure optimal kinematics. A good example of kinematics in the fit process is setting saddle height. An ideal saddle height creates a 30- to 40-degree angle at the knee. This leg extension angle is adjusted based on the cyclist's flexibility, type of riding, and how their ankle adapts to pedaling. Cyclists with poor flexibility have their saddle set to produce an angle close to 40 degrees (leg less extended), while those with excellent flexibility end up with an angle close to 30 degrees (leg more extended).

Saddle pressure mapping provides information on how the rider is interacting with the saddle. This data quantifies the pressure points and assists in making precise adjustments. This technology can significantly enhance the comfort and performance of the cyclist and help identify the root cause of saddle sores, low back pain, and groin discomfort.

The handlebars and shifters on a bike (the controls that enable a rider to change the gear ratio) are customized for the rider. Handlebar width and shape depend on shoulder width, type of cycling, and the rider's goals. Shifters are positioned to ensure easy shifting and braking in all positions, and that the sensitive nerves in the wrist are not in a position that produces pain or numbness.

The Bike Fit Session

A bike fitting session typically lasts 90 to 180 minutes, depending on the fitter's process and technology. Cyclists should bring their bike, cycling clothing, shoes, bike-specific proprietary parts, and any equipment they think might solve their comfort issues. Specific types of fitting often require helmets and glasses as they impact posture in triathlon and time trial positions. During the session, fitters may suggest purchasing items for optimal positioning. For example, stock bike saddles are often unsuitable for long-term comfort. Saddles are the most replaced item in a bike fitting.

Scheduling a Bike Fitting

Professional bike fittings require advance scheduling, and good fitters are often booked weeks in advance. Unlike a simple bike sizing, a fitting is a comprehensive process that ensures every aspect of the bike is tailored to the cyclist's needs.

Bike Fit Outcomes

There are three outcomes the fitter seeks. The first is the fit dimensions. Fitting details are recorded of the final bike position and notes for possible future adjustments are added. These records provide a reference for maintaining the optimal setup. Second, posture and off-bike recommendations are made. Good cycling posture isn't intuitive; fitters will help "find" the right way to sit on the bike. Recommendations may include exercises or stretches or even a physical therapy recommendation. And third, bike recommendations may be made. Fitters can provide valuable insights into the best bike models and components for the cyclist's specific needs and preferences.

Choosing a Bike Fitter

Selecting the right bike fitter is crucial for achieving the best results. Look for a fitter who is experienced, thorough, and well-reviewed. Find a fitter who performs detailed physical assessments, and analyzes both sides of the body while you are riding. Many professional fitters have certifications from reputable organizations, which may indicate a high level of expertise. Investing in a professional bike fit is a crucial step for any cyclist looking to improve their riding experience, enhance training outcomes, and achieve their goals.

Paraic McGlynn, the CEO of Cyclologic and VelogicFit, has worked with elite cyclists and triathletes for 30 years. His passions are developing scientific approaches in bike fitting, cycling aerodynamics, and motion analysis.

BREAKTHROUGH TRAINING

I've been using the word "training" quite a bit in these first two chapters and I'll continue to mention it on most of the following pages. What exactly does that word mean? It's often taken to mean workouts, the physical things you do to prepare for a race, such as riding your bike and lifting weights. It certainly includes these, but to me there's a lot more to the word than that. I use it to mean everything you do in preparing to race, and the higher the goal, the more things I would include. For the high-performance cyclist I believe it includes all your workouts along with nearly everything else in your daily lifestyle—eating, sleeping, resting, recovering, planning, and even thinking. All these things are closely related to how you will perform on race day. But many athletes consider these lifestyle matters inconsequential when compared with riding the bike. That's too narrow a view to produce a truly successful athlete. High-performance training is complex and involves a lot more than time on the saddle.

What are the most important factors for high-performance racing in endurance sports? It's common to start answering that question with what the best physiological producers of endurance fitness are. That's usually where most coaches start when talking with an athlete about their preparation for a high-performance season. While I don't disagree that physiological fitness is certainly important, and even critical, I prefer to start with lifestyle matters that will greatly increase your chances of becoming race-ready at the highest level.

If you can combine on-the-bike fundamentals and the lifestyle determiners of fitness, then you are on your way to an exceptional season.

Without these, even if you focus your training only on physiological race preparation, fitness just doesn't fully develop. These seemingly insignificant factors are often overlooked and taken for granted. They are often disregarded as being trivial by comparison. I believe the following, however, are essential to your success in endurance sport. I'll come back to the physiological essentials of high-performance racing later in this chapter as they are obviously important. If you can combine those on-the-bike fundamentals and the following lifestyle determiners of fitness, then you are on your way to an exceptional season.

TRAINING BASICS

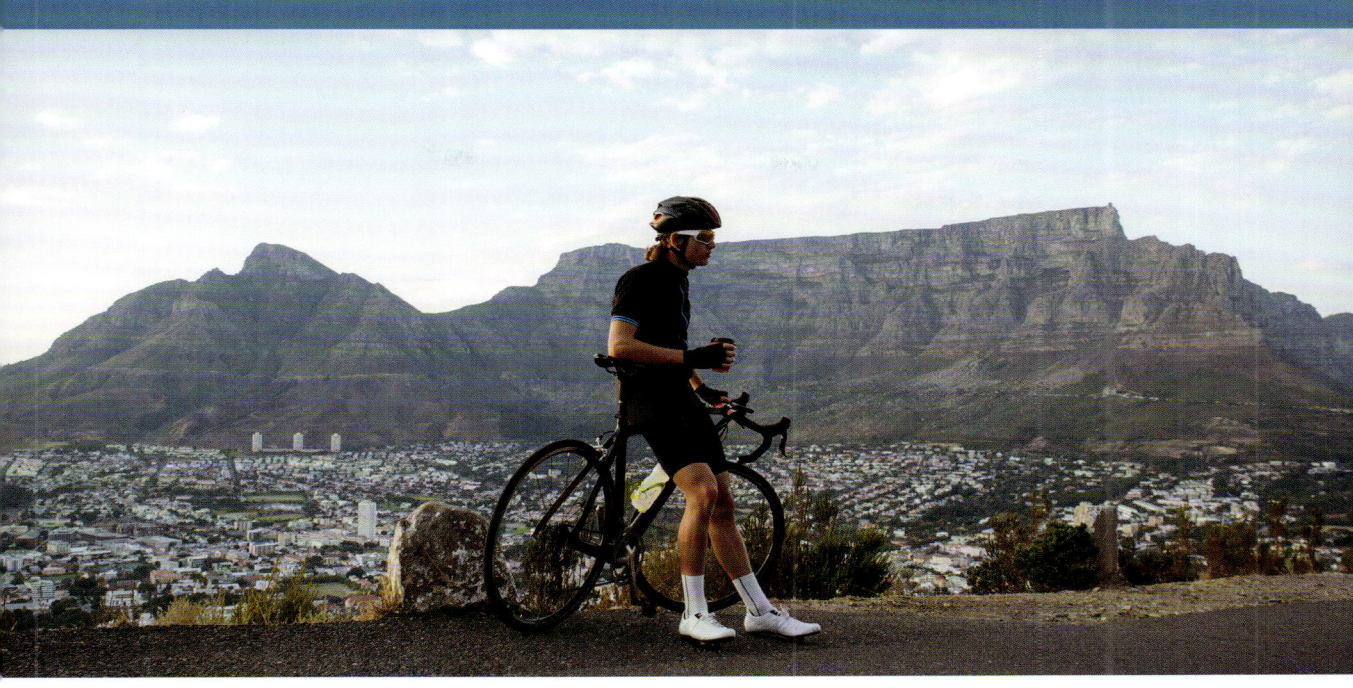

CONSISTENCY

Above all else, the foundation for high performance is consistent training. Not a very sexy topic, is it? But there's nothing more important. Ride *consistently* and you're sure to improve. Ride *inconsistently* and much of your bike time will be wasted.

Before we get too far into this, let's make sure that we agree on what the word "consistency" means. It *does not* mean doing the same workout day after day as many believe. That's repetitiveness. Consistency means having a persistent devotion to your purpose and training steadily. Put another way, it simply means showing up for work every day—not missing workouts. That doesn't mean you must never miss a workout. There are good reasons why you should sometimes skip a workout, and the best cyclists in the world occasionally do that, just don't miss too many. Having days when you miss workouts is simply the way life is and can't be avoided. But the more workouts you miss, the more unlikely you are to achieve your high-performance goal. I'll return to this throughout the following chapters. *You must be consistent in your workouts.*

Consistent riding results in greatly improved fitness. After a few weeks of consistent riding, you'll probably be aware you are somewhat fitter, but nothing big at first. Perhaps just a slight feeling going up that hill on one of your usual routes that it was a little easier than a few weeks ago. You probably won't have a strong sense that you are more fit for about six to eight weeks. Changes that affect performance, even when working out exactly as you should, happen very slowly—weeks, not days.

This, however, is a two-sided coin. When missing a workout, you also won't be aware of the physical losses right away either. Missing several workouts, however, will be noticeable. That slight sense of less effort on the hill will backslide to where it was a few weeks earlier. A single missed session is not a big deal.

39

Missing several is problematic, however. Riding consistently is so important that you would likely perform at a higher level if you did the *wrong* workouts consistently rather than if you did the *right* workouts inconsistently. There is simply nothing more important that you'll learn in this book than the significance of being consistent with your workouts, but what should you do if you miss a workout or, heaven forbid, more than one? That's an important question given the likelihood of that happening. We'll come back to this topic in Chapter 8.

Consistency was largely the reason for Dirk's success. He came a long way—from limited activity to state junior champion—in a little over three years. The primary reason he was able to pull this off was simply his devotion to riding. It wasn't that he had exceptional talent or did hard workouts. He simply rarely missed a day of riding for year after year. He patiently built his "talent" from the ground up, one workout at a time.

MINDSET

Pick up any cycling magazine or book, or search "success in endurance cycling" online and you'll find lots of discussions on topics such as intensity, duration, heart rate, power, speed, biomechanics, nutrition, and more. You'll find very little on what goes on between the cyclist's ears—mindset. And yet study after study has shown that the psychology of endurance sport is at least as important as the physiology of sport. After all, your most basic performance tool is your brain. How you think is critical to your performance. For example, a rider who lacks confidence or thinks negatively is likely to find a way to produce a poor performance regardless of physical fitness. Or, at a key moment in a race when a split-second decision must be made, the rider with a poor mindset is apt to be overwhelmed with negative thoughts decreasing their chances of doing what's needed to succeed. Your brain must be trained, much as you train your physiology, to perform at a high level.

As Dirk matured, I occasionally talked with him regarding what he thought about during races. This was part of our father-son conversation. My purpose was not just to hear his random thoughts, but to help him think positively and constructively when racing, and hopefully remove distractions from his mind. We sometimes even used the same type of conversation regarding his hard workouts, especially group rides. "What were you thinking when the speed increased?" or "What were your feelings climbing that last hill repeat?" I wanted him to be aware of his thoughts, both positive and negative, and how they could influence his performance. I also wanted him to believe in himself. Another goal was to harness his emotions so he could think more clearly. This last one is a big challenge for racing. Did such discussions of his workouts and racing mindsets make a difference? I don't know. These things are not easily measured. But if I had to do it all over again, I'd do the same thing. We'll dig quite a bit deeper into this topic of mindset in Chapter 7.

LISTENING TO YOUR BODY

I've been coaching endurance athletes for more than 40 years. Those athletes have had several weaknesses in common, but one weakness really stands out for me. In the middle of a workout, many of them paid very little attention to precisely how they were feeling. They ignored their physical sensations, no matter how serious they were. Athletes who have a high level of motivation, which is most of those I've coached, rarely place value on the signals their bodies send them during workouts. Most ignore their feelings.

A good coach will ask you how you felt during a hard workout, while you were doing intervals, a hard climb, or a fast group ride, or, of course, how you felt during a race. This is to get into how you think and to talk about different ways of engaging your mind positively while, perhaps, you are suffering at a high intensity. A good coach wants to make sure you are aware of your body and the messages it is sending you.

Unfortunately, unless the coach raises the topic, riders seldom do this. For example, if a knee doesn't feel quite right, or the back is tight, or there is a slight feeling that a cold may be coming on, or something else is amiss, most will ignore the messages from the body and press on with the planned workout. They will push the problem to the back of their mind and, if necessary, deal with it after the ride. *Maybe it will go away*. There is little thought about what that unusual sensation means and the possible consequences if the workout continues. Pressing on with the hill repeats when a knee keeps saying it's slightly tender is a good way to wind up injured. Continuing the planned hard workout when a cold may be coming on is a big mistake. An injury or illness is likely to mean missed workouts. And by now you know what that means, I'm sure. It's much smarter to decide to abandon a hard workout and replace it with an easy one, or even to take the day off, than to miss several days of riding due to a physical breakdown.

If you don't have a coach to raise such questions, you must do so yourself. Listen to your body. When it says something is wrong, back off the intensity, shorten, or abandon, the ride. Don't make it worse. Call it quits. Take care of your body. Your entire season may hang on how closely you pay attention to its messages on any given day and how you respond. And the closer you get to the race, the more critical this advice becomes. That's because the more race fit you are, the greater your risk of a breakdown due to having pushed your body to its limits for weeks or even months. It's only one workout. Don't be afraid to pull the plug when something isn't right. That's the smart thing to do. Consistency doesn't mean pushing yourself beyond your limits. Train smart.

REST AND RECOVERY

R&R days are not optional. They are just as important as any long or hard rides. Why? I'll explain, but first let's make sure we are on the same page with what "rest" and "recovery" mean. I take "rest" to mean a day off from riding your bike. You kick back and relax. And, hopefully, there's no mental stress on that day either, although I realize that this could be a work or school day for you with some emotional, or even physical, pressure you must manage. We're certainly not going to significantly change what happens in your normal daily activities off the bike when dealing with the world around you, but I'd strongly encourage you to keep your stress levels as low as possible. Mental stress management is at least as critical to your performance as physical stress management.

I will mention "recovery" throughout the following chapters as meaning when doing something physical, such as riding or cross-training, doing it very gently to allow your body to recuperate. The purpose, of course, is to recover from the previous day or days of hard riding so that you are ready to ride hard again on a subsequent day.

With your experience in the sport, it's obvious that every ride can't be an all-out effort. There need to be times when you allow the body to unload the previous day or days of accumulated stress from workouts or races. Without doing this it's clear that you will soon find yourself experiencing overreaching and possibly overtraining (see Chapter 6). R&R are very important for your performance.

> **R&R days are not optional. They are just as important as any long or hard rides.**

What I've found with many self-coached riders is that they don't take R&R days seriously. They soldier on because they *don't want to lose any fitness*. If they use an online training app, such as TrainingPeaks, with a tool that estimates current physical fitness, they soon discover that backing off for a few days or even one day results in a loss of fitness. But this "loss" is only a mathematical calculation using an algorithm. Even if the app's math is based on 100 percent accurate data, it's looking at only a couple of markers of what's happening to your training, and offers no measures of actual physiological loss. It's just an assumed estimate, not a true measure of what your body is experiencing. Even if it was accurately measuring your physical status, you still need to reduce workouts for a few days periodically or you are just digging a hole you can't get out of without taking an extremely long break from riding. That's why R&R days are not optional. They are a requirement of high-performance training. In Chapter 6 I will go into much more detail on this topic and show you how to arrange these breaks from serious riding using both subjective and objective determiners.

SLEEP

Are you seeing a pattern here: listening to your body, R&R, and now sleep? These are probably not the topics you expected to read about in a chapter on training basics. Sleep, however, is another of those underappreciated elements of racing success. In fact, it's more important than anything I've told you about so far, except consistency. Why? Because sleep is *when* you become more fit. Workouts only provide the *potential* for fitness gains. You're not more fit after

Training is made up of two components. One is quality workouts, and the other is deep sleep.

a ride. Without sleep you would never improve your fitness. In fact, you would only go backward in terms of fitness—and health.

This topic is so important that I usually bring it up very early in the first conversation I have with an athlete inquiring about my coaching services. This part of our meeting starts with me asking how much sleep the rider typically gets at night. If the answer is less than seven hours, I start digging into the details of the athlete's life. *Why is it less than seven?* The reason I ask is because sleep is foundational for high performance. It's during sleep that anabolic (tissue-building) hormones are released into the body to help it rebuild by improving muscle strength, repairing cells, increasing bone density, cleaning the nervous system, increasing the heart's stroke volume, improving the brain's ability to adapt and think clearly, improving immunity to disease, and a lot more. It probably takes a minimum of seven hours of actual sleep, not simply being in bed, for all of this to occur. So, an athlete's average sleep should be at least seven hours. Eight is better.

If the athlete I'm talking with seems to be chronically or frequently short on sleep, the next question is *what takes most of your time during the day?* What I'm looking for is what are they doing that cuts into sleep time. This is a common problem in our society. People simply don't get enough sleep because they try to cram too many things into their days. I can't help everyone on this issue, but I can help the athlete I'm coaching. What I tell the rider who has a high-performance goal but is frequently short on sleep is that they should have only three important, time-consuming things in their lives in the months leading up to their very important race: family, career, and training. More than these three usually means that something else must give, and the way most people resolve this problem is to go to bed later. Then they're awakened early by an alarm clock. That means too little sleep to reap all the benefits of the previous day's workout. Anabolic hormones, such as growth hormone, testosterone, estrogen, insulin-like growth factor, and many more, are released throughout the night in waves. Get too little sleep time and you are likely to miss one or more of those waves. The athlete must also understand that they can't make up for lost sleep time on the weekend. The sleep average needs to be greater than seven hours *every* night, not just on the weekends. If your riding is not going well, this is one of the first causes I'd suggest considering. Are you getting enough sleep?

Another way of thinking about this is that sleep is when adaptation takes place. It's the time when your body "absorbs" the benefits of the day's workout. Not getting a full night's sleep is much like not doing the entire workout. You get a few positive results, but not all. Some amount of the ride was wasted. Training, in the broader sense, is made up of two components. One is quality workouts, and the other is deep sleep. You must ride well, and sleep well, to become more fit.

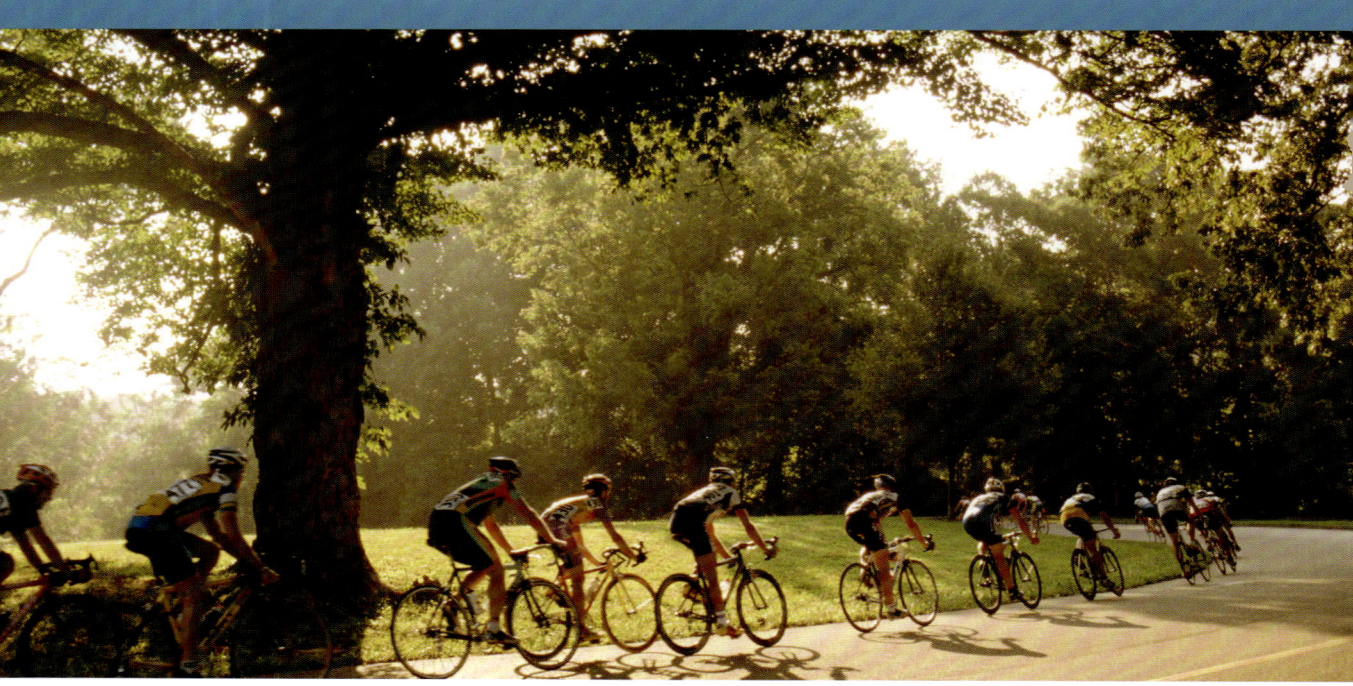

TRAINING INTENSITY

You're not going to like this, but here goes anyway: You are *probably* riding too hard. You undoubtedly need to ride slower—sometimes. In fact, most of the time. I'll stretch that just a bit more. Riding slower most of the time will make you faster. I know, you don't believe me. I've been told many times, *I'm already good at going slow. I need to ride fast to race fast*. Unfortunately, that's a naïve way of viewing the physiology of high-performance training. And while I try to keep training relatively easy, it's much more complex than pushing yourself to go a bit harder on almost every ride. *The workout calls for zone 2 now, but I'll push a little harder to zone 3 to get faster.* It doesn't work that way. Always pushing your limits just slightly won't help you to race faster. That's a sure way to have mediocre workouts and wind up racing poorly. It comes down to what's happening in your body during a ride. As mentioned, this is not always a popular topic with athletes. Let's take our first dive into this topic of getting intensity right in riding a bike (I'll come back to it repeatedly in the following chapters as it's essential to your success).

You have two overarching goals in preparing to race. The first is to build aerobic, or low-intensity, fitness. The second is to increase your high-intensity fitness, sometimes called "anaerobic." If all you do is concentrate on high, or even throw in moderately high, efforts, you are not developing the most basic aspect of fitness—your aerobic system. This is putting the cart before the horse. Aerobic endurance, the most essential part of cycling fitness, must be built before you start to work on the truly hard stuff. And then this basic fitness must be constantly maintained. After all, endurance cycling, especially in mass start events, is largely an aerobic sport in which outcomes are often determined by relatively brief high-intensity efforts—sprinting, climbing a hill, staying off the front, or closing a gap.

However, the aerobic side of fitness is what gets you to the moments of high effort and usually makes up well over 90 percent of the race. One without the other leads to poor performance. And the one aspect far too many riders cut short in their workouts is their aerobic fitness. They tend to take it for granted that it will just happen on its own, and so try to ride at a moderate or high intensity as often as they can. They usually see slow, easy rides as a waste of time. Nothing could be further from the truth. Most of your rides should be on the easy end of the intensity spectrum with only a few that push your limits (more of the details on this in Chapter 3). Self-coached riders tend to spend too much time in the middle of the intensity curve—not quite fast enough to help them race faster and not quite slow enough to build aerobic fitness. That doesn't really accomplish much, although most think it does, because it makes them feel tired.

To become a high-performance cyclist, the starting point is to get faster by riding easy. How do you do that? By spending a lot of time riding at low intensities—zones 1 and 2. And we can measure your progress here much as we do with high-intensity rides. Here's how. After a low-intensity ride compare your power-heart rate ratio to that of similar rides done a few weeks earlier. I call this ratio the "efficiency factor" (EF). After an easy ride in which you spent most of your time in zone 2, for example, divide your normalized power by your average heart rate (TrainingPeaks does this for you) and compare the resulting quotient with that of a similar ride done several weeks earlier. Eight weeks prior is usually a good reference point. "Similar" here means comparable course, duration, and intensity. You are, essentially, comparing your output (power) and your input (heart rate). When output and input are compared, you're expressing efficiency. If you are early in your season, the Base period, you should find this number rising gradually and steadily over the course of a few weeks. It will likely change very slowly and not be a linear rise. It typically ratchets up. But by eight weeks, it should be clearly higher if you are doing a lot of easy rides in zones 1 and 2. How about doing moderately hard rides instead? Not so much. Zone 3 rides just don't boost the aerobic system nearly as well. That increase in EF is a sign that you are becoming more powerful by riding easily.

Why is this happening? Why are you becoming more efficient? There are a lot of physiological changes taking place. For example, if EF is rising, one reason is that you have developed more capillaries in your working muscles. That means more blood is being delivered along with oxygen and fuel. The muscle doesn't have to work so hard to drive the pedals. Another is that you're becoming better at using fat for fuel. Fat is the energy source we most want to harness, especially early in the season. The primary alternative, of course, is carbohydrate, the fuel source you use for moderate- to high-intensity rides. In a long and steady, low-intensity ride you are training your body to utilize its stored fat to fuel your muscles.

As the intensity increases beyond zone 2 your muscles begin to significantly shift their fuel source to carbohydrate as lactate production increases. Lactate, which increases in your blood during moderate- to high-intensity rides, has been shown to inhibit the muscles' use of fat for fuel (I'll tell you more about lactate below). This is but one reason why I want you to do a lot of low-intensity riding. Besides building capillaries and burning fat, it will ultimately make you faster even at higher intensities. And there are many other benefits of easy, aerobic rides that I'll point out below and in the chapters that follow. Going slow is going to help you race faster.

Don't get me wrong here. I'm not going to have you riding in zones 1 and 2 all the time. That would be a sure way to ruin a race season. As you'll see in later chapters, I intend to have you ride in all zones. There is a time for each. Each has a purpose and a benefit which you will learn about as you read. But I'm placing an emphasis here on easy rides because years of experience tell me that self-coached riders underappreciate the importance of low-intensity exercise and so don't reap the many benefits.

FUEL

Athletes usually pay lip service to healthy eating. They've been told so many times how important healthy nutrition is that they usually give in and agree that it's critical to riding and race performance. But then most go right back to eating less-than-desirable food. Why? It's because they work out regularly. That makes them immune to the health-related consequences of a poor diet, or so they believe. This is normal, and an obligatory argument when it comes to this topic. Why? Because it's very difficult in our society to eat a healthy diet. Unhealthy "food" is ubiquitous, it's cheap, quite tasty, and it makes for a quick and easy meal on days when we have way too much stuff crammed into our 24 hours. That's very common. However, it's hard to be a high-performance rider if you fuel your body with junk.

As with most things in life there are some caveats when it comes to dietary importance. For example, the younger you are, the more likely you can get away with making poor food choices and still compete well. How young? Teenagers come to mind. In fact, that age group can make lots of mistakes in their lifestyle and still manage to perform well in sport. They are very fortunate—temporarily. But as we get older, what we put in our bodies becomes more important to not only our performance, but also to our long-term health and lifespan. If you still want to be around, physically and mentally fit, and racing in your 60s, 70s, and beyond you need to start by eating a healthy diet now. You can't put it off. That will catch up with you and it will be too late. Yes, it's more expensive and time-consuming to eat well. But the money and time expended now will pay you back later in life in many ways. The clock is ticking. You can't put it off to a later age. Add a healthy diet to your already healthy lifestyle and you'll be around a long time and still having fun riding a bike well into the future. With regards to your life and health in general, eating nutritious food is the single most important thing you can do besides riding a bike consistently.

In Chapter 8 we will go much deeper into this topic. I'm not going to overwhelm you with a lot of scientific mumbo jumbo about nutrition or precise foods you should, or shouldn't, be eating. You can find plenty of that online from nutritionists who know a lot more about the science of eating than me. I'm going to look at it in terms of how your diet affects your workouts and race performance, and what you can do to improve them. In fact, it's quite simple—and you probably already know the solutions. Diet also plays a key role in body composition, which is a challenge for some riders. I'll touch on that, also.

Sport nutrition doesn't have to be complicated. I won't tell you exactly what to eat in Chapter 8, but rather how small changes—more small gains—can make a difference.

TRAINING PLAN

Do you need a written plan? Probably. Having a written training plan can be quite beneficial to how you train and race. There are, however, some athletes who don't need a written plan. These are the highly experienced, self-coached riders, with a deep understanding of sport preparation and who also understand what they're doing because they've done it so many times. They know how much workout load their bodies can handle, and they understand the timing of their loading and unloading to produce a high performance at just the right time. This balancing act is a rather complex topic which borders on being a science. Such wise athletes are few and far between. Most riders, however, would benefit from having a scripted seasonal plan they could view on a regular basis to see what the direction ahead is for workouts. When a written plan is viewed weekly it reinforces your direction and purpose in riding. It's also motivating to frequently review your goals and objectives, otherwise they tend to move to the back of the mind. Without a written plan we are likely to forget the *hows*, *whats*, and *whys* of our training. The training plan is also a lot of details to store in your brain. Having it in writing is very beneficial. We'll go into considerable detail on this topic in Chapter 4.

KEY TAKEAWAYS

- High-performance is both physical *and* mental.
- Lifestyle has more to do with race success than you probably realize.
- Nothing is important than consistent training—*nothing*.
- How you think about yourself, and your world, is as important as anything you do on the bike.
- Something you *must* learn to do is to listen to your body.
- How well you train and race, and how fit you can become, are mostly determined by R&R.
- Sleep is when fitness happens—don't artificially shorten it with an alarm clock.
- You are probably riding too hard—slowing down will sometimes make you faster.
- You train and race according to how well you eat (see Chapter 8).
- Coming up with a training plan is just like having a map for a cross-country drive—it's essential (see Chapter 4).

HIGH-PERFORMANCE FUNDAMENTALS

So far in this chapter I've briefly touched on several aspects of race preparation that are usually not taken seriously by athletes. Many of these, if not all, may be things you have never considered important or you perhaps showed only a passing interest in them. I often sense resistance from athletes on those suggested lifestyle changes above, such as: *Ride easy? I don't have time for that. Sleep a lot? Not possible with how busy I am. Eat healthily? Get real! Take days off? Pay attention to my thoughts? Ain't gonna happen.* So let me tell you again: these little things that are often ignored by riders can make or break you when it's time for an A race. Individually they may not be a big deal, but combined they can make a huge difference. While they may not be easy at first to meld into your lifestyle and training, they will pay off in the long term if pursued. I guarantee that. To perform at the highest level, you must be willing to do the demanding, tedious, and disliked things that others won't do. These are the ultimate markers of your dedication to your goal.

   Now let's move on to a topic that you may be more concerned about in your training—the three most important fitness markers. There are no small gains to consider here. These are what I consider to be the fundamentals of high-performance training—aerobic capacity, stamina, and sprint power. These are required. You can't decide not to train for these as you might with the above topics. Oh, I suppose you could, but then there would be no reason to race. Without an investment in these three you are doomed to failure. That may sound a bit harsh, but it's true. The following are what truly determine if you are a high-performance rider or not.

AEROBIC CAPACITY

Aerobic capacity, commonly referred to as VO_2 max (meaning *maximal volume of oxygen*), is in many ways the most important product of training. It is a measure of the maximal amount of oxygen you can deliver to the working muscles via your lungs, heart, blood, arteries, and more. The greater the amount of oxygen you deliver, the greater your muscular energy production and potential for power and speed. While the outcome of a race is somewhat dependent on the aerobic capacities of the riders, this is not the only physiological determiner of performance. Stamina, which I'll explain below, also has a lot to do with how well you perform when it comes to endurance. And, of course, there are other race outcome determiners besides your fitness such as nutrition, hydration, strategy, tactics, and lots more.

   Aerobic capacity is usually all about your VO_2 max number. This is measured in a laboratory with equipment that measures inhaled and exhaled gases during a step test in which the intensity is increased every few minutes until the rider is unable to continue. Your VO_2 max is expressed as the volume of oxygen utilized (in milliliters) divided by your body weight (in kilograms). It is expressed in a single number as milliliters per kilogram per minute. The higher the number, the more aerobically fit the athlete is.

VO_2 max varies quite a bit among athletes. It's highest among young cyclists who ride a lot. As we age up, or if we significantly reduce our training load, or add considerable body weight, aerobic capacity declines. Regarding age, it is typical for a serious rider to see a drop of around 7 to 8 percent per decade. For sedentary people, the drop is more on the order of twice that per decade. The VO_2 max is typically higher for males than for females, everything else being equal. Elite male riders generally have aerobic capacities in the 70s and elite females in the 60s. Of course, there are outliers. The highest VO_2 max ever measured for a male was 97.5 (Norwegian cyclist Oskar Svendsen) and for a female 78.6 (American runner Joan Benoit).

While it's not necessary for your training, being tested for VO_2 max can be a real eye-opener. You'll learn a lot about yourself as an athlete. It will also serve as motivation to work out consistently by training with the appropriate intensities at the right times to improve it. In later chapters I will tell you of a field test that helps gauge the progress of your aerobic capacity power, but it won't determine your actual VO_2 max number. You may, however, get a ballpark estimation of your aerobic capacity if you have a wearable device, such as a watch, ring, or strap. But realize that it is only a rough estimate and could be way off. It may, however, give you feedback on how your VO_2 max is trending.

What does it take to increase your VO_2 max, to get a lot of blood to your muscles, therefore increasing your aerobic capacity? And how can purposeful workouts raise it? I will only touch on a few of these as there are many, but you will notice that most of the following result from low-intensity rides.

The first VO_2 max determiner is your heart's stroke volume. That's how much blood it pumps with each beat. High volume is good. One way of judging your stroke volume is counting your resting heart rate. A low resting heart rate is a sign of a high stroke volume. Very fit riders typically have resting heart rates in the 40s and 50s. Untrained people generally have resting heart rates in the 60s, 70s, and 80s. Since so much blood is being pumped per beat by the athlete's heart, it doesn't take a lot of beats to meet your body's needs if the stroke volume is high. How can stroke volume be improved? The starting place every season is with low-intensity riding—zones 1 and 2. That will produce the bulk of your stroke volume improvement for the season. Much later in your season, high-intensity interval workouts will take it up just a bit higher. Much more on this in later chapters.

Another reason for the rise in an athlete's aerobic capacity is an increase in blood volume that comes with training. Top-end cyclists have been found to have twice as much blood in circulation as sedentary, non-athletes of the same age and size. The high blood volume, besides raising aerobic capacity, also improves heat dissipation through sweating, as well as ensuring that the heart quickly refills with blood after each beat. How does an increase in blood volume happen? The biggest contributor is low-intensity, aerobic riding.

One change I mentioned above is an increase in the capillaries of the legs' working muscles. Let's go a little deeper into that. Capillaries are the smallest blood vessels in the vascular system. They are the final stop in delivering blood from the heart to the working muscle. This is where oxygen and nutrients are released into the muscle. As noted above, this aerobic capacity benefit comes largely from easy, aerobic rides. A few weeks of aerobic exercise have been shown to significantly increase the size of the capillary beds, thus increasing aerobic capacity.

Once the blood is delivered to the muscle, the primary nutrients, fat and carbohydrate, are taken up by little organelles in the muscle called mitochondria. These are often referred to as the "powerhouses" of the muscles as this is where the energy is produced that allows the muscle to contract. The more mitochondria you have, the higher your aerobic capacity. How does your body accomplish this mitochondrial growth? Aerobic, low-intensity exercise causes your body to build more mitochondria. With a few weeks of such riding done consistently a rider can make significant increases in mitochondria and therefore aerobic capacity.

Remember the doping incidents with pro road cycling in the 1990s and early 2000s? Some riders were using a banned drug, erythropoietin (EPO), which increases the body's red blood cells. These are the cells that carry oxygen to the muscles. In effect, the dopers were artificially increasing their aerobic capacities. The more oxygen you can deliver to the muscles, the faster you ride. The good news is that the body produces the EPO hormone naturally. It's one of the normal physiological changes sport scientists observe in exercise research subjects over a period of a few weeks of exercise. What intensity range is most responsible for producing this natural increase in red blood cells? You guessed it: low-intensity, easy aerobic exercise increases your EPO levels and therefore increases your red blood cell count, which boosts your aerobic capacity.

> **If you can combine on-the-bike fundamentals and the lifestyle determiners of fitness, then you are on your way to an exceptional season.**

I hope you are seeing a pattern here. The bottom line is that if you want to increase your aerobic capacity for high-performance racing, which is highly recommended, the starting place is low-intensity, aerobic workouts. In other words, you must ride easy to get faster. That's the workout type most athletes don't think does much for them. In fact, it's just the opposite—such training is the key to racing well. But that doesn't mean that high-intensity rides won't help build aerobic capacity. They will, but the bulk of the improvements come from riding easy. Low-intensity, easy workouts build your engine; high-intensity, hard workouts fine-tune it (more on this topic of "easy" and "hard" in Chapter 3). Figure 2.1 illustrates this point. This is why I will continually make the case throughout the following chapters that riding easy is of primary importance to your performance.

TRAINING BASICS

Figure 2.1 Low-intensity training vs. high-intensity interval training and their contributions to aerobic capacity (VO$_2$ max) for one season

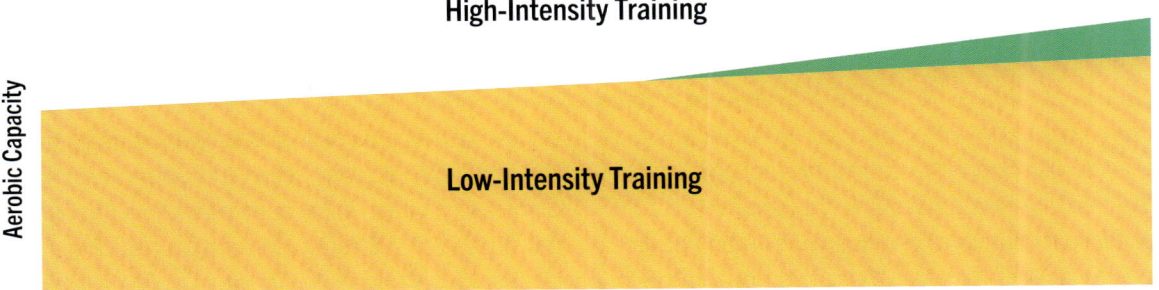

Courtesy of Alan Couzens

STAMINA

I want to begin wrapping up this chapter with a training topic that is at the heart of race performance as much as aerobic capacity, but you don't hear much about it. "Stamina," sometimes called "durability," is closely related to endurance. The key to having good stamina is continuing to ride at a relatively high intensity despite the onset of fatigue. The rider is resilient and determined while coping with suffering, something that's often talked about in our sport. Stamina implies some degree of misery and the willpower to stay focused and working as the effort becomes increasingly more challenging. It's not the sort of thing that an untrained rider can do on the initial exposure to such a situation. You must train for this.

Let's shift gears here momentarily so I can make an important point about stamina. Let's examine lactate, as it's closely related to stamina. Lactate is perhaps the most misunderstood topic in endurance sports when it comes to discussing exercise intensity and performance with cyclists. The way lactate is commonly described by television announcers and athletes in general is that it causes muscle fatigue during exercise and muscle soreness the day after a hard workout.

Neither is true. These mistaken conclusions have been around since the 1920s and refuse to go away. Lactate is a very efficient fuel that some tissues, such as the heart and brain, prefer even more than the glucose produced by your high-carbohydrate meal. The working muscles also rely on lactate for fuel. And it has no part at all in muscle soreness. Your heavy breathing on a hard ride, your increasing leg fatigue, and how you feel the day after have nothing to do with lactate (or "lactic acid") either.

Why did I insert this brief explanation of lactate? Because with stamina we are getting into a performance determiner that is closely related to fatigue. And I want to make sure we're on the same page before getting into the details of high-intensity training to head off any confusion. So, let's draw some conclusions about what *may* cause fatigue during a hard ride—and how little science understands all of this.

Now, about a century since lactate was falsely accused of triggering muscle fatigue, we still don't know the precise causes of withering performance. Why do we slow down? It's certainly related to the workout's intensity and duration along with the athlete's level of fitness. That's a given. But it may have something to do with other obvious causes such as the athlete's heat adaptation, nutritional status, hydration, sleep, mental stress, and muscle fiber composition (your unique mix of fast and slow twitch muscles). These are a few big-picture causes of fatigue. At a more cellular level, fatigue *may* have to do with hydrogen ions, depletion of muscle glycogen (the stored form of glucose), the central nervous system, the sodium-potassium pump in the muscle, or many other deeply scientific possibilities. The bottom line is that muscular fatigue is a complex subject. It's simply not fully understood yet, except that it's not as closely tied to lactate as we have been led to believe for more than a hundred years.

We're not going to solve this centuries-old dilemma about fatigue here. I just want you to understand how little is known about this topic. With that in mind, let's move on to the subject of training your stamina for high performance based on what we *do* know about fatigue.

How do you improve stamina? The starting place is (you probably guessed it) low-intensity aerobic rides. Having a lot of mitochondria in your muscle cells is the initial step to take in building your stamina. The more mitochondria, the more energy you can produce. As explained above, mitochondrial growth is accomplished with long-duration, low-intensity, aerobic workouts. But once you have increased your mitochondria there's another benefit from aerobic exercise that boosts your *high-intensity* power. This has to do with the movement of lactate from outside the muscle cell to the mitochondria inside, where the lactate can be used as a source of fuel. It takes a special protein called MCT-1 to move the lactate into the muscle-bound mitochondria. Aerobic exercise increases the number of these key transporters so that when you are riding at high intensity, the mitochondria can use lactate in addition to glucose to fuel your muscles. This gives you two readily available sources of energy—glucose and lactate. Every little bit helps when you're suffering.

The key here is doing long-duration, low-intensity rides early in the season, and over the course of many weeks, gradually increasing the intensity while staying below the upper threshold of intensity, which is sometimes referred to as the "anaerobic" threshold (more on this upper threshold in Chapter 3). To begin building your stamina, do one or two long rides weekly, starting in the Base period. This will build stamina if you start at a low intensity and slowly increase it as the season progresses, including doing some sub-threshold intervals along the way. There are many benefits that come from such training. One that's often mentioned but seldom taken seriously enough is the ability to use fat for fuel. This initially results from long, easy rides. While you have relatively little carbohydrate stored, you have hour after hour after hour of fat at your disposal to be used for fuel regardless of how skinny you are. What you want is to train your body to rely heavily on fat so that when you are seriously using your stamina in a race, it's being fueled by your largest energy source. Having excellent stamina means that, eventually, you'll be able to do rides of greater than one hour at a relatively high intensity while still using fat for fuel. Stamina, along with a high aerobic capacity, greatly improves your race performances.

Let's look at some real-world examples of stamina in action. Regardless of your specific cycling sport, I'm sure you watch pro road racing. These athletes are the pinnacle of their sport and have not only high aerobic capacities, but also well-developed stamina. As with everything else in sport, some pros have greater capabilities at these two race outcome determiners than other athletes. I've already mentioned the high VO_2 max numbers for such athletes. If two riders are racing head-to-head and they have similar aerobic capacities, the eventual winner will probably be the one who has more stamina and the motivation to use it. For example, the top road racers, when in a breakaway, are typically capable of holding at least 75 percent of their functional threshold power (FTP—more on this in Chapter 3) for an equivalent number of minutes. Here's an example of that. Assuming the pro rider's FTP is 400 watts, 75 percent of that is 300 watts. The best breakaway riders can maintain 300 watts for 300 minutes—five hours. The 300 watts isn't the hard part, it's the 300 minutes that is grueling. That is a tremendous level of stamina and is why, in addition to their aerobic capacities, they are pros.

I know we haven't reached this yet, but if you know your FTP, multiply it by 0.75. Are you able to hold that power output for an equivalent number of minutes? Let's say your FTP is 300 watts, which multiplied by 0.75 is 225 watts. A challenging goal would be to ride for 225 minutes (3 hours and 45 minutes) at 225 watts. If you can do that you are at the starting point for boosting your stamina and on the threshold of high-performance cycling. In Chapter 3 I'll explain how we will go about measuring your stamina and improving it.

The starting place for both aerobic capacity and stamina is developing your aerobic endurance with long, easy rides. It's during these workouts that you are establishing the physiological changes necessary to eventually boost your aerobic capacity and stamina. But you must be patient. It will take a few weeks to realize the most basic gains. Once your endurance is at a high level you will then start increasing the intensity of these long rides. Along the way we'll also blend in some interval workouts to prepare you for the higher intensities you'll need to race at a high output. The result will be a higher aerobic capacity and greater stamina.

SPRINT POWER

So far in this section I've been explaining training basics for endurance-focused racing. Aerobic capacity and stamina are both closely tied to the endurance aspects of cycling. Most of the sports this book is focused on fit neatly into that endurance category. But there are times, even in relatively long events, when sprinting for a few seconds at high power is necessary for position, a win, or high placement. The ability to instantly produce a high-powered sprint, even if you aren't a pure sprinter, is certainly necessary for high-performance racing. All cyclists, regardless of their exact sport, must be prepared to do that. Climbing or time trialing may be your strength, but you must also be able to sprint. You may not be as good at it as a rider who focuses primarily on that ability, but you must nevertheless have a powerful sprint for when it's needed. We will work on your sprint throughout the course of your training season just as we will work on aerobic capacity and stamina.

Training to sprint differs greatly from aerobic capacity and stamina training. While pure sprinters may not be the best in the endurance-focused realm of cycling, it is obvious that they must still get to the finish to unleash their sprint power. Some endurance is still necessary to get to the finish or wherever the sprint will happen. Pure sprinters, therefore, can't focus solely on a few seconds of power. They must also have some endurance. Just as climbers and time trialists must also be able to sprint. Sprinters typically have an abundance of fast twitch muscles which are good for quickly producing speed. But there are two types of these fast twitch muscles. One of them—type 2a—can take on some of the characteristics of slow twitch muscles with the proper training, which means they don't fatigue quickly. They aren't as fatigue resilient as type 1, slow twitch muscles, however. The other fast twitch muscle—type 2b—doesn't take on slow twitch muscle characteristics. It's powerful but fatigues very quickly. So, for an endurance sport like cycling, sprinters typically have a good deal of 2a, which gives them a bit of the best of both worlds. Climbers and time trialists have a lot of type 1 slow twitch muscles which are made for endurance. Due to the unique physiological characteristics of these two broad categories, no one is going to be a top performer in both endurance and sprinting. Those cyclists who come close to being good in both categories are called "all-rounders." They are a unique athlete subset in cycling with an intriguing mixture of muscle types. Figure 2.2 provides a general overview of how climbers, sprinters, time trialists, and all-rounders perform relative to power and duration.

Figure 2.2. Common power-duration curves for climbers, time trialists, sprinters, and all-rounders

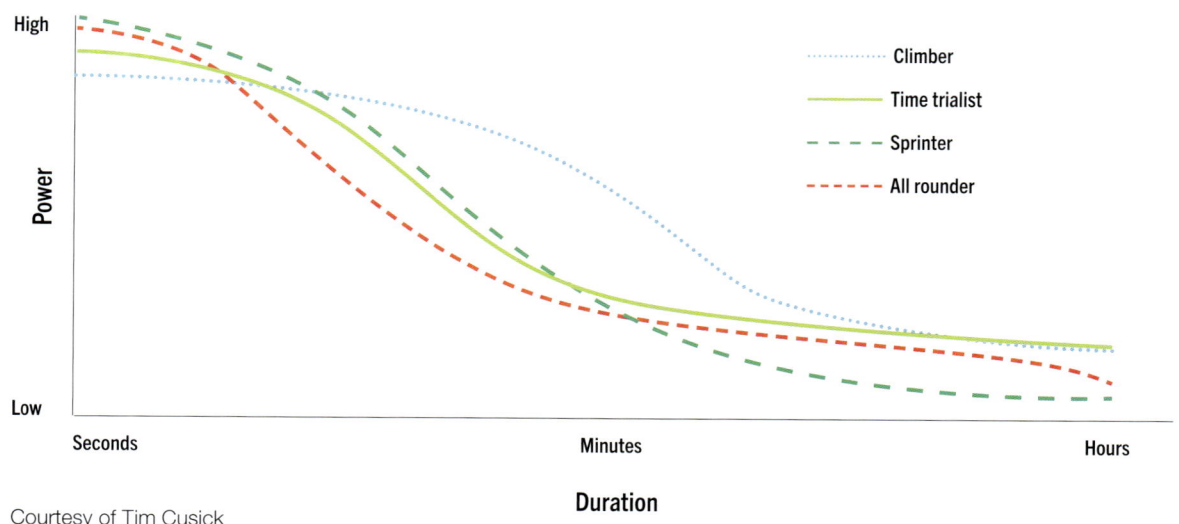

Courtesy of Tim Cusick

Whenever there are variables that are critical to high-performance racing, it is necessary that they are measured regularly to gauge their progress. This includes sprint power. I'll address that topic in Chapter 3.

In this chapter we touched on many of the areas that contribute to high-performance training and racing. The training for aerobic capacity, stamina, and sprint power will be especially challenging, but if you are up for it, I'm ready to coach you.

KEY TAKEAWAYS

- The fundamentals of high-performance training are aerobic capacity, stamina, and sprint power.
- In many ways, aerobic capacity is critical to your racing success, especially for short races.
- Wearable devices that suggest your aerobic capacity (VO_2 max) may not be accurate, but can give you trends.
- VO_2 max is largely determined by your heart's stroke volume.
- Other determiners of VO_2 max are blood volume, capillary bed size, mitochondrial count, and natural EPO levels.
- Low-intensity training is largely the creator of your VO_2 max.
- Stamina is the ability to ride for a relatively long time at a relatively high intensity.
- As with aerobic capacity, stamina initially improves with low-intensity riding.
- To improve stamina, start with long rides and later add intensity.

THE REST OF DIRK'S STORY

Dirk went on to win the Colorado State Junior Cycling Championship when he was 17, beating second-place Bobby Julich (third at the 1998 Tour de France). By this time cycling was the singular focus of his life. He lived and breathed riding and racing. He traveled around the country going to races in his old car with a training buddy. During his high school years, he set a goal of racing in Europe after graduation, turning pro, and finding a team that would support him. Everything in his young life centered on cycling. For example, in those days French was the language of the peloton in Europe. So, of course, he took French classes in high school to prepare for racing there. His senior year he managed to get his course credits early so that he could fly to Belgium in February to race with a Belgian-based amateur club for one month. That worked out well for him and he was invited to stay the rest of the season in Belgium. That left one goal.

The biggest goal was to turn pro and race throughout Europe doing the races he had only read about. A couple of years later Dirk signed with a Swiss pro team, which allowed him to race some of the biggest races in Belgium. In fact, in Dirk's first semi-classic, Het Nieuwsblad (Het Volk back then), he found himself in a breakaway with the likes of another young American—Lance Armstrong—and a few other big-name stars of the day. I'm glad I took that kickstand off for him on that warm day in June many years ago.

3.
EXERTION

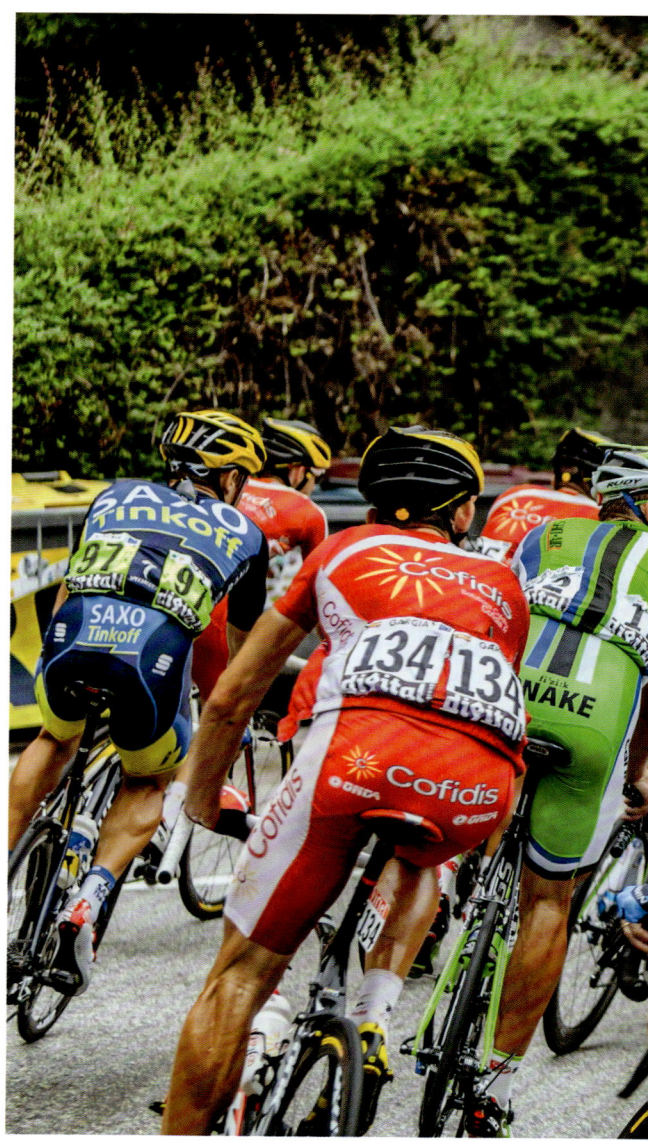

This chapter is about intensity—how great your exertion is during a workout or race. This is probably the most complex topic there is in any endurance sport. I get more questions from athletes about this than any other. Why? Because it can be confusing. I am going to throw a lot of new information at you here, but I'll try to keep it simple. Most of the confusion has to do with setting "training zones." Here I'll give you some options for how to go about doing this. Then I'll tell you about basic and advanced abilities that help to tie your workout purposes to the intensities of your workouts. Pay close attention here as I will refer to these two workout categories in most of the remaining chapters. And finally, I'll tell you about when you should use heart rate and power to get the most out of your workouts.

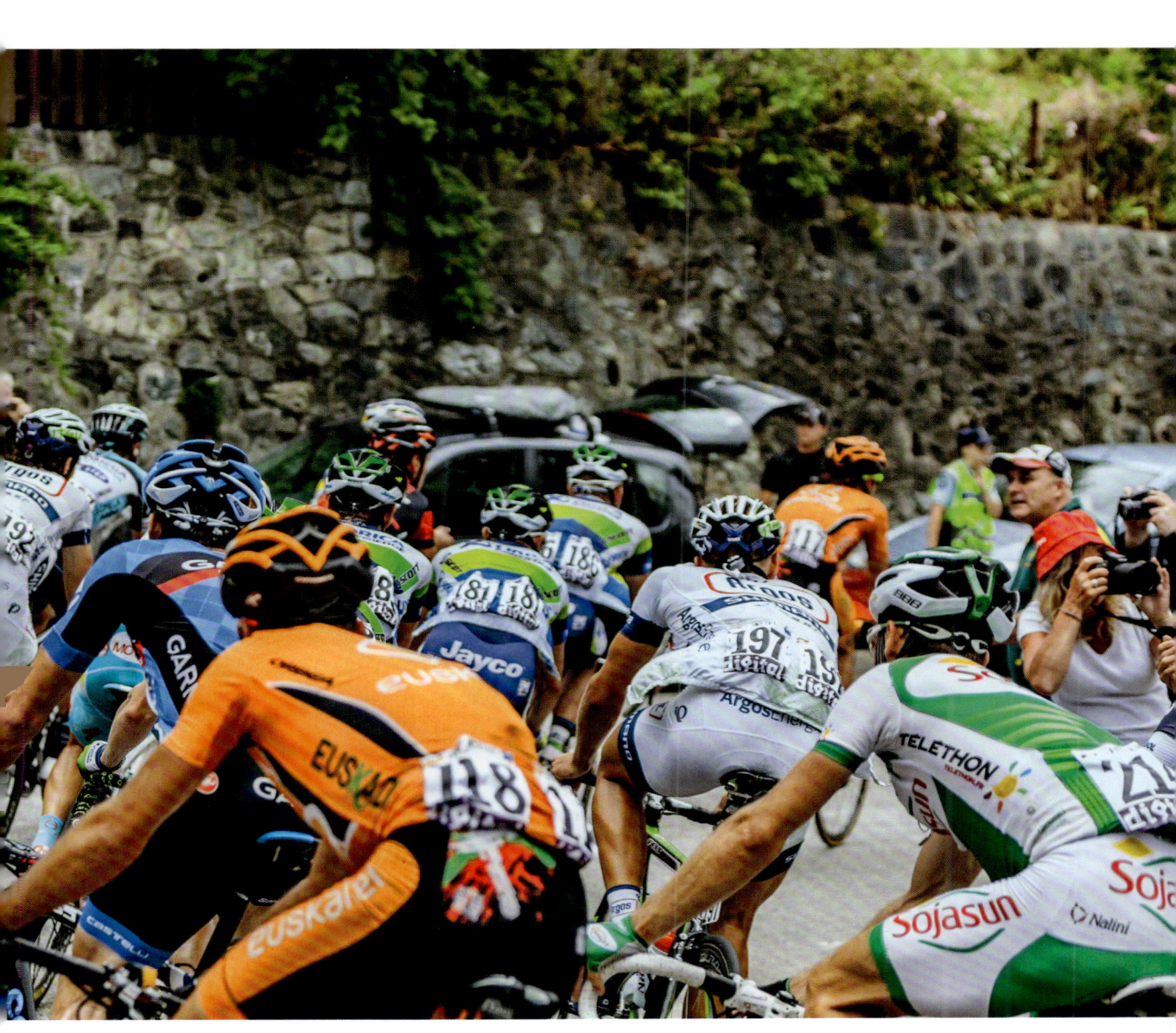

LYNDA'S STORY

Although we were both cyclists and lived in the same city we had never met. I had heard the name before in local bike shops, but knew little about her, other than she was from Scotland and had a lot of natural talent as a mountain bike racer. She called me one day and we agreed to meet at a local coffee shop. It was a soggy, late-fall day. We talked about her background in the sport, especially her most recent season, which had just ended. It hadn't gone as well as she had hoped. Now in her late 20s, she felt time closing in and was obviously serious about improving. She hoped I might be able to help her.

Lynda was a pro and had shown quite good results in the past. She came across as somewhat reserved, but very knowledgeable about sport and the athlete's lifestyle in general. "Reserved" may not be the right word. It seemed like I had to pull information out of her. When successful, I often found a much deeper person than expected. She had a few strong ideas about training with which I sometimes disagreed. It would be challenging to change her views on some of these differences. But she had all the other key ingredients for success in endurance sport.

First, she had a high goal for the coming season—to win Scotland's National Mountain Bike Championship in late summer the following year. She had raced it before and finished top 10 a couple of times. I could tell by her increasing enthusiasm as she talked about her goal that she was fully committed. Her motivation was apparent. Motivation is the starting place for any athlete I coach. Not a problem here.

Following some initial testing to establish training zones and base levels of fitness, I started working on a training plan for Lynda's season. She proved to be fully dedicated to training, despite the nasty winter weather in northern Colorado. Nothing stopped her from doing a workout. I also learned over the next few weeks that she was also very consistent with her training. That's the second characteristic I look for in an athlete. We were well on our way to a good season.

There were only two things about Lynda that concerned me. The first was that I had to dig deep to get information from her when we talked every week. It wasn't that she was shy, she just didn't answer my questions fully. Her answers were always guarded and brief. One-word replies were common. Me: How did your workout go yesterday? Lynda: Okay. I had to do a lot of asking to find out how things were going. The daily diary with training data helped me fill in the gaps on how her training was progressing. But the key thing I always look for after a ride is how it felt to the athlete. That's when I had to do the heavy prying.

The second matter was much more concerning. She often wanted to ride harder than I scheduled. And since I included several low-intensity, easy rides in her weekly schedules that presented a problem. She would frequently do them just a little harder than called for. A couple of times she even inserted very hard rides when I had planned very easy ones. She seemed to want me to schedule more higher-intensity sessions in a week. Then I'd suggest to her in our weekly conversations that she hold back a little on her intensities. There was a reason for my doing this. She would hesitatingly agree, but when I saw her next week's diary the workouts were often just a bit too hard. Over the first several weeks, I frequently commented on this to her and suggested she needed to follow the planned intensities more closely. But she often deviated from the planned intensity. I was becoming a bit perplexed. My talks with her became more serious. After a few weeks of this I casually mentioned that perhaps our coach-athlete relationship wasn't working out. Maybe I could help her find another coach who was more in line with her training philosophy? That seemed to work. From that point on Lynda followed the plan much more closely, although somewhat reluctantly, I could tell.

By late winter that first season her training was going as I had hoped. In the spring races she did quite well with a few podiums. We were getting along great now. The only significant problem I saw was that she was overly conservative at the start of a race. She would hang out at the back of the pack. If the course was such that there was lots of room for passing and moving up, she would do well. But when it was mostly narrow single track she was often caught up in a crowd and unable to advance. After seeing this a couple of times, I suggested she needed to be just a little more aggressive at the gun, especially when the course was mostly single track. She agreed to do that in the next race.

We spoke after that race. "It was a disaster," she said. "I went out fast and was leading but had to stop after a few minutes because I was out of breath!" It was obvious we had to work on how to pace at the start. That became the next challenge. But it would be an easy one compared with our chat about intensity.

Lynda went on to be one of the best riders I ever coached. After a bit of a shaky start in our relationship, she became a joy to work with. We got along great, and best of all, she won the Scottish National Championship late that summer. It mostly came down to getting the intensity of training rides straightened out. After that, she excelled.

HOW LOW-INTENSITY RIDING PREPARES YOU TO RACE: ALAN COUZENS

Training as a cyclist involves both low- and high-intensity sessions, each serving distinct purposes and leading to unique adaptations in the body. Low-intensity training, which occurs at or below the first rise in lactate, is primarily fueled by fat, can be sustained for long periods, and allows for quick recovery due to minimal stress on the nervous system. In contrast, high-intensity training relies heavily on glycogen/carbohydrates, causes quick fatigue, and significantly stresses the system.

A common mistake among "time-crunched" cyclists is to over-rely on high-intensity workouts, thinking they can substitute for missed low-intensity training. This approach is flawed because should be high- and low-intensity training stimulate different physiological adaptations. The key question cyclists should ask before starting any session is, "What physiological adaptations am I seeking with this training?"

Low-Intensity Adaptations
- Increased mitochondrial density: particularly in type 1 (slow twitch) and type 2a (fast twitch) muscle fibers. This can be seen in lower lactate levels for a given power.
- Enhanced cardiac capacity: low-intensity training leads to changes in heart size and structure over time, increasing the heart's end-diastolic volume. These changes can be seen in a higher power output for a given heart rate, i.e. a higher efficiency factor (EF).
- Fat utilization: increased liberation of free fatty acids into the bloodstream, providing an extensive energy source for endurance and aiding in body composition by utilizing fat stores. This adaptation enables the athlete to go further at a given power before glycogen stores are emptied.

High-Intensity Adaptations
- Increased mitochondrial density: mainly in type 2x muscle fibers, but this is limited.
- Improved cardiac output at maximal efforts: enhances the heart's ability to pump a large proportion of its total capacity, in other words, its "ejection fraction", especially at high outputs.
- Enhanced glycolytic power: utilizes sugar quickly and efficiently for short bursts of energy.
- Acidosis buffering: improves the muscle's ability to buffer and tolerate increased acidity during intense efforts.

During high-intensity efforts, fast-twitch fibers produce large amounts of pyruvate, which can be processed by the mitochondria-rich, slow-twitch fibers, preventing premature acidosis and fatigue. Additionally, a well-developed slow-twitch fiber base enhances high-intensity performance during race periods.

Additionally, the oxygen supply to muscles during high-intensity efforts is dependent on the heart's stroke volume. While high-intensity training can maximize the percentage of the heart's capacity per beat, the absolute size of the heart, built during the low-intensity Base period, is the more critical factor.

Similarly, glycogen stores, essential for high-intensity work, are conserved by the ability to rely on fat as the primary energy source during low-intensity training. This is true, not only of high-intensity work during training, but also racing. For longer races, the ability to generate energy from fat significantly influences stamina during a race. Athletes who fail to build a strong fat-burning capability during their Base period will struggle with time to exhaustion during longer race efforts. Moreover, low-intensity adaptations can improve over long periods, while high-intensity adaptations plateau quickly.

Type 2x muscle fibers, designed for short, fast efforts, can improve their fatigue resistance, but their endurance capacity is limited. In contrast, the slow-twitch fibers can greatly enhance their mitochondrial density through sustained low-intensity training. Heart improvements also differ. While high-intensity training has limited effects on the heart's ejection fraction, low-intensity training can significantly increase the heart's size and end-diastolic volume over time.

Finally, increased mitochondrial density in slow-twitch fibers and higher free fatty acid availability enable cyclists to fuel extensive aerobic training primarily from fat. This adaptation is crucial for elite cyclists who train for over 1000 hours or 30,000 or more kilometers annually.

In summary, cyclists, especially those with limited training time, often skip low-intensity training, which is crucial for developing slow-twitch fibers, cardiac capacity, and fat-burning metabolism. By focusing on low-intensity training, athletes build a foundation that maximizes the benefits of high-intensity, race-specific work. Reducing overall intensity and prioritizing low-intensity systems prepares cyclists for peak performance when it matters most.

The bottom line for low- and high-intensity adaptations is that low-intensity training is crucial, because it underpins the high-intensity adaptations.

> **Low-intensity training is crucial—it underpins the high-intensity adaptations.**

Alan Couzens has been an exercise physiologist since the 1990s, working as a sports scientist and coach to world-class swimmers, professional triathletes, and cyclists.

TRAINING ZONES

The three elements that are central to your workouts and that ultimately determine your race performance are frequency, duration, and intensity. A big challenge you face as a serious rider is getting the mix of these three right every time you mount your bike. The first two are easy to measure. *Frequency* is simply how often you ride. High-performance cyclists typically get about six rides weekly. Then comes *duration* which is a measure of how long—in hours—each of those weekly rides are. It is just slightly more complex. An individual workout is likely to be anything from about an hour to several hours depending on your highest priority race, how long you have until that race, your available time for riding, the purpose of the workout, and what you are capable of handling at a particular time in your season. That's certainly not difficult to figure out. I'll address frequency and duration in more detail in Chapters 4 and 5.

The third workout element is intensity—how easy, moderate, or hard your workouts are. This one is very intricate. Getting it right every time you ride can be a challenge. It's also the one that riders are most likely to get wrong—intentionally—thus upsetting their training and, eventually, their race performances. My purpose in this chapter is to help you not only understand the nuances of physical exertion, but also to guide your training intensities, so they are appropriately dialed in for your workouts.

MORE ON LOW INTENSITY

I've touched on some of this in Chapter 2. Part of my purpose there was to kill the myth that the only important workouts are those that are high intensity. Having read that chapter, I hope you now accept the importance of low-intensity workouts. There I made the point that easy rides do more over time to boost your aerobic capacity, which is one of the best markers of your endurance fitness, than hard workouts do (see Figure 2.1). The bottom line for that portion of the last chapter is that you will get tremendous benefits from the easy rides which should make up the largest portion of your training (more on that in Chapter 4). Those rides are not just throwaways. Nor are they only for recovery. They have a significant and measurable impact on your fitness and race performance. If that weren't so I would have instead made a case for simply not riding on a day that wasn't high intensity. You would recover much more completely when taking a day off rather than going for an easy ride. But that wouldn't work. Those easy, aerobic rides account for the bulk of your fitness. They should be taken very seriously and not disregarded as insignificant nuisances standing between you and your next hard ride.

My point here is that when I use the word "intensity," I'm not referring only to the higher effort ranges of your workouts. Every workout you do should have a precise purpose for the intensity, ranging from extremely easy to a maximal effort. In this chapter I will introduce you to how I group heart rate and power intensities into unique zones.

MATCHING INTENSITIES AND WORKOUTS

This idea of intensity zones is nothing new. They have been used for five decades and I'm sure this is something you are already familiar with. How I assign the zones, however, may be a bit different to what you are used to. I'll get to that shortly. To realize the best possible results from the workouts described in the Appendix you need to follow my guidelines for setting your personal intensity zones. Using a different set of zones, no matter how familiar you are with them, along with my workouts is likely to have you doing the wrong intensities and not fully realizing the intended benefits. I appreciate that this may be somewhat of a hassle for you if you have all your previous zones memorized from years of use, but

it's necessary that we are on the same page when it comes to the intensities of your workouts. Let's get started down this new intensity zone path by closely examining Table 3.1.

I realize that at first glance Table 3.1 looks quite complex and perhaps even confusing. I've shared it with other coaches who tell me it's too complicated for athletes to grasp, but I disagree. I suspect you are fully capable of understanding it. Once you fathom the basic concepts it becomes quite easy to work with. And it also gives you room to customize your zones to better fit your unique needs.

Table 3.1 Training intensities

Zones	Training Triad Ability	Rating of Perceived Exertion	Description	Time to Exhaustion	Heart Rate			Power		Workout Type
					Maximal (MHR)	Functional (FTHR)	Lactate (LTHR)	Functional (FTP)	Lactate (LTP)	
1	Aerobic Endurance 1	1	Really really easy	Many hours	Less than 72% MHR	Less than 78% FTHR	Less than Z2 LTHR	Less than 56% FTP	All watts less than Z2	Very Easy Recovery Ride (LIT)
2	Aerobic Endurance 2	2	Very easy	5–8 hours	73–82% MHR	78–86% FTHR	LT1 -10	56–75% FTP	Watts at LT1 -10	Long, easy ride (LIT)
		3	Easy	3–5 hours						
							LT1		LT1	
3	Stamina 1	4	Somewhat hard	2–3 hours	83–87% MHR	87–93% FTHR	HRs between LT1 and LT2	76–90% FTP	Watts between LT1 and LT2	Steady ride or very long intervals Short recoveries (HIT)
		5								
							LT2		LT2	
4	Stamina 2	6	Hard	1–2 hours	88–92% MHR	94–99% FTHR	LT2 +10	91–105% FP (FTP is in this range)	Watts at LT2 +10	Long intervals short recoveries (HIIT)
		7								
						FTHR				
5a	Aerobic Capacity 1	8	Really hard	Less than 30 minutes	92–100% MHR	100–102% FTHR%	HRs higher than Z4	106–120% FTP	All watts higher than Z4	Short intervals long recoveries (HIIT)
5b	Aerobic Capacity 2	9	Really really hard	Less than 6 minutes		More than 102% FTHR				
					MHR					
5c	Sprint Power	10	Max effort	Less than 30 seconds	Not applicable	Not applicable	Not applicable	Max power	Not applicable	Short repeats Sprints Very long recoveries

KEY TAKEAWAYS

- Setting your intensity zones using my methods in Table 3.1 may seem confusing at first, but once you get started it will make sense.
- Easy workouts are just as important as hard workouts, perhaps more so.
- If you use my workouts in the Appendix, you *must* use my zones to reap the benefits.

SETTING YOUR ZONES

The main point here is that Table 3.1 is all about giving you options for setting your training zones. The system I used previously, while simple to understand, gave the rider no other options. There was only one way of setting up your zones: my way or the highway. I'll help you set your zones using this new table. But before we get into the details of this table let me explain the basic idea behind training zones.

Why do nearly all coaches and athletes use zones to establish the various intensities they use in training? Why not, for example, just tell you a given heart rate or power to maintain during your ride? The short answer is that just doesn't work. Heart rate and especially power are both stochastic, meaning they change frequently during a ride. You can't possibly hold a one-beat heart rate or single-watt power output for a few seconds, let alone for an entire ride. Heart rate and power both go up and down constantly during a ride. That's due, in part, to changes in terrain, surfaces, shifting wind, how you sense the effort, what's going on around you, and your mental focus. It's obvious that you must have a broader range of intensities that give you similar physiological outcomes.

I should post a disclaimer here: all is not perfect in the world of training zones. Something you must come to accept is that the zones in Table 3.1 are not magic. For example, each zone has a rather limited range from top to bottom. That does not mean that if you go outside the zone that you no longer reap the intended benefits of the workout. It simply is not that precise. There's a bit of estimating that goes into the settings for each zone and the zones overlap. The numbers and percentages you see in Table 3.1 under "Heart Rate" and "Power" are based on what seems to work across the board for most riders. There are certainly outliers for whom the zones leave something to be desired. For the zone system I used previously, I had several athletes over the years tell me, for example, that the upper end of zone 1 felt too hard for recovery. That's quite possible. It's also likely a reflection of their unique physiological characteristics. And with the zones shown in Table 3.1, that, or something similar, may be the case for you also. In other words, you may need to make slight adjustments to the zones to better fit your needs. I'll soon give you a few examples of how you can do that with simple "tools."

ZONES

Let's get started examining the details in Table 3.1. We'll start with the left column and work our way across to the right. Note that there are seven zones in column 1 on the left side. This is a common way of organizing training intensities around both heart rate and power. What is unique for my five-zone methodology is that zone 5 is broken into three subzones—5a, 5b, and 5c. The last one, 5c, is a bit of a wildcard and doesn't exactly fit the way the other zones do. More on that later.

TRAINING TRIAD ABILITIES

The "Training Triad," mentioned in column 2 of Table 3.1, and shown in Figure 3.1, will make all this a bit easier to understand. The six abilities in Figure 3.1 that make up the sides and corners of the figure are tied directly to your zones and your workouts. Each of the key workouts in the Appendix is categorized under these abilities.

On first examining this figure you should immediately notice the three high-performance essential workouts described in Chapter 2—aerobic capacity, stamina, and sprint power. Those, along with aerobic endurance, muscular force, and speed skills, are the workouts you will build into your training plan in Chapter 4. Going forward I will refer to these workout categories as the "six abilities." I'll come back to these abilities frequently in the coming chapters. Let's get to know them a little more closely.

At the corners of the Training Triad in Figure 3.1 are the three "basic" abilities—aerobic endurance, muscular force, and speed skills. They are referred to as basic because all three of the advanced abilities are based on them. They form the foundation of your fitness. On the sides of the triad are the "advanced" abilities—aerobic capacity, stamina, and sprint power. The basic abilities are

Figure 3.1 The Training Triad illustrating the six workout types: basic abilities (corners) and advanced abilities (sides)

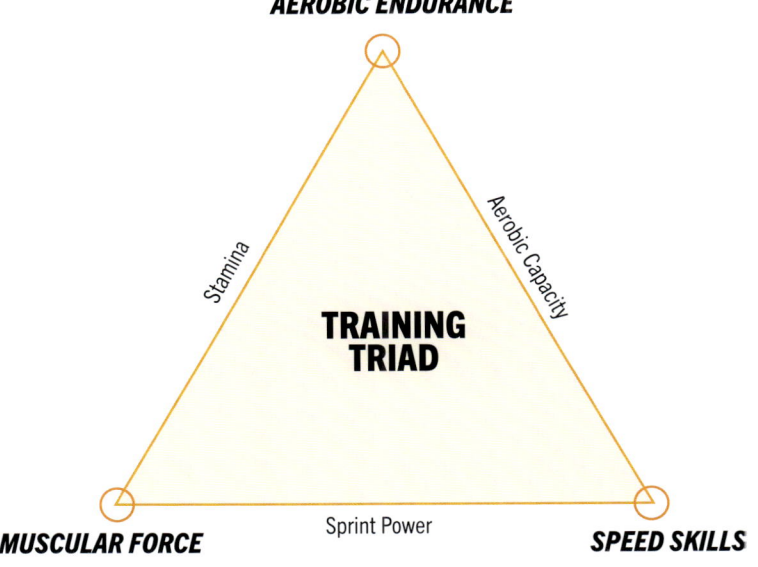

the ones we will focus on in your Preparation and Base periods early in the season and work to maintain in the Build, Peak, and Race periods later (more on these periods in Chapter 4). I've already said quite a bit about aerobic endurance—low-intensity training—in Chapter 2. In that chapter I went into a lengthy discussion of the many benefits of zones 1 and 2. Aerobic endurance should not be taken lightly, as it too often is, by self-coached riders. While all six abilities contribute to your race performance, the advanced abilities will have a tremendous impact on it. While the basic abilities make up the bulk of your training throughout the season and account for the foundation of your general fitness, the advanced abilities are the icing on the cake that get you ready to race. The advanced abilities are the focus of the Build, Peak, and Race periods of your season while you maintain aerobic endurance, muscular force, and speed skills in those periods.

In the Appendix are all the fundamental workouts you will do in the coming season. They are organized by the six abilities. There you will also find the field tests you will do during the season. More on these later in this chapter.

I've already described in Chapter 2 some of the many details of the advanced abilities. Let's look now more closely at the basic abilities.

As mentioned in Chapter 2, aerobic endurance is literally at the heart of your training. There I told you of its many benefits. As you may recall from that chapter, aerobic endurance training is likely the single most important workout type of the early season. Without this nothing else that has to do with race performance happens. It is the starting point for most of the abilities. You will devote a lot of time, especially in your early season, to fully developing this critical ability. Then we will include workouts in the later stages of training, as you approach race day, to maintain the benefits you've gained. For all of this, the focus will be on low-intensity training as this is the wellspring for your aerobic endurance fitness.

Muscular force is a basic ability that has to do with building strength. Improved strength means you will have the potential to drive the pedals with greater force, thus increasing your power output. This type of training is generally done in a weight room, especially in the Base period with maintenance workouts in the Build period. It will be explained in greater detail in Chapter 5.

Speed skills are drills and exercises intended to improve skills such as pedaling, descending, climbing, sprinting, and cornering. As you become more skilled at each of these your speed increases. That's because improving your skills means that you become more economical. That means less wasted energy due to ineffective movements. Basically, economy has to do with how much stored energy it takes for you to drive the pedals and maneuver the bike. Poor skills mean energy leaks resulting in riding slowly or running low on fuel while trying to go faster. A good example of this is what you have probably observed in novice cyclists when pedaling. They typically turn the pedals in squares, wasting a tremendous amount of energy. By working on your skills, you can become more economical and ride faster. This is also a focus of the early season Base period.

The one category of workouts not listed here or on the Training Triad are those that have to do with field testing. Later in this chapter I will explain the testing necessary to establish your current levels of fitness in the advanced abilities and to set your training zones.

All the suggested workouts for each ability and the field tests may be found in the Appendix.

RATING OF PERCEIVED EXERTION AND DESCRIPTION

When I started serious training in the 1970s there were no intensity-measuring devices such as heart rate monitors or power meters. Intensity was defined by how you felt during a workout or race. It was either easy, moderate, or hard. And there were variations on those labels such as "very easy" and "somewhat hard." This allowed us to communicate to others what we were experiencing. It wasn't the least bit scientific, but it worked. And it also forced us to pay close attention to how our bodies were reacting to the stress.

Of course, there were speedometers on bikes then, but the nature of cycling with head and tail winds, drafting, climbing, descending, tight corners, and variable surfaces made them interesting but irrelevant. They were mostly used to measure how long the ride was.

Then along came a Swedish researcher by the name of Gunnar Borg. In 1982 his idea for a scale of intensities was introduced in a sport science journal and it immediately caught on with both sport scientists and athletes. It was also used in the medical field during tests for the severity of diseases. His original scale was from 6 (very, very light) to 20 (very, very hard). The reason for this strange scale was that athletes could multiply their perceived position on the scale by 10 and have an estimate of heart rate. Of course, not all athletes have the same range of heart rates, so he eventually introduced the 1-to-10 scale, which you see in Table 3.1 in column 3. The descriptions of the Ratings of Perceived Exertion (RPE) for Borg's 10-point scale are shown in column 4.

I would suggest that as a cyclist, Borg's 1 to 10 scale is your most important gauge of intensity. Not only does it force you to continually consider how you feel in a workout or race, but also in a mass-start race you can't be looking at your handlebar device or wristwatch for heart rate or power. You must often make quick decisions based on how you feel. RPE is all you have once all electronic devices are ruled out. I highly recommend using the 1-to-10 scale during workouts, in addition to power and heart rate, to define more closely what you are experiencing. Comparing a RPE number with heart rate or power will also serve as a very important learning session for you. That newly developed workout skill will come in handy during races: "When it feels like a RPE 8 in a workout, what does that mean in regard to my power, and how long can I hold an 8?"

TIME TO EXHAUSTION

Speaking of "how long can I hold an 8?" brings us to a critical element of racing—your time to exhaustion at the various zones. Column 5 on Table 3.1 is an attempt to offer some possible answers to such a question. The numbers you see here are based on what I've typically seen riders do in race-like situations. These numbers are certainly not expected of every rider. And the real numbers for you may be significantly different to these. For example, you may be able to hold low zone 2 for more than five hours, but in zone 4 you can't hold on for an hour. These numbers are largely ballpark estimates. Part of the challenge for any rider is to come to know their expected times to exhaustion for each zone. Nice to know, but this probably isn't going to happen. The time-to-exhaustion durations are somewhat of a moving target. They change considerably, both up and down, over time due to fitness, fatigue, and form. I'll come back to these three "Fs" in Chapter 4 as they have a lot to do with how well you perform when it comes to keeping exhaustion at bay.

HEART RATE—MAXIMAL (MHR)

We've finally gotten to an intensity marker for which you will eventually be able to set your training zones. But first, a little background on the heart rate monitor which is a necessary tool for this metric.

In 1977, Seppo Säynäjäkangas, a professor at the University of Oulu in Finland, invented the first wireless heart rate monitor for Nordic skiers that could be used in the field during a workout. Professor Säynäjäkangas went on to found Polar Electro, probably the most recognized manufacturer's name in heart rate monitors to this day. He changed the world, including mine. I got my first Polar in 1982 and after I thought I had figured out what all the numbers meant, I came to rely closely on the data from it—and, sadly, then I slowly began to slip away from relying solely on how I felt. That is one of the common costs of all new technologies. Such devices give us much more precise information, but they come with a price: we become much more externally focused. I have at times had riders put a piece of tape over their handlebar devices when doing workouts, especially hard ones, so they are forced to gauge their intensity on feel. After the ride we would compare their feelings with their intensity data. You can learn a lot about yourself by doing this on occasion.

As mentioned above, one purpose of Table 3.1 is to give you options on how you set your zones. For heart rate, it gives you three options. The first is based on maximal heart rate, the second on functional threshold heart rate, and the third on lactate threshold heart rate. I'll explain the use of thresholds in the following discussions of heart rate zones.

Maximal heart rate, column 6 of Table 3.1, is the only zone metric on the table not based on a threshold. So it's simple to use—*if* you have a known maximal heart rate. If you don't know what yours is, *do not* go out on your bike and bust a gut trying to get your heart rate as high as possible. That's not a good idea. What you can do instead is look back in your training diary or online data for the past year and search for the highest heart rate you produced. It will

EXERTION

probably have come in a race, hard group ride, or interval session. We'll assume that number is your maximal heart rate unless it's raised in the coming months.

Once you have a maximal heart rate (MHR), go to column 6 on Table 3.1 and multiply your MHR by each set of percentages listed for each zone. I'd suggest penciling these in on the table for future reference.

Notice that zone 5c does not have a maximal heart rate percentage. It's marked as "Not Applicable." That's because zone 5c is for sprint power training and the efforts are so brief that heart rate doesn't have time to rise significantly. And as you look across to the right, you'll see that the only 5c zone that does have a metric is under the header, "Power—Functional (FTP)" and is listed as "Max Power." More on that later.

HEART RATE—FUNCTIONAL (FTHR)

If you have a known maximal heart rate you now have one set of heart rate zones you can use for workouts. But if you don't have an MHR, or the number seems too low, then consider using the functional threshold heart rate to set zones. There are two things here I need to explain so we are both on the same page. The first is why there are so many zones on the table based on "thresholds." In fact, all the remaining zones for both heart rate and power are derived from thresholds. The second matter has to do with the word "functional."

As an endurance athlete (and human) you have one or two thresholds for the intensity of your movement based on how they are determined. The reason for these thresholds is that reference points are needed to set up your zones since riders have unique heart rates (and power outputs). The thresholds have different names based on the method used to identify each of them—for example, "functional threshold" and "lactate threshold." For the lactate-based methods there are two thresholds —"lactate 1" (LT1) and "lactate 2" (LT2). LT1 is the lower threshold at the border between zones 2 and 3. LT2 is the higher threshold between zones 3 and 4. The functional threshold heart rate column also has a threshold, but only one. It's in the range between zones 4 and 5a. We'll come back to this shortly.

What is a "functional" threshold? This is an idea that was developed by exercise physiologist Andrew Coggan, PhD, and cycling coach Hunter Allen, and described in their book, *Training and Racing with a Power Meter*. Since lactate testing is historically one of the most accurate ways of setting zones and yet most athletes don't have access to the equipment or the skill necessary to do such testing, Coggan and Allen wanted to come up with a field test, rather than a lab test, to determine a threshold reference point more easily. They referred to this reference point as the "functional" threshold. Their test is a practical way of establishing a reference point without any physiological data such as heart rate or lactate. Using their field test, you can find both your functional threshold heart rate and functional threshold power in a single test. The field test is described in detail in the Appendix under Field Tests—see T1 Functional Threshold Power (FTP) and Heart Rate (FTHR) Test. It requires doing a 20-minute, time trial-like ride. From that an average heart rate is determined from which 5 percent is subtracted to give you a functional threshold heart rate (FTHR). That's the magic number. Use it to set the percentages in column 7 to establish each of your functional heart rate zones.

HEART RATE—LACTATE (LTHR)

Heart rate zones determined by using lactate testing are potentially more accurate than either of the methods described above (see Chapter 2 for more on lactate). By measuring the lactate in single-drop blood samples, which are usually taken from a finger prick, thresholds can be established from which to set zones. There are two thresholds that can be determined using this method. The lower one, usually referred to as "lactate threshold 1" (LT1), defines the border between zones 2 and 3. From the drop of blood analyzed, LT1 is determined as the heart rate where two millimoles per liter (2mmol/L) of lactate is measured. That's a tiny amount. LT2, the higher threshold at the zones 3 and 4 border, is determined when the lactate measurement is four millimoles per liter (4mmol/L). Twice as much lactate, but still tiny. Once you have these thresholds follow the instructions in column 8 to set your zones.

Zones set in this manner are the gold standard for setting heart rate and power zones. You can purchase the test gear (search online for "lactate measuring devices") and learn to self-test, which a lot of athletes do. Or you can find someone who has the test equipment and is more experienced in such testing to do the finger pricks and lactate measurement for you. This latter option, of course, will come with a fee. Lactate testing may be done at universities, at health clubs, or by local coaches.

OTHER HEART RATE OPTIONS

I've now offered three alternatives for defining your heart rate zones. The first is quite easy if you have a known max heart rate. The second entails doing a very challenging field test. And the third, while the most accurate, requires purchasing lactate-measuring equipment and learning how to use it, or paying a more-experienced tester to do it for you (I expect we will have a wearable "continuous lactate monitor" on the market soon).

Having three different methods raises the question of accuracy. Would you get the same zone results if you completed all three of these options? It's highly unlikely. In fact, there may be a considerable difference between them. The more precise you want your zones to be, which is a worthy goal, the stronger the argument for using the lactate-testing method. But you may not want to spend the money to do that several times each year—at the start of the training season and at various times throughout the remainder of the year. Assuming you want to use the max heart rate method or functional threshold test, which are probably less precise than lactate testing, let me give you a couple of simple and easy "tools" you can use to *help* confirm which is more accurate for you.

Heart rate and power are always changing throughout a ride and that's why we use zones.

There is significant research (see References) showing that a "talk test" or ventilatory threshold method is a rather accurate determiner of your heart rate thresholds. This is based on the idea that as the intensity of a ride increases you can say fewer words aloud without taking a breath. There are many ways of doing this described in the research—singing, reciting a poem, saying a common phrase, and more. An easy one involves counting. After warming up, while riding with a slowly increasing intensity over a few minutes, when you are at your "ventilatory threshold 1," which is like LT1—at the border between zones 2 and 3—without taking a breath you should be able to count like this: "One thousand one, one thousand two, one thousand three, one thousand four, one thousand five, one thousand six." If you count to one thousand seven, then you *probably* have not yet reached VT1. In this case, your threshold heart rate is a bit higher. If you can't reach one thousand six without breathing, then your threshold heart rate is lower. As your intensity increases, when you reach VT2 at the border between zones 3 and 4, you should only be able to say, "one thousand one." If you can say more than that then your VT2 is *probably* a bit higher. Choose the heart rate method—max or functional—that comes closest to your talk test thresholds. The talk test combined with the max heart rate or functional threshold heart rate methods is not nearly as accurate as lactate testing, but it gives you some options for helping to confirm your heart rate zones with the other two methods, without spending any money or pricking your finger (as I write, a product is being introduced that will continuously check your ventilatory threshold while wearing a mask).

POWER—FUNCTIONAL (FTP)

Let's move on from heart rate to setting your power zones. But first, a quick history lesson on the origins of power-based training. In 1986, Uli Schoberer, a German cyclist who was also an engineer, was looking for a better way to measure bicycle intensity than simply heart rate. Due to his engineering background, he knew that the answer was figuring out how to measure the power a cyclist produces. From this quest a very rough power meter model was created and eventually refined. He received a patent for his device the following year and founded the business SRM to manufacture and sell his new power meter worldwide. It took about 15 years for his invention to catch on with cyclists, but now the power meter is considered a staple piece of equipment for serious riders, and he has many manufacturing competitors worldwide.

Herr Schoberer loaned an SRM to me to try as I was writing a cycling book in 1994. I eventually purchased a power meter and, once again, it changed my world. Now I had two precise markers of training intensity, giving me more options but also decreasing my reliance on perceived exertion. That would change a few years later.

Let's get back to setting power zones. Worldwide, the most common way to set power zones is with the 20-minute, functional threshold test described above in the heart rate section. Doing one such test allows you to set both your heart rate and power zones. Again, it's not a physically easy test, the effort is that of a short time trial, but it's easily repeated—and costs nothing. There is, however, a learning curve when doing such a test. It is very common the first time a rider does the test to start at too high a power output. This results in the rider rapidly fading over the next several minutes, and poor power and heart rate data are produced. When doing this test, I recommend starting conservatively, easier than you think you can maintain for 20 minutes, and then every five minutes decide if you need to ride slightly harder or slightly easier. The more times you do the test, the more accurate your results become.

Heart rate doesn't change nearly as much as power does over time. And that's the way you want it to be. What you would like to see happen is that your power increases throughout the season as you repeat this test, but heart rate remains relatively stable. Because of the power changes, you should probably test every six to eight weeks.

A common problem with setting training zones based on this test, as with most of the other intensity-determining options above, is that the common way to define zones is to estimate the percentages to use in mathematically setting individual ranges. Notice in the columns for MHR and FTHR in Table 3.1 that each zone is set by multiplying MHR or FTHR by a proposed range of calculations. While the individual ranges may work well for many athletes, there is no guarantee they are right for you. This is one of the problems commonly associated with setting zones—each is essentially an estimate. We are stuck with this incongruity. The most I can say in support of these percentages is that they are likely close to what your physiological zones should be if determined in a lab. There is no perfect measurement system, although lactate testing comes quite close.

You may have noticed that I didn't put "FTP" on a zone border as I did with MHR, FTHR, LT1, and LT2. Instead, it is included in zone 4. The reason for this is that the limited research done on FTP relative to other physiological markers such as maximum lactate steady state, critical power, ventilatory threshold, and lactate threshold have been contradictory.

You can find out more about the functional threshold test in the Appendix under Field Tests—see T1 Functional Threshold Power (FTP) and Heart Rate (FTHR) Test.

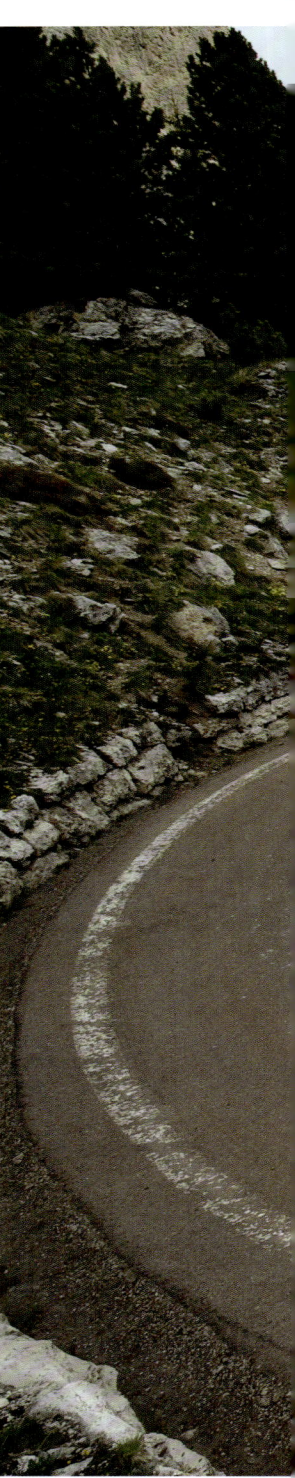

EXERTION

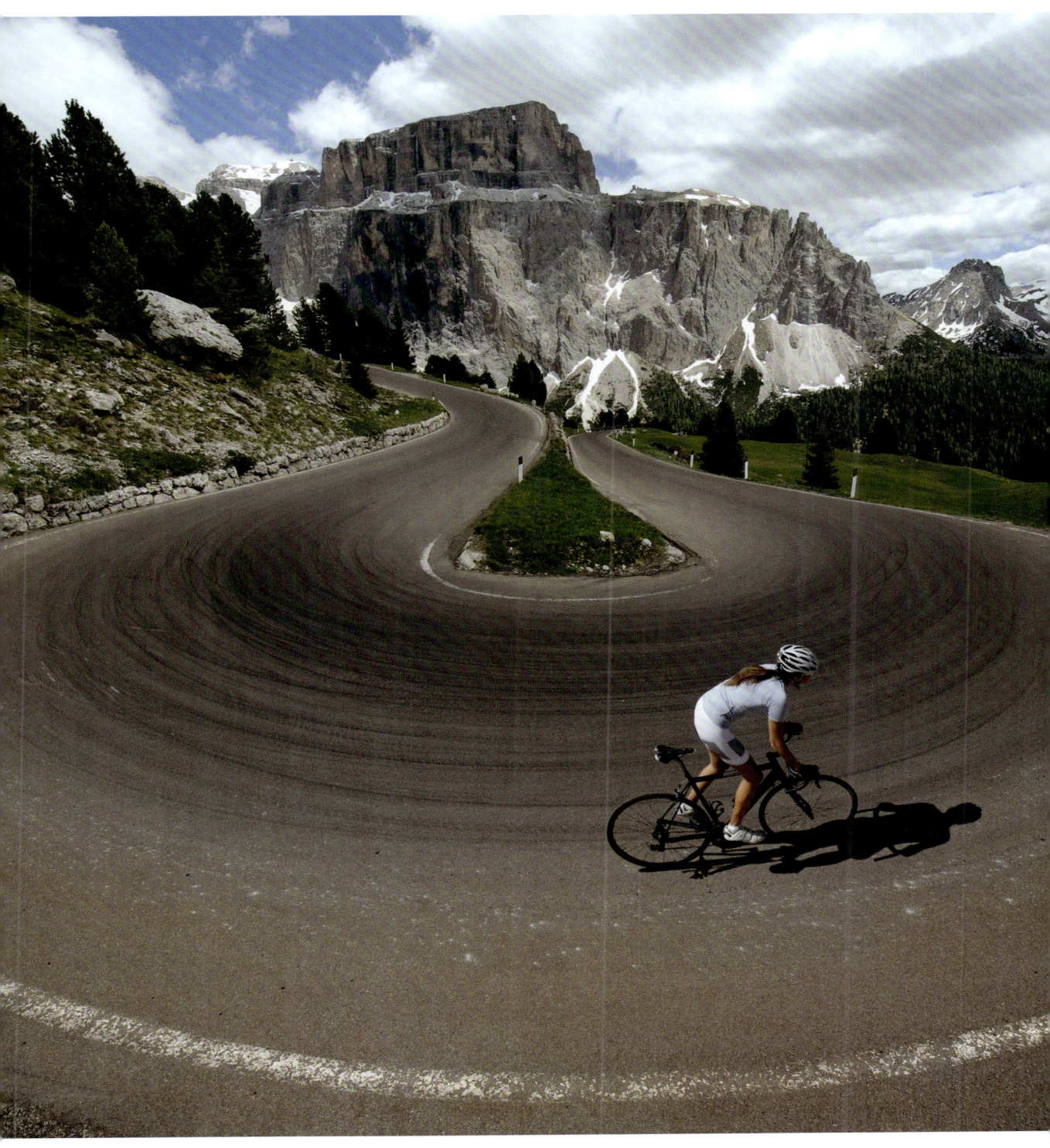

POWER—LACTATE (LTP)

While the functional threshold test is well established as the standard method of setting power zones, it's not without problems. The most common has to do with the many details of the test ride. Such variable matters as the bike you test on, the course you use, weather, wind, temperature, your warm-up, tire pressure, motivation, traffic, and lots more can affect your test results. That brings us back to commonly accepted proven standard—lactate testing.

As mentioned above in the discussion of heart rate measurement using lactate testing, this method for setting power zones is also considerably more accurate than the FTP test, *if* the tester knows what they are doing. If you are the tester and doing it for the first time, there are likely to be errors made that affect outcomes. A highly skilled person would likely do a much better job, at least compared with your first few attempts, but the skill can certainly be developed.

Lactate testing for both heart rate and power is best done on an indoor trainer using your bike—not a standard indoor cycling machine. And as with all indoor rides, there are many conditions to be controlled. The biggest issue is typically heat, which is usually resolved by having a couple of fans aimed at you. Another issue is that the lactate testing equipment must be easily reached and carefully used while riding. This test is usually done as a "graded" test, meaning that every two or three minutes the effort is slightly increased until failure. Having to be precise with the testing equipment while also straining to maintain the effort is not easy.

That's why I suggest having someone who has carried out the test many times as the tester. Such knowledgeable people can likely be found at a university lab, a health club, or with a local coach. You can then concentrate on riding. But just as described above, this means another expense in an already costly sport. And such testing needs to be done every six to eight weeks due to the strong likelihood of power changing throughout the season.

WORKOUT TYPE

The last column on the right side of Table 3.1 describes the type of workout associated with each zone. Examples such as "Very Easy Recovery Ride" at zone 1 to "Short Repeats/Sprints/Very Long Recoveries" at zone 5c give you a general idea as to the type of workout to be done for each zone. Most of them also have in their titles "LIT," "HIT" or "HIIT" in parentheses. These are common terms I will use throughout the book. LIT is "low-intensity training." That means riding in zones 1 and 2. HIT is "high-intensity training"—zone 3. HIIT is "high-intensity interval training" for zones 4, 5a, 5b, and 5c. Zones 3, 4, 5a, 5b, and 5c also generally describe what the recovery durations should be when doing intervals—"Short Recoveries," "Long Recoveries," or "Very Long Recoveries." These terms are used relative to the durations of the work intervals for each workout. A general rule of thumb is that when doing intervals (or repeats), as the work intervals get longer, the recoveries get shorter. For more details on specific workouts go to the Appendix, where workouts are listed by ability.

KEY TAKEAWAYS

- Heart rate and power are always changing throughout a ride and that's why we use zones.
- Training zones are not perfect; you may need to adjust yours based on experience.
- Your Base period will be focused on the basic abilities: aerobic endurance, muscular force, and speed skills.
- The Build and Peak periods will be focused on the advanced abilities: aerobic capacity, stamina, and sprint power.
- Of the zones, the most important for your aerobic endurance are zones 1 and 2, and you will spend a considerable amount of time there.
- Muscular force training builds strength, an early season contributor to your power.
- Speed skills will improve your economy and will help you ride faster without working harder.
- I strongly suggest becoming adept at using Borg's 1-to-10 Rating of Perceived Exertion scale, which is the primary determiner of intensity in a bike race.
- Time to exhaustion varies considerably between riders and is highly trainable.
- Your heart rate zones can be based on maximal heart rate, functional threshold heart rate, or lactate threshold heart rate.
- Use the "talk test" to confirm your heart rate zones.
- The 20-minute field test can be used to set your functional threshold power and functional threshold heart rate zones.
- Heart rate zones are rather stable once accurately set, but power zones can (and should) vary throughout the season as fitness changes.
- Lactate testing is the gold standard for setting zones for both heart rate and power, but requires some expertise.

MEASURING HIGH-PERFORMANCE PROGRESS

Besides testing to establish zones, you should also periodically test the progress of your advanced ability in the high-performance fundamentals—aerobic capacity, stamina, and sprint power. These were explained in Chapter 2 and are illustrated in Figure 3.1. The purpose of the testing is to measure changes in those key determiners of your race performance. Although fitness is always changing throughout the season, both up and down, it typically takes six to eight weeks to see measurable differences in physical readiness to race, so there is no reason to do such testing more frequently. The first of such high-performance tests is not necessary until the late Base period (however, you will do heart rate and power zone testing in the Base period). Otherwise, throughout the Base period the focus is on the basic abilities of the Training Triad—aerobic endurance, muscular force, and speed skills.

The following is a brief explanation of the three advanced ability tests. You'll find more details on these in the Appendix under Field Tests.

FUNCTIONAL AEROBIC CAPACITY TEST

Let's refresh your memory before getting into testing this advanced ability. You may recall that the key to laying the foundation for a high aerobic capacity (VO_2 max) is easy, low-intensity training (LIT) in zones 1 and 2. There are many physiological changes that take place when training this way that high-intensity interval training cannot accomplish. That does not rule out doing hard rides. They are still critical to your performance by bringing your fitness to a high level (see Figure 2.1). You won't be doing HIIT until we start the Build period in the last couple of months of your race preparation. At that point in the season such training will play a pivotal role in how you perform for most race types. As for the LIT in the Build period, you will be doing maintenance rides to keep your aerobic fitness high. This combination of maintenance through LIT workouts and additional fitness-building with HIIT will bring you to a peak of aerobic capacity fitness by race day.

A key issue here is how you will know that your aerobic capacity is improving. One way would be to go back to the lab every few weeks to have a VO_2 max test done. But that's not necessary. You can do a field test to gauge progress and save a lot of money. The test is quite simple. When you are well-rested following a break from training (more on this in Chapter 6), and after a good warm-up, do a five-minute, all-out time trial. Your average power for that test is a very good indicator of your *functional* aerobic capacity. In the Appendix see Field Tests and T2 Functional Aerobic Capacity Test. This test will be done every few weeks.

What should happen over the course of several weeks is that your aerobic capacity power rises. That serves as an excellent indicator of how your training of this ability has been going. Be aware that there may be times when there are downturns in your test results. There are many possible reasons for this, including rested status, lifestyle stress, motivation, change of test course, using a different bike, and the fact that you are human and not a machine.

STAMINA TEST

Stamina is central to your high-performance racing. It is necessary when you are trying to stay away from a charging field of riders, you are at your limit trying to close a gap, you are hammering to maintain your position in a race, or you are all-in climbing a long hill. This is when suffering, which cyclists, regardless of their specific sport, all like to talk about, occurs. You are at your top-end power given the duration of the effort and yet must hang on for what seems like an eternity. Either you have the stamina to keep going or you throw in the towel. There is nothing more mentally and physically demanding in our sport than being called upon to produce stamina. That's why we need to test it to see how yours is progressing throughout the Build period.

You may recall from the last chapter that training stamina starts with long, easy endurance rides early in the season. Then near the end of the Base period, when endurance is well established, the intensity of the long rides is gradually increased. By the time of the peak period, just a few weeks before your race, your stamina must be at a high level. You should be able to hold relatively high power for a relatively long time.

For this test we're going to consider percentages of your functional threshold power (FTP) or your lactate threshold power (LTP) from Table 3.1, whichever you will use for setting power zones. If you use TrainingPeaks this percentage is referred to as the "intensity factor" (IF). On that app the percentages that describe your workout, or interval-like portions of it, are displayed on the post-workout analysis page as your IF for the ride that day. So, by glancing at that page, you can easily see the data you need without doing any math yourself

The stamina test is challenging but simple. It's based on doing a hard effort for 90 minutes. This is best done in the latter part of a workout, for example, following an hour of aerobic endurance riding. Your most basic goal for the 90-minute portion is to maintain an IF of 88 to 92 percent for the duration. That's a basic level of stamina fitness. An IF which is higher than 92 percent is excellent. If your IF is in this range, then stamina is not a limiter for you. This is outstanding and puts you into an exceptional group of riders.

The stamina test will also be done every few weeks in the Build period when you are rested and ready. The first such test will be done at the end of the Base period to establish a fitness standard before you progress to the Build period. Again, you can find the details for the stamina test in the Appendix under Field Tests and T3 Stamina Test.

SPRINT POWER TEST

The third high-performance fundamental is sprint power. It doesn't matter if you are a pure sprinter or not—every rider must be able to produce a good sprint. You never know when you may need that ability. Besides producing a powerful sprint at a finish line, you must also be able to close a gap, jump out of a corner, maintain your position in a group, and many more situations when you must quickly accelerate. As with aerobic capacity and stamina, you need to measure your sprint power regularly and work to improve it. Besides being able to quickly pounce on the pedals, you must also refine your position on the bike to maximize power while reducing drag. Handling your bike skillfully, especially in a pack of riders, is critical not only for a strong finish but also for your safety.

Improving your sprint starts with the ability muscular force—developed primarily by weightlifting—in the early part of the season. Next you will refine your aerodynamic and bike-handling skills. That's also in the Base period. And finally, we will bring it all together by working on your sprint in a group of riders. We won't be able to measure your aerodynamics or group-sprint skills, but we can measure your power. In the Appendix, under Field Tests you will find T4 Sprint Power Test. The purpose of this test is to measure your top-end power over a five-second jump and a 20-second sprint. We should see improvement in both by the last few weeks before your A-priority race.

Besides strength and sprint skills, position on the bike during a sprint has a lot to do with how fast you are. There are several key points you should focus on, especially in the early part of the season when you are refining technique. You are probably already familiar with them but let me refresh your memory. Here are the critical body positions for sprinting that must be mastered in the Base period. Your most powerful sprints are done standing with your butt over the saddle. Your hands are in the drops with elbows bent. This lowers your torso to reduce drag. But for safety and maneuvering reasons, in this position you must have your head up and eyes looking forward.

Another key skill to be developed early in the Base period is pedaling cadence. Pure sprinters can't grind out sprint finishes in a high gear. Their cadence should be high—probably well over 100 RPM. However, there is room for difference here for riders for whom sprinting is not their primary ability. Time trialists and climbers when working on their sprint skills may find that using slightly higher gears and lower cadences is more effective.

KEY TAKEAWAYS

- It takes six to eight weeks to see a measurable change in fitness.
- Aerobic capacity (VO_2 max) is the product of both low-intensity aerobic training and high-intensity interval training.
- You will test functional aerobic capacity with a field test every six to eight weeks in the Build period.
- Stamina, maintaining a relatively high intensity for a relatively long time, is often the determiner of race outcome.
- Testing for stamina indicates how long you can hold a relatively high-power output.
- All riders must be able to sprint regardless of their primary ability.
- The speed skills associated with cadence and position on the bike are both important for sprinting success.

HEART RATE OR POWER?

In Chapter 1 I told you that you should have both a heart rate monitor and a power meter. And by now you've read through a very detailed explanation of how to set zones for both devices. I'm sure that has raised some questions for you: *Should I use a heart rate monitor and a power meter every time I ride? Or should I use just one, and if so, which one, and when?* Before digging down into those questions I'd like to offer my view on what the differences are between using heart rate and power in training, and how this determines which you use in workouts.

Here's my take on this. When measuring the basic ability aerobic endurance, use heart rate in zones 1 and 2. You will do a lot of this type of training, much more than any other zones. This is when you are looking strictly at the physiology of *input*—exactly how the body is responding as you become more aerobically fit. The heart rate monitor is an excellent measure of the aerobic, internal progress you are making. On the other hand, performance is all about *output* and is best measured with power—an external indicator of change. Output, and therefore performance, is aligned with the advanced abilities. And this output marker is closely tied to all of the other zones—3, 4, 5a, 5b, and 5c.

Will you ever use both at the same time? Yes, when doing low-intensity rides. That's your Aerobic Endurance 1 and 2 sessions. What you want to know then is how your "efficiency factor" (EF) is progressing. As I briefly explained EF in Chapter 2, in the world at large, especially in business, efficiency is measured by dividing output (production) by input (cost). In cycling EF is calculated by dividing your power ("normalized" power if using TrainingPeaks, which does the math for you) by your heart rate for a workout or a portion of it. What you are doing is calculating how many watts you put out per heartbeat (production divided by cost or output divided by input). Of course, what you'd like to see happen is that over time (typically six weeks or more) EF increases for similar types of aerobic endurance rides. This means you are producing more watts per heartbeat than for previous, similar rides. You're becoming more efficient. That's always a very good thing to happen and something you should watch for in the early part of the season, the Base period. That's when you will be heavily focused on aerobic endurance. EF is not a concern when doing high-intensity workouts in zones 3, 4, 5a, 5b, and 5c. Due to the nature of these types of hard workouts, EF is not a good indicator of high-intensity fitness progress. It's for strictly aerobic rides—below the lower thresholds of LT1 in Table 3.1.

KEY TAKEAWAYS

- Use your heart rate monitor when training calls for zones 1 and 2.
- Power is the preferred intensity-measuring tool for zones 3, 4, 5a, 5b, and 5c.
- After zone 1 and 2 rides, compare your efficiency factor (EF) with similar rides from eight weeks before
- EF should slowly increase over several weeks indicating improving aerobic fitness.

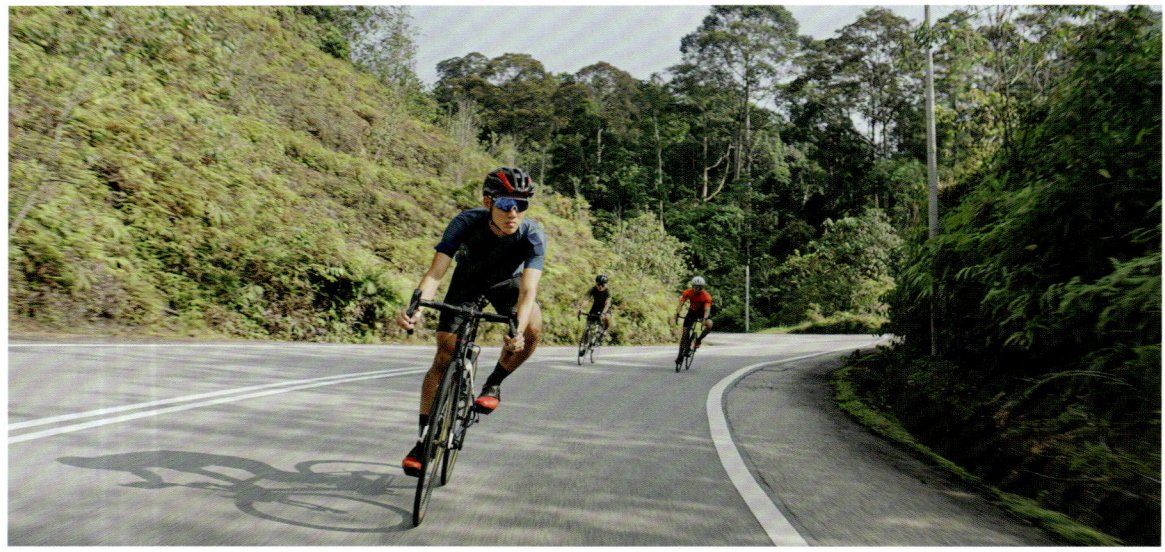

PUTTING IT ALL TOGETHER

There's a wealth of important training information in this chapter. I hope, however, that the heavy chore of reading about intensity hasn't overwhelmed you. Unlike the other workout components, frequency and duration, intensity is a complex topic. I expect you may need to go back and review key topics, such as how to set your zones using max heart rate, functional threshold heart rate, lactate threshold heart rate, functional threshold power, and lactate threshold power. Then decide which you are going to use to set your personal zones. As mentioned frequently above, using lactate testing to set heart rate and power zones is generally the most accurate of all the methods, but it comes at a cost—literally. If you decide not to do lactate testing, I'd highly recommend the functional threshold test which gives you basic data for setting both heart rate (FTHR) and power (FTP) zones. As for heart rate zones determined this way, you may want to confirm the zones 2 and 3 border and the zones 3 and 4 border by doing the counting talk test described above. It will also help to confirm your max heart rate-based zones.

You may recall that in the Prologue I told you about the basic "principles" of training. The first was "individuality." The key point here was how as athletes we are quite similar, but each of us is also unique in many ways. Some of those ways have to do with the intensities of your rides. That's why I gave you lots of options for setting your zones. And you may decide you need to adjust the zones to better fit your unique needs by using the talk test. Also, bear in mind that your intensity zones will vary day to day based on your freshness and fatigue.

That's one of the reasons the zone ranges are wide. If a bit leg-weary in a workout, you may decide to ride in the lower portion of the called-for zone. If feeling good, you will probably want to stay at the higher end. And, as mentioned earlier in this chapter, the zones are not magical nor carved in stone. They are my suggestions for what *may* work for you in a workout. It's okay to go slightly above or below the zones. My concern in suggesting this is that you will opt for doing most of your rides in the middle of the intensity range, probably zone 3. That's a common mistake made by self-coached riders. Assuming your zones are correct, zone 3 is too hard to reap the aerobic benefits of LIT and doesn't do much to boost aerobic capacity. There's a place for zone 3 training, but it should be saved for those times when you are focused on boosting your stamina. The only other time zone 3 is important to your performance is when you are in the final weeks of preparing for an event that will be largely conducted in zone 3, such as a gran fondo or century ride. Other than that, it's best avoided, especially when concentrating on aerobic endurance.

KEY TAKEAWAYS

- The first principle of training is individuality and must be considered when setting training zones.
- Zones vary from day to day based on how fresh and rested or fatigued and rundown you are.
- With a few exceptions, as in the Base period, zone 3 training is best avoided.

THE REST OF LYNDA'S STORY

I coached Lynda for two more seasons. In our second season together, she won the Scottish National Championship again. She was an exceptional athlete. We had a very good working relationship. Lynda retired from racing after our third season together. She went on to become a coach whose athletes have also done quite well. I still have a lot of respect for her as a person, rider, and as a coach.

4. PLANNING

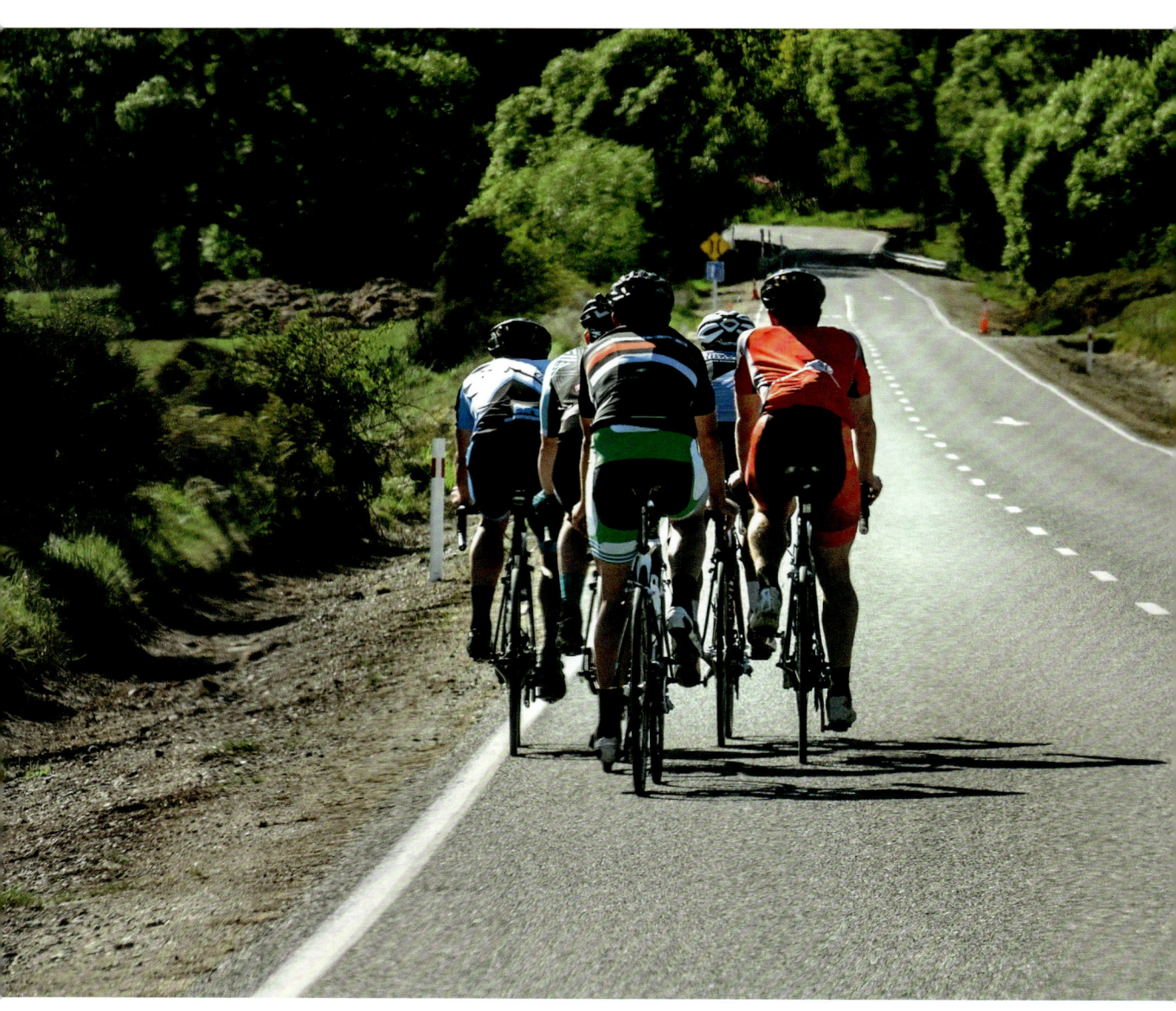

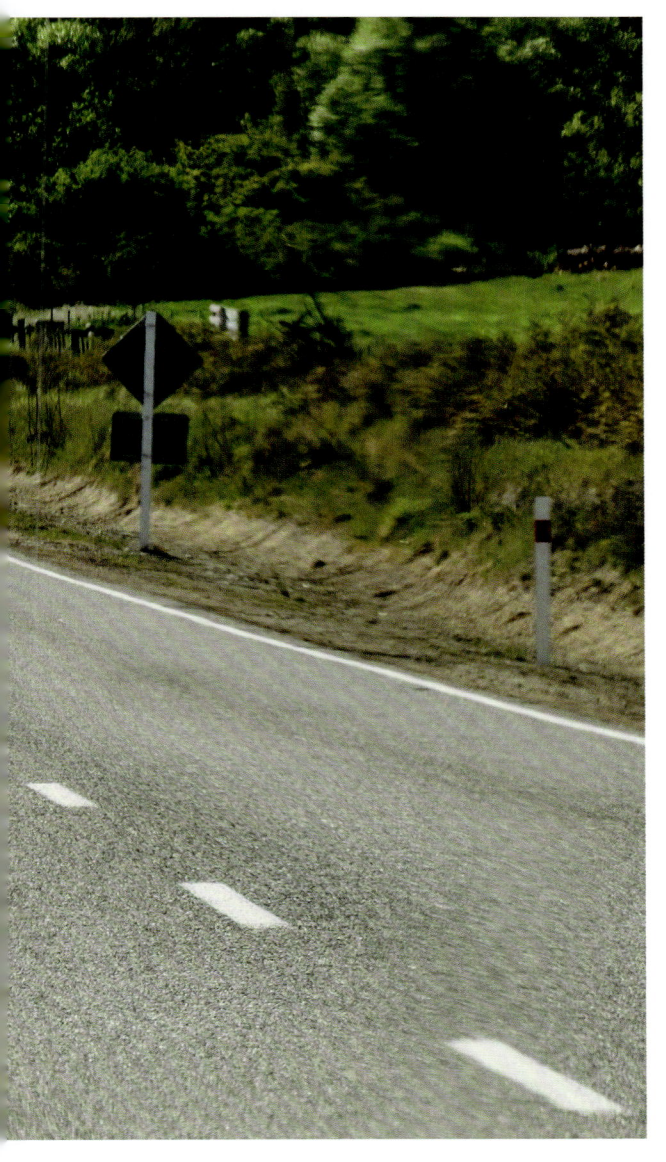

In this chapter we will start putting together your training plan for the season. And we'll finish it in Chapter 5. I will keep this as straightforward as I can using only one periodization model and a simple way of organizing it. Otherwise, this can become a rather complex topic. However, should you want to dig into this subject in greater detail by viewing more of the periodization options available, see my book, *The Cyclist's Training Bible* 5th edition, as it goes deeply into the many ways you can build a training plan.

Planning is the primary purpose of that book. I wouldn't recommend, however, getting overly deep into this topic. Most riders can put together a well-thought-out, and effective, *linear* periodization plan, which is what I will describe on the following pages. I will help you develop a broad and general understanding of seasonal training before we dig into the specifics in Chapter 5.

Let's start by getting a basic understanding of the essential components that make up a training plan. Then we will lay out the basics of your custom training plan.

TOM'S STORY

Our paths crossed again at a local race that fall. I had met him before as he was on a team that frequently competed with my son's team. And I also learned that day that they went to the same university. After his race he asked if we could talk. He wanted to know if I would coach him. I already knew quite a bit about him as I had been to several local races, and he was frequently racing. He was a decent sprinter but lacked the stamina to hang in there late in a long road race. His forte was criteriums.

I liked Tom a lot, and since he raced locally where I could easily attend, I agreed to coach him. And because he was a full-time student, I gave him a break on my coaching fee. I think he probably could have afforded it, with his parents' help, but I have a soft spot in my heart for students.

We met at the university cafeteria a few days later so we could talk about where he wanted to go with his racing the following season. Tom lived up to what I had learned of him at the few races I'd seen: a nice guy, enthusiastic about racing, a strong desire to perform at a higher level, and very open to learning new ways of doing things. I could tell that motivation was not a problem. Motivation can be a positive or a negative when it comes to training. Too much and the rider becomes greedy wanting even more fitness than planned. But if motivation is in check the rider will figure out ways to meld his lifestyle and training.

As Tom and I talked over lunch, however, he threw a monkey wrench into the works. He had just started his senior year and was in the early stages of a very challenging class schedule. On top of the classroom work, he was training to be a teacher and in a couple of weeks he was to start three months of an internship at a local high school. He was going to be up to his ears in work. Training would have to take a backseat to his school commitments. That would mean limited time on the bike until, probably, second semester. But he still wanted to get started training. He asked if I could lay out a basic plan with light volume that he could follow through the fall semester until things opened for more training time later in the school year. "No problem," I said.

From having seen him race as a sprinter the past summer I had a good idea of what he needed. I would schedule a lot of indoor training for late fall and winter with an emphasis on strength development in the school's gym. He'd do a total body strength program with an emphasis on the legs in addition to hip flexibility and mobility work. As for the bike, he needed to focus on his basic pedaling and bike-handling skills. That wouldn't take much of his time as it would be mostly drills he could do on campus or even on his indoor trainer. In the winter we would also include some running for cross-training to help build aerobic endurance since he wasn't riding much and the weather was often a factor. Easy, short runs would accomplish in a half hour what would take an hour on the bike. That fit very nicely for a time-crunched rider this time of year. Then when his schedule became less challenging in the second semester, he'd start getting in some longer rides to build aerobic endurance and, later, stamina. By next March he'd be ready to do team rides and start working on group sprinting, which I knew was very important for him.

All I needed to know to get him started was the weekly internship and classroom schedule and when he would have time for the gym and bike skills work. From that I put a get-started plan together for the next few weeks. He was to provide me with his daily training diary so I could see how he was progressing. We would talk weekly about what I was seeing in his diary, if he was able to fit in all the weekly workouts, how he was feeling, what his off-the-bike stress load was like, how much sleep he was getting, his appetite, and what he thought he needed to work on going forward. From his feedback and my sense of his progress, I would adjust his plan for the coming week while we were on the phone. After the conversation I'd put together a one-week practical training plan to continue where the current one ended. These plans were always subject to change if we saw problems. And they frequently did change with regards to the demands on his time. This weekly process continued throughout the first semester, which ended in January.

The second semester would be somewhat easier for Tom with the internship over and a lighter classroom workload. He then stopped running and began to get in longer rides with an emphasis on aerobic endurance. We included "form" sprints near the ends of many of these early rides. In March he began stamina training along with hill work as he cut back on weightlifting. By now he was only in the gym once a week.

From the testing he did throughout the winter I could tell his early season race preparation was coming along well. He had stayed focused on fitting in workouts all winter, his motivation was excellent, his stress level was manageable, sleep was consistent, and he seldom missed a workout. His spring group rides with the team also went well, and sprinting seemed to be making great progress once he started riding with the team. I had a good feeling about his first C-priority race in late April, a one-hour criterium on a mostly flat course.

He came away from that first race with a second-place finish, just a half wheel from winning. When we talked after the race, he was ecstatic. He had never started a season with such a strong race. I expected even better results for him as the season unfolded. His A-priority race for the season was still several weeks away and this first race was a good predictor of the coming season. We were off to a good start.

Great endurance coaches know that success is not about epic workouts or ever-increasing intensity. Success is achieved when athletes stay healthy and successfully execute most of their training sessions with intent, discipline, and with quality.

A POLARIZED TRAINING APPROACH:
DR. STEPHEN SEILER

Twenty years have passed since I first introduced the term "polarized training" in a scientific research paper. It is fair to say that this term has taken on a life of its own since then. I have spent the last 20 years trying to better understand the "why" behind the training intensity distribution I observed in elite endurance athletes so long ago. Data from three types of "laboratories" all contribute to our understanding of the endurance training process today.

The Darwinian-ish laboratory of thousands of coaches and endurance athletes iterating their training methods over time remains where the rubber meets the road, where effective training practices emerge, and ineffective or even harmful training practices eventually go extinct. Secondly, the traditional systems physiology laboratory that I have spent a lot of time in has helped us to understand how brain, heart, lungs, muscles, and more all interact and collectively respond to changes in exercise intensity and duration in training or racing. Finally, in the last 25 years or so, molecular exercise biology laboratories have dived into the inner workings of muscle cells and other molecular components of the training process. By combining the findings from all three of these experimental arenas, we are now able to speak with some clarity about how training frequency, intensity, and duration interact to generate both cellular level signals for adaptation inside and around different types of tissue, and the systemic stress responses that come along with those adaptive signals.

I now see *polarized* training fundamentally as a day-to-day management system evolving in the real world of high-performance endurance. This training approach helps ensure that the balance between adaptive signal and systemic stress is appropriate and manageable over time. Endurance athletes play the long game. If the training process is not sustainable, the results will not be attainable. This training sustainability criterion is the same for the Olympian and the age-grouper trying to find time to train for their first triathlon while working full time and coaching their daughter's soccer team.

What are we "polarizing" in our endurance training programs? It is not heart rate, power, or pace. Twenty years on, I am convinced by the data from all three of those laboratories I described above that we are polarizing *stress*. Put another way, *no pain, no gain* is a catchy slogan, but it is a terrible training philosophy! Joe Friel is a coach who truly understands this and the methods clearly presented in his book reflect that understanding. Great endurance coaches know that success is not about epic workouts or ever-increasing intensity. Success is achieved when athletes stay healthy and successfully execute most of their training sessions with intent, with discipline, and with quality. This is true for three-hour low-intensity training sessions, 75-minute threshold sessions, and 45-minute high-intensity interval sessions. All these types of sessions generate important molecular signals for adaptations, like increasing the synthesis of mitochondrial proteins or building more capillaries around skeletal muscle fibers. However, threshold and HIIT sessions also generate a lot more systemic stress that appropriately prescribed and executed lower intensity, longer duration sessions do not. Staying under the stress radar while inducing lots of adaptive signaling is what the 80 percent is all about!

Intensity can only be understood in the context of duration. Threshold intensity (slightly lower intensity but longer accumulated work duration) and high-intensity sessions (shorter total duration but higher intensity) are both HARD and require longer recovery, because of the physiological and mental stress they induce. They are both part of the 20 percent in the 80-20 session intensity distribution we see so often among the best endurance athletes across sports.

So, threshold sessions are NOT bad for you, but the most common mistake endurance athletes make is letting their training intensity distribution "regress toward the mean." We tend to let the intensity become too hard on planned easy days, so we are not recovered enough for planned hard days. The result is too much threshold intensity training—an effective recipe for stagnation and burnout, whether you are an elite athlete training every day and 25 hours a week, or a recreational cyclist getting out the door three to four times a week.

I have learned a lot of what I know from thoughtful and systematic coaches like Joe Friel. I can also see when perusing his writing that Joe keeps up with the science. This is a great combination and one you will benefit from throughout the pages of this book.

Dr. Stephen Seiler of the Department of Sport Science and Physical Education, University of Agder, Kristiansand, Norway, is well-known for his research and teaching on the organization of endurance training and intensity distribution. He has published around 125 peer-reviewed publications and given over 100 international lectures on the endurance training process.

TRAINING METHODOLOGIES

Since the early 2000s two conflicting methods for distributing daily workout intensities have developed. Until this conflict appeared there had not been much thought given to how easy, moderate, and hard workouts should be allocated in a weekly training plan. How much of each was appropriate and effective? In this regard, training was more art than science.

POLARIZED TRAINING

Then in the early 2000s Stephen Seiler, PhD, a Norwegian sport science professor, discovered that elite athletes in many endurance sports distribute their workouts so that roughly 80 percent of the sessions are easy and 20 percent hard. Later, he and other sport scientists determined that this 80-20 distribution of workouts was effective for athletes at all levels of competition—not just elites. The significant take-home here is that avoiding workouts that fall into the middle intensity, the "threshold" zones 3 and 4, and ensuring that easy workouts are truly easy and hard sessions are hard, may produce greater fitness and better race results than the more common method of intensity distribution. Since then, I've found this "polarized" method of training has proven effective at the right time of the season for the athletes I've coached.

Note that in this description of polarized training the emphasis is on the workout type, not on precise measurements of intensities by zone during a workout. This is a very important point in understanding polarized training. For example, an athlete may do a workout they call "hard" because it involves high-intensity intervals. But of course, there was a warm-up in which the workout intensity was low and, perhaps, slowly rose to a moderate intensity as the heart rate went up. Following the warm-up, the athlete completed several very high-intensity efforts. Between those hard efforts were recovery intervals during which the athlete's heart rate gradually came down by passing through moderate and into the low-intensity range. Here's where Dr. Seiler's research makes an important distinction. The workout, regardless of the up and down progressions of the heart rate throughout, was classified as "hard" because that was the intent and focus of the session, and it was executed in keeping with that intent. In other words, it was the highest intensities (heart rates, in this example) that caused the entire workout to be described as "hard." The same was done with the easy workouts. So, polarized training is not referring to the specific and detailed distributions of the workout's intensities, such as heart rate or power, but rather to the distribution of the training *sessions*. They are either very hard or easy.

PYRAMIDAL TRAINING

In a polarized approach to training the athlete avoids *moderate* workouts ("somewhat hard" and "hard"), and instead focuses on doing either really hard or easy sessions. This, of course, implies that moderate workouts are not necessary for developing race readiness.

PLANNING

This brings us to the other common training method, called "pyramidal." In this method the athlete, essentially, does three broad types of workout—easy, moderate, and hard. This is much more in line with the classic way of preparing for a race by using all the available intensities with, perhaps, an emphasis on a particular intensity in each workout. Training intensity in this case is distributed according to how much time was spent in the training zones, not what the purpose of the workout was.

WHEN TO USE EACH

I've found there are times when both are beneficial. I prefer to use pyramidal training for riders in the early season (Base period) when the emphasis is on establishing general fitness, especially aerobic fitness, which is "easy" training. But the athlete will devote some training time to moderate efforts as fitness is developing. I make this progression to more moderate-intensity rides (zones 3 and 4) after the aerobic system is well developed. This involves a lot of middle zone rides to boost stamina. Then, once the athlete progresses to the next period of training approaching the race (which I call the Build period), we begin to follow a more polarized approach—easy or hard workouts with very little in the moderate range. The exception to this in Build period training is for riders who will be performing on their event day in the moderate intensity range—for example, gran fondo or century riders. In that case, an athlete's workouts will remain pyramidal in their training intensity distribution throughout the season. But in the Build period, road cyclists, mountain bikers, gravel racers, and others whose race outcomes depend on very high intensities, will train polarized.

This discussion is leading us to a point where you will be ready to create your training plan for the season. But before we can do that there are a couple more periodization topics you need to fully understand.

KEY TAKEAWAYS

- To polarize your training, 80 percent of your workouts will be easy and 20 percent hard.
- The 80-20 split is not based on heart rates or power, but rather on the purpose of the completed workout—hard or easy.
- When using polarized training avoid moderate-intensity (zone 3) workouts.
- In pyramidal training do easy, moderate, and hard workouts based on measured intensities (heart rate or power), not the "intent" of the workout as in polarized training.
- I recommend following a pyramidal plan in the early season (Base period) and a polarized plan later in the season (Build and Peak periods).
- The exception to this Build and Peak method of training is if you are training for an event which is contested primarily in zone 3—if so, then use pyramidal training throughout the season.

GENERAL AND SPECIFIC TRAINING

Besides polarized and pyramidal training, workouts on the bike are divided into two broad types—general and specific. General training happens early in the season in the Preparation and Base periods. These are the periods when you are *not* doing workouts that mimic the race. In other words, the intensity is low—not race-like—and you are lifting weights. The latter is also something you don't do in a race. These types of workout are therefore termed "general." They are not "specific" to the race you are preparing for. The specific workouts come later in the season in the Build, Peak, and Race periods, when training gradually comes to reflect the demands of the event.

The final period of the season—Transition—is also general and serves as the physical and mental shift from the previous race season to the next season. This is, essentially, the "off season."

The idea of this general and specific training concept is to help you understand exactly what your purpose in training is at various times. When the training is general you are doing things that are unlike the race—for example, cross-training, riding slow and easy, lifting weights, improving weak skills, and lots of solo workouts. When training is specific your workouts increasingly take on the characteristics of the race you are training for—workouts at high intensity, improving limiters, riding on race-specific terrain, training in conditions like those expected in the race, doing group rides, and refining race strategies and tactics.

KEY TAKEAWAYS

- Do "general" training early in the season (Preparation and Base periods) with workouts that are mostly *unlike* the goal race.
- "Specific" training simulates portions of the race and is done later in the season (Build and Peak periods).
- The period between seasons—Transition—is general training and is often called the "off season."

TRAINING PROGRESSION

You should now have a good understanding of how your workouts will be distributed relative to intensity and type—pyramidal and general in the early season and polarized and specific later in the season. But there's more. Before we get into the details of the training plan we'll use for your next race season, I'd like to go into a bit more detail as to why your season will be structured in a certain way. The following is an overview of what I'll guide you through later in this chapter as you develop your training plan. I think it will help you understand the *whats* and *whys* of your plan.

As your season progresses from the start to your eventual A-priority race and beyond, we will manipulate the workout frequencies, durations, and intensities to progressively bring you to a peak of readiness by race day. The order of the following three-fold progression is important as it allows your body to gradually adapt to the stresses of training throughout the season.

Athletes all too often decide that they are somehow significantly different from other humans who ride bicycles and so none of this applies to them. They jump right in to doing high-intensity intervals and hard group rides several months prior to their A-priority race and skip all the earlier stages that develop the basic abilities (aerobic endurance, speed skills, and muscular force). All this early season training, though it might seem like a waste of time to some, prepares the body for the more advanced training of the final weeks before the race that eventually produces high-performance, race-specific fitness. Diminishing the importance of workout frequencies and durations, and skipping ahead to the high-intensity sessions, precludes the body from fully absorbing the intended benefits of, for example, aerobic training.

High-performance fitness is the accumulation of the many different components of training. It's not simply high-intensity workouts. In fact, when it comes to high performance, that won't take you very far. Training solely that way will not produce excellent fitness. That way of thinking is more common for back-of-the-pack riders. Riders that believe high intensity is the *only* key to successful racing simply don't grasp what training is about. The bottom line is that by skipping all the early season basic abilities, pyramidal, and general training you will have less fitness on race day than if you had followed a full-season plan. There are no shortcuts to high performance. It takes patience and persistence for weeks and months. Trying to rush race readiness by leaving out the basics always leads to disappointment. I'm going to show you a much more effective way of training.

Besides polarized-pyramidal and general-specific, there is a third key element of successful training—the seasonal progression. The following discussion of frequency, duration, and intensity explains the progression I strongly suggest you follow throughout the season. It's another important overview of your training plan, which we will get to shortly. The following progression produces peak fitness at the right time. Here we will break your training down into three broad stages. The following is a deeper explanation of the intensity and Training Triad topics shown in Table 3.1 and Figure 3.1.

THE FIRST TRAINING STAGE: PREPARING TO TRAIN

The purpose of this early season stage of training is to gradually increase the volume of training without riding long durations by increasing the *frequency* of workouts. To do that you can either do two short rides daily or, and this is the preferred method, you can do one ride daily along with one cross-training session. The ride (or rides) early in the season are relatively short compared with what you'll be doing later. This doesn't have to be your typical ride. It could, for example, be riding your bike to and from work for your daily workouts. If that doesn't fit your situation, then just do a shortish ride every day. Such a ride could be about half the duration you typically do in the summer or less. That's one of the two daily workouts. The other is a cross-training session.

The cross-training sessions are also similarly short and could be any other aerobic activity that appeals to you. That could be running, hiking, rowing, Nordic skiing, snowshoeing, rowing, or using an aerobic exercise machine such as a stair climber or any other machine that you enjoy. Variety is good for motivation at this time of the season so you may want to use several aerobic cross-training workout types. An often-overlooked option is walking briskly. For such a session, male and female riders with aerobic capacities greater than about 50, which is likely to be those under age 50, can walk wearing a weighted backpack—10 percent of bodyweight or less is usually adequate. Older riders or those with lower aerobic capacities will get the aerobic benefits we're seeking here just by walking briskly. Again, the purpose is *not* to push your limits—no heavy breathing—but rather to build aerobic endurance with lots of low-intensity training.

There are a couple of reasons I want you to cross-train at the start of the season. One is that it is likely to be winter and so getting a lot of time outdoors may be quite challenging due to the weather where you live. Another option here, however, is to ride indoors using a trainer. The downside of that for some riders is boredom. Of course, you could use one of the many available apps for virtual workouts and even online group rides. The only problem I see with this is the urge to compete with other riders using the app by riding at an overly high intensity. You need to keep *all* workouts at this time of year in the aerobic endurance range—low-intensity training in zones 1 and 2. Higher intensities at this time of year are counterproductive and will *not* improve your race performances later in the season. Keep it easy!

Another reason for cross-training now is that your season is probably long and the boredom from too much of the same thing over and over for the entire season can easily lead to burnout. You may be enthusiastic now, but that eagerness is likely to wane when you're several months into your season and not quite as keen anymore, perhaps leading to inconsistent training.

All your workouts at this time in the season, both cross-training and on the bike, should be in heart rate zones 1 and 2 (see Table 3.1). You are unlikely to have zones set for your cross-training sport, so instead use the talk test as explained in Chapter 3. The talk test will determine your lower threshold at the upper end of zone 2. Stay just a few heartbeats below that during the cross-training sessions. Check frequently to make sure you are. Your aerobic system (heart, lungs, blood, and more) will benefit from a wide variety of endurance sports in addition to riding the bike. But it must all be easy.

Besides boosting aerobic endurance with short rides and cross-training, the other element of building your fitness we want to work on now is muscular force (see Figure 3.1). That calls for doing some type of resistance work. This is typically done by weightlifting in a gym, but it doesn't have to be done that way. There are many strength-building devices available on the market that will help you make muscular gains without spending a lot of money. One such commonly used device is a heavy-duty, elastic stretch band. Bodyweight can also be used for many strength-building exercises. Chapter 5 goes into greater detail on muscular force.

In this frequency stage of training, which is all aerobic, your purpose is to build aerobic endurance without doing long rides. You'll get plenty of that later. By doing two daily, relatively short workouts on most days of the week, you will be preparing for what comes next in training—longer duration rides.

THE SECOND TRAINING STAGE: TRAINING TO TRAIN

The next stage of the season begins with a gradual transition from two daily workouts to longer, single-ride, daily sessions done on the bike. The purpose now is to keep the daily and weekly training volume about the same as in the previous, frequency stage of training, only to gradually shift to doing it all by riding. That means the emphasis now becomes workout duration. This requires progressing from relatively short two-a-day workouts to only one longer ride. After three or four weeks you should have phased out all cross-training in favor of increased time on the saddle. And, hopefully, the weather is starting to break, making outdoor rides more enjoyable. If not, continue cross-training or ride indoors.

Your rides will now follow a pyramidal intensity distribution. That basically means that your workouts will include some zone 3 along with occasional zone 4 rides. This will put you in the early stages of stamina training, which is one of the advanced abilities (see Table 3.1 and Figure 3.1). By the end of this stage, you will test your stamina to see how well developed it is. That will help to determine how you train in the following stage.

Also, in the first few weeks of this stage your strength training for developing muscular force will reach its pinnacle. It will have advanced from low resistance and high reps in the first stage of training to high resistance and low reps. Your strength should be at a seasonal high by this point. After that we go into a strength maintenance mode for the remainder of the preparation for your first race.

THE THIRD TRAINING STAGE: PREPARING TO RACE

In this third stage of training, we begin to introduce race-like intensity workouts as you slightly cut back on high-volume training, allowing for more energy to be used in high-intensity training. Training now becomes all about getting ready to race. That means your hard workouts will be devoted to aerobic capacity, stamina, and sprint power. How these are prioritized depends on your race type, goal, and limiter. This is the stage of training which is most customized to your unique needs. As you approach the end of this stage you will taper the training, meaning you will cut back on volume by reducing durations even more, while intensity remains race-like. That will be your final preparation for the race.

Your training progression will now be polarized with key workouts being either high-intensity, challenging sessions or low-intensity sessions primarily intended to maintain aerobic endurance and speed skills. If you are preparing for an event which is done in a lower intensity zone, such as a gran fondo or century ride, you will train using a pyramidal structure with a greater emphasis on stamina. Strength training in this stage is strictly for muscular force maintenance (more on this in Chapter 5).

This stage is much shorter than the previous one, because the previous duration stage of training is, in many ways, the most important of the season. In fact, it could be extended for several more weeks without any problems, and that's what you should do if you are starting your event preparation more than 48 weeks prior to race day. However, this final intensity stage of training is very different from the previous two in one important way. If this last stage is appreciably extended it will eventually result in a *loss* of fitness. The body can only handle this level of high-stress intensity for a few weeks before breakdowns begin to occur, followed by a drop in fitness and race readiness. This is a common problem for self-coached riders who believe that months of high intensity is the key to racing well. The bottom line here is that if you make a mistake, make it on the side of too much time in the duration stage and too little in the intensity stage.

KEY TAKEAWAYS

- In the first stage of training do frequent, short workouts—two a day is perfect.
- Cross-train early in the season—run, hike, walk, row, Nordic ski, snowshoe, or whatever aerobic activity you enjoy.
- In the Base period, when riding indoors using a virtual training app, do *not* compete with other riders.
- Do all workouts in the *frequency* stage of the season in zones 1 and 2.
- In the second stage of training—duration—increase the length of your rides as you phase out cross-training.
- In the latter portions of the second stage, train pyramidal with some zone 3 stamina workouts (see Appendix).
- Early in the second stage of training, maximize your strength and then begin strength maintenance.
- In the third stage make the workouts increasingly like the race.
- Polarized training—either hard or easy—is the way to train in the third stage.
- Do not extend the third stage beyond eight to 11 weeks of race-like workouts as you are likely to lose fitness.

TRAINING PLAN OVERVIEW

We are finally at the point where I believe you are ready to put a seasonal training plan together, so we'll now examine a very popular and successful method for organizing your workouts. What is described below I've successfully used with athletes at many levels. In the rest of this chapter, I will explain how you can go about designing your custom seasonal training plan by following a *periodized* structure. This simply means that your season will be divided into short periods of one to four (or more) weeks, each with a purpose that is gradually integrated with the others based on what you've read above. You don't have to follow my suggestions here if you know of a unique organizational training method that has proven successful for you in the past. There is no arguing with success. But I'd strongly recommend giving what I suggest here some thought as it may be just the breakthrough you need. If you are disappointed with how your racing has gone in past seasons, this could be the change that gets you back on track.

PERIODIZED TRAINING

There are many ways to organize your seasonal plan, but linear periodization, while not perfect (none are), is easily understood and has a long history of success for athletes at many different levels of competition. Now that you have a good understanding of the basics of planning, we will start laying out a linear plan for your season.

But first let's take a step back to make sure we are on the same page. I keep using the word "periodization" in this chapter. What, exactly, does that mean? Periodization is simply a way of organizing the frequencies, durations, and intensities of your workouts along with including R&R breaks at appropriate times over the course of the season. There are many ways to periodize a training plan. In the following I suggest laying out your season using what is called a *linear* periodization model. "Linear" means that it simply follows a direct pattern from the time you start training all the way up to race day with no undulating, blocks, inverse or reverse periodizing, or any other complex planning variations. I have used this with most of my client-athletes at all levels of performance for years, including for Tom in his story at the start of this chapter. This classic model has been used in sport for decades. It is the most common way of laying out a training plan across a wide spectrum of sports and athlete talents. In this model, as described above, you start the season focused on workout frequency followed by boosting workout duration, and gradually progress to an emphasis on workout intensity as you approach your A race. Also, of significance is how the R&R periods are distributed. We will get to those in Chapter 6. Other planning details will also be described in Chapter 5.

Table 4.1 lists the linear periods and a broad description of each based on what you read earlier in this chapter.

Table 4.1 The training periods, training types, progression emphasis, purpose, and common lengths in days and week

Period	Training Type	Progression Emphasis	Purpose	Common Length Prior to First A Race of Season
Preparation	General	Frequency	Preparing to train. Start the season with an emphasis on aerobic endurance using cross-training along with introductory strength.	3–6 weeks (can be longer)
Base	General – Pyramidal	Frequency/ Duration	Training to train. Phase out cross-training. Gradually increase ride durations. Develop the basic abilities. Introduce basic stamina and sprint power skills workouts.	12 weeks (more is better)
Build	Specific – Polarized	Intensity	Training to race. Workouts gradually become more race-like as the emphasis shifts to advanced abilities while maintaining basic abilities.	8–9 weeks (not longer)
Peak	Specific – Polarized	Intensity	Training to race. Taper weekly volume. Gradually reduce workout durations to shed fatigue while keeping intensity race-like. Avoid distress.	10 days–2 weeks (not longer)
Race	Specific – Polarized	Intensity	Training to race. Sharpen race readiness. The week of the race do short, race-like efforts with an emphasis on avoiding fatigue.	5–7 days (not longer)
Transition (Off Season)	General	Rest and Recovery	Rest and recover. After several weeks of heavy loading for the race, take a rest and recovery break to unload. The break is longest after the last race of the season.	1–4 weeks (can be longer)

KEY TAKEAWAYS

- If your racing has not been up to par, a purposeful and well-designed training plan may be just the change you need.
- I strongly suggest using a simple linear periodization structure to plan your season.
- Periodization is a refined way of melding workout frequencies, durations, and intensities, along with R&R, into a training plan with a focus on an event.
- The linear periodization planning structure is both simple and effective.

YOUR TRAINING PLAN

There are two important points I want to make about periodization before we get into the particulars of your training plan. The first is that the plan we come up with must be flexible. Following the plan without deviating when it's apparent that change is needed is the biggest reason why periodization fails to work for some athletes and why it often gets a bad rap. You must treat the plan as merely a strong suggestion that must be constantly rethought or you are doomed to failure. For the plan to be successful, you must always be willing to make changes. They can even be big changes. There will be days when you are unmotivated, tired, sore, or feeling on the edge of burnout. If you don't make a significant change to the plan on such a day, I can guarantee that you are starting down a rabbit hole from which there is little relief (I'll describe how to make such changes in Chapter 6). Your plan *must* be flexible.

The second point that you must come to accept for your periodization plan to work is that the body can't be *forced* into fitness. You have a race goal which you are 100 percent committed to. That's understandable. And that race has a fixed date. Race day is approaching, and you are mentally focused on it. You obviously want to do well. But can your body arrive ready to go on that day? It depends. It all comes down to timing and physiology. Each rider responds in a unique way to training (the principle of *individuality*, again). Some respond very quickly to workouts. They achieve a high level of performance in a few weeks. Others respond moderately fast. And still others respond slowly, taking many weeks to be race-ready. This seems to be built into our DNA (but there may be lifestyle matters that affect this). You can't force your body to adapt at a rate that it is incapable of achieving. This means you must, first, know what to expect from your body, and, second, design your training plan to fit your likely response time. Trying to force the body to an overly quick pinnacle of race fitness never works. It just leads to frustration followed by a poor race performance. You must know how your body responds to different types of training—especially high volume, long durations, and high-intensity workouts—before laying out the plan.

Have you used a periodized training plan that simply didn't work out for you? Its failure was more than likely the result of one or both cautions above—it was inflexible, or you didn't give it enough time. Of course, there could be other causes, such as aiming too high, overtraining, injury, low motivation, inconsistent training, a poor diet, inadequate sleep, or any number of other obstacles. These are all problems a hands-on coach would address with you right from the start and continually follow up on. Since I can't be there with you, you'll have to do some self-assessment to decide what typically gets in the way of your success. And then vow to correct the problem and move on. Not knowing where that will go, I'm going to assume you're being held back by one or more of your basic or advanced abilities (see Figure 3.1). I'll help you come up with a plan with these limiters in mind.

YOUR GOAL

The starting point for laying out your plan is your goal (or goals) for the season. The most-important goal should be a key event you are doing—an A-priority race. Your goal should be based on the SMART method described in Chapter 1— Specific, Measurable, Achievable, Relevant, and Timed. Also, I'd strongly recommend having only one A race for the season. This will allow you to develop the fitness to excel in the coming season as you've never done before. The more A races you have, the less likely you will be to achieve *any* goal as you will be unable to fully develop your race readiness for each one. The reason for this is that for every A race you will taper (Peak period). That means cutting back on workout durations and volume for a couple of weeks as you taper. With multiple A races often there is not enough time between races to fully regain the lost fitness (yes, *fitness* is lost when you taper but you gain *form*—more on this later in the chapter). As a result, you are likely to slowly become less fit as the season progresses and you'll always be trying to catch up. If you have two A races, they must be separated by several weeks to rebuild race readiness. How many is "several?" I'd suggest no fewer than 12 weeks, and that makes for *very* limited preparation. More is much better.

Other races that may be almost as important as the primary A race are called B races. They are important to you, but you will not peak for them. Instead, you will cut back on training workload for three days prior to these races. There could be, perhaps, three or four of these in a season. Any other races you may do are C races. These are much like group rides. There is no tapering or peaking before a C race. You simply show up and give it your best effort. They are viewed as hard workouts.

YOUR LIMITER

Now comes the truly challenging part. This is a critical decision you must make to ensure your goal success. It has to do with what I call "limiters." A limiter is what is standing between you and the achievement of your goal. There are many possibilities. Common limiters are often related to the layout or terrain conditions of the race. For example, if the course is hilly and climbing is a weakness, then that's a limiter that must be addressed in training. Or if the course is flat and the race often comes down to a sprint, and your sprinting is woefully lacking, then that's your limiter. An obvious fix for such dilemmas is to select races that better match your strengths (such as endurance, climbing, or sprinting), assuming such race options are available to you. They may not be.

Another common limiter could be that your stamina is lacking, which causes you to slow down as fatigue gradually sets in. You may also come to realize from how last season went that your limiter is related to too little saddle time. Or perhaps your limiter has to do with one of the basic abilities, such as poor aerobic endurance, lacking in a particular skill such as descending, or the need for greater strength to drive the pedals more forcefully. It could also be that you have not raced well in the heat in the past. Perhaps you need more heat exposure (see Chapter 9). Or it could be as simple as not having taken in enough fuel in the past in long races (see Chapter 8). Inconsistent training is another very common limiter, as is mindset. In fact, everything mentioned above as a possible limiter is minor compared with the psychological challenges facing many athletes (Chapter 7 addresses the mental side of racing).

The bottom line is that your limiters are your weaknesses relative to the demands of the race. To do well the limiters must be enhanced. Otherwise, your training is largely a waste of time, and your results will not improve. After selecting an A race, you must keep your limiters uppermost in your mind while designing your training plan. "Fixing" your limiters is the key to a successful race.

Now it's time to lay out some of the key training details for your training plan. Start by writing your goal where you are likely to see it every day. For example, write it on the cover of your paper training diary, record it prominently in your online diary, or write it on a piece of tape and stick it on to your handlebar stem. Wherever you put it, it should be front and center every day. Once your goal is nailed down, determine the primary limiter standing between you and success in achieving that goal. Determining what is limiting your performance is the most important decision you will make and will ultimately have a big impact on how your season goes.

Let's circle back to this most critical of topics: what is standing between you and success? The bottom line here is that whatever your limiter or limiters, your training must focus on this throughout your training for the race. It could be as simple as your advanced abilities—aerobic capacity, stamina, or sprint power. One of these is likely to be the restraint that is holding you back. Whatever you decide about this becomes the primary focus of your training leading up to your A race. I understand that your limiter may take a lot of thought and is unlikely to pop into your mind right away. That's always the way it is for me when coaching a new client-athlete. If that's the case for you, give it deep consideration. There's no need to rush the decision, but you must eventually determine what it is. Your limiter must be decided by at least the start of the Build period about three months prior to your A race. If you already have a sense of what it may be, record it in your diary or wherever you go to see what the day's workout is. As with your goal, keep your limiter front and center as the focal point of your training. "Fixing" your limiter, or at least greatly improving it, is central to your success this season.

KEY TAKEAWAYS

- Your training plan must be flexible—it is *not* carved in stone.
- Do not try to force your body to become fit with an overly short, artificially designed schedule—it won't work.
- The probability of your goal success is greatly increased if you have only one A race for the season.
- You *must* know your limiter—whatever stands between you and goal achievement.
- Training must focus on your limiter, not your strengths which you are already good at, but which must be maintained.

YOUR WEEKLY PLAN

Let's start planning your season from the bottom up by deciding what your weeks will look like. For the Base periods I suggest using a 4+3 routine with four short and easy days and three long, easy rides. If using the 5+2 plan in the Build and Peak periods, which I strongly recommend, you will train hard for two days and easy for five days a week, including a day off the bike. Note that you will do gym workouts including weightlifting twice weekly in the Preparation and Base 1 periods. After that, gym sessions will be done only one day each week (more on this in Chapter 5). The central purpose here is to design a training week that fits your lifestyle while keeping the daily gaps between hard workouts manageable, so that you can adequately recover before the next hard ride.

The following is a description of how to organize a plan that matches your lifestyle for each period of the season. Each of the following periods is based on Table 4.1. Again, always keep your limiter relative to your A race goal uppermost in your mind when planning each week. It should be addressed in some manner every week of the season. By the Peak period your limiter must be significantly better for race-day success. It may not be a strength by then, but it should be greatly improved. For the details of suggested workout types mentioned in the following, see the Appendix.

PREPARATION PERIOD

The Preparation period should start no fewer than 26 weeks prior to your season's A race. Having many Preparation weeks is beneficial as that will increase your aerobic endurance, which is ultimately the key to your performance in the coming season. In this period you will be *preparing to train* for a bike race. In other words, your training will be unlike your goal race, which is several weeks in the future. Workouts now are relatively short but frequent. Two-a-day sessions are perfect. These workouts are largely or completely cross-training. Such workouts are best done as endurance activities, such as running, hiking, walking, Nordic skiing, snowshoeing, rowing, or whatever endurance activities you most enjoy besides cycling. Another good option is bike rides in another cycling sport, such as a road cyclist doing trail, velodrome, or gravel riding. Other than being easy, any on-bike workouts you do now are unstructured. Riding to and from work or using the bike for errands are what many of your rides should be like now, *if* you do any riding at all. Strictly cross-training is always an option.

Your cross-training and bike workout durations now are each less than half as long as your usual rides done during periods of high training volume. Start the season with an emphasis on aerobic endurance along with introductory strength and other gym work. The strength workouts are usually called "weightlifting," but it doesn't have to be a traditional gym session with free weights or strength machines. Most of what you need to accomplish can be done with body weight and inexpensive equipment such as heavy-duty elastic cords or even a backpack filled with books or other heavy objects. We'll get to gym workouts, which include weightlifting, core strength, and mobility exercises, in Chapter 5.

The following are the weekly workouts I would like you to do for the Preparation period. Near the end of this chapter you'll decide how to arrange the days to fit your lifestyle. The only point of concern for this period is making sure to separate gym sessions by two or three days. Otherwise, aerobic endurance workouts—both on the bike and cross-training—are "easy" and done strictly in zones 1 and 2. Here are the three components of the Preparation period:

- Gym: two gym sessions separated by two or three days.
- Very short Aerobic Endurance (AE): 10-11 sessions per week as cross-training with only a few bike rides if so desired.
- Off: one day off from both cross-training and riding (this may be a gym day).

BASE PERIOD

Many endurance coaches, including me, consider the Base period to be the most important time of the season. This is when you develop a great depth of fitness, especially aerobic endurance, which is the single most important determiner of how the coming Build period will progress. In Base you are *training to train* by not only maximizing aerobic fitness, but also refining skills and optimizing your strength. These are the foundations of the advanced abilities—aerobic capacity, stamina, and sprint power. Workouts now shift toward more time in the saddle as cross-training is phased out early in this period. Gradually increasing your ride durations is critical for the development of aerobic endurance, and for aerobic capacity and stamina, both of which will be important for your race performance in a few weeks. The workouts are still *not* specific to the demands of your A race, so training is *general*. The training routine is *pyramidal*, meaning you will now begin to include slightly higher intensities (zones 3 and 4) in your rides. Later in this period, zone 3 workouts will become common. This is a critical period in the season which many riders consider a waste of their time since it's so easy. Nothing could be further from the truth.

Start your Base period no fewer than 23 weeks before your A race. More is better. In fact, you could make the Base period many weeks longer than that minimum, which would greatly enhance your performance on race day. I've known of athletes who spent an entire year in the Base period to fully prepare their bodies for a very challenging year ahead. Don't be afraid to do more. It will pay off later in the season.

The early weeks in the Base period are a mixture of what you did in the late Preparation period (frequent aerobic endurance workouts, cross-training, twice-a-week weightlifting) and what you will do in the last few weeks of the Base period, as shown here. The suggested Base period week that follows is what you will do late in this period. The weeks of early Base 1 training detailed below still include some two-a-day cross-training sessions, while increasing bike time and weightlifting to maximize strength, before going into a strength maintenance mode with only one strength session weekly. The late Base period should be at least eight weeks long. Again, longer is better.

In the Base 1 period include the following workouts each week:

- Gym: two gym sessions (details in Chapter 5) separated by two or three days (Max Strength phase).
- Short Aerobic Endurance (AE): six AE workouts (primarily bike but some cross-training is okay). One session daily.

- Speed Skills (SS): include near the end of AE rides as needed.
- Muscular Force (MF): include near the end of an AE ride as needed.
- Off: one day off from both cross-training and riding (may do a gym session on day off).

In the Base 2 and 3 periods include the following sessions each week. Note that "long" and "short" are used relative to your needs and weekly volume, which will be addressed later in this chapter:

- Gym: one gym session (Strength Maintenance phase).
- Long Aerobic Endurance (AE): three long, easy AE rides.
- Short Aerobic Endurance (AE): three short, easy AE rides.
- Speed Skills (SS): include near the end of AE rides as needed.
- Muscular Force (MF): include near the end of an AE ride as needed.
- Off: one day off from riding.

BUILD PERIOD

Up until now, your training has been general—not like your A race. In the Build period that begins to change as workouts become increasingly specific to the demands of the race, especially the expected intensities and duration, but you should also make the terrain, weather, group dynamics, strategy, tactics, refueling, equipment, and anything else that defines your event (more on these topics in Chapters 8 and 9), as similar as you can. Again, with all these race details in mind—no small task—you must also stay focused on your limiter. This is critical to your race performance. Training is now polarized—workouts are either easy or hard.

After many weeks of general preparation, you are now specifically *training to race*.

Note that when training for a stage race, the Saturday and Sunday rides in the following suggested week could both be races, or one race and one aerobic capacity, stamina, and/or sprint power ride on the other weekend day. If the weekend has both hard training or race days, the following Tuesday should be an "easy" AE1 ride (zone 1).

Be aware that how long the Build period lasts is much more of a concern than in the previous periods. More is *not* better now. The body can only handle so much high-intensity stress before things start going the wrong way. I'd strongly recommend no more than eight or nine weeks in the Build period with frequent R&R breaks throughout (see Chapter 6 for more on this).

Here are the workouts to be completed in a standard 5+2 training week in the Build 1 and 2 periods with two hard rides and four that are easy, plus a day off the bike and one gym session.

- Gym: one gym session (Strength Maintenance phase).
- Limiter: one hard ride focused on your limiter (Aerobic Capacity, Stamina, or Sprint Power) or group ride focused on limiter.
- Strengths: one hard ride focused on your strengths (Aerobic Capacity, Stamina, or Sprint Power), or B or C priority race, or group ride.
- Long Aerobic Endurance (AE): one long, easy AE ride.
- Short Aerobic Endurance (AE): three short, easy AE rides.
- Off: one day off from riding.

PEAK PERIOD

In the Peak period you start reducing the durations of workouts. You are "tapering." While the rides get shorter, the frequency of your rides remains just as it was in the Build period, while each hard-day intensity is still race-like.

This brings us to an important point that I mentioned earlier in this chapter, to do with the loss of fitness when tapering. There are three matters central to what goes on in the Peak period as you are tapering your workout durations: fitness, fatigue, and form. "Fitness" here refers to your physical race readiness. Nothing new there. "Fatigue" is what you've been experiencing in various degrees throughout many of the previous weeks of training. Your legs were often heavy, sitting down felt good, and you may have sometimes wondered if you were on the edge of burnout.

Fatigue was with you frequently. Some days were better than others, but you may have thought that this fatigue was fully dismissed every time you took a few days' break from hard rides (see Chapter 6). It wasn't. It's just that you have become so used to it lingering in the background that you aren't aware that deep down, you are at least slightly tired all the time. You simply aren't as sensitive to it now. Some days are worse than others, but it's always there. It has never fully gone away, because you've been training consistently for weeks with only brief breaks from riding.

In the Peak period we are going to get rid of it—mostly. There may be just a little bit that hangs on that you won't be aware of. How do we get rid of most of the fatigue? By cutting back on the durations of rides—tapering your volume. As this gradually eliminates the fatigue, you are coming into "form," which is just another way of saying "freshness"—the absence of fatigue. But the unavoidable result of increasing form is losing fitness. Whenever you reduce the training load, fitness takes a loss. This should be obvious. Reduced training ultimately means reduced fitness. You can't improve your fitness by training less. If that was possible, you'd just stop riding altogether and develop great race fitness. That obviously doesn't happen. What's happening during a taper is that by reducing the training load (workout durations and therefore weekly volume), you are coming into form. You begin to feel fresh and ready to race. Yes, you will lose a tiny amount of fitness but the loss here is more than made up for by the increase in form—the significant decrease in fatigue. The bottom line is that you will be *fresh, on form,* and *ready* on race day—if we get the taper right.

The following training details for a 5+2 routine in a week of the Peak period include two race-like rides and four that are easy, plus a day off the bike and a gym workout:

- Gym: one gym session (Strength Maintenance phase).
- Aerobic Endurance and Sprint Power: ride one AE session this week finishing with a few sprints.
- Limiter: do two race-like group rides (or B or C races); or do Aerobic Capacity intervals, a Stamina session, or Sprint Power repeats, whichever is a limiter for you.
- Aerobic Endurance (AE): complete three AE rides.
- Off: take one day off from the bike.
- Taper volume: reduce training volume in Peak week 1 by 30 percent and Peak week 2 by 40 percent *of Base 3 weekly volume* (see Table 4.2).

RACE PERIOD

You're now down to the week of the race with the event on either Saturday or Sunday. The workouts are short, meaning half or less of your longest rides in the Build period. The emphasis is on R&R to ensure freshness. Your purpose now is to sharpen your race abilities by doing brief workouts with intermittent high-intensity intervals, and repeats for aerobic capacity and sprint power maintenance. Training is now very specific to your race, but avoid Stamina workouts as they are overly fatiguing for this week, and weightlifting is left out this week for the first time in the season. Should you decide to take another day off this week, make it two days prior to race day:

- Gym: no gym workouts this week.
- Hard ride: ride one *short*, race-like workout early or midweek (group ride, Aerobic Capacity or Sprint Power intervals).
- Aerobic Endurance: do four short AE rides including sprints near the end.
- Taper volume: reduce weekly volume by 50 percent of Base 3 volume (see Table 4.2).
- Race.
- Off: take a day (Monday) off.

TRANSITION PERIOD

This is your "off season." It is scheduled for the period starting immediately after an A race. This time off could be only a week if there is another A race planned for your season, but it is still an off season. If this was your last race of the season the Transition period may last four weeks or more. The purpose is to rest and recover both physically and mentally. After several weeks of focused loading for an important race you need to take a break to fully unload the fatigue. Will that mean you lose fitness? Yes, you will. And that's a good thing. You can't be highly fit and race-ready all the time. Such an "always ready to race" attitude is why athletes wind up sick, injured, burned out, or overtrained. Fitness *must* be set aside at the end of the season. Your physical and mental stress during the year is like a bank account from which you are always making withdrawals. In the Transition period you begin to make deposits again.

The only purpose of the Transition period is to regain your physical and mental health along with lifestyle normalcy while renewing your relationships with family and friends. This is your chance each year to be a somewhat "normal" person who isn't always training for a race and who has time for others. Take it easy. Don't work out unless you simply can't stand it. And even then, it must be brief and embarrassingly slow and easy. In fact, it's best not to ride your bike. This, again, is where cross-training can be beneficial.

As you may have guessed, there is not a standard weekly plan for the Transition period. Do what you feel like doing, but mostly take time away from the bike and focused training. Enjoy life.

WEEKLY VOLUME

We are finally at a point where we can determine what your training volumes should be for each week of the season. Once we've decided how many hours you train weekly, the next major step is laying out your plan, including workouts and their durations, using Table 4.3. This can be quite a complex topic. I'll streamline it as best I can.

The starting place for scheduling weekly hours is determining what your highest-volume weeks of the season will be. That will serve as a reference point for scheduling daily and weekly volumes for the entire year. The highest volume weeks of the year are in the Base 3 period (and Base 4 for "older" riders, as will be explained in Chapter 6). Once you know the number of hours for that period, you can schedule for the other weeks of the season as they will all have fewer hours. Base 2 will have fewer hours than Base 3, as will Build 1 and 2 (and for some, Build 3, also to be explained in Chapter 6). The Build periods will have about the same number of hours as the emphasis here is on the intensity of training, not the weekly volume. There's a reason for that. Whenever weekly intensity rises, duration must drop, which is why you ride fewer hours in the Build periods as compared with Base 3. To have both high intensity and high duration could be a disaster. The Peak and Race periods will have the least amount of scheduled volume, as training then is focused on tapering duration to come into form on race day.

Table 4.2 provides an overview of what your training week volumes in each period may look like. To use this table, start in the Base 3 column and find the weekly hours that come closest to what you expect your highest volume of the season to be. Be realistic. Start by asking yourself what your typical high-volume weeks in the Base period should look like. It's alright to add up to 10 percent more weekly hours over what you've done in the past, but that should be your limit. Thinking you can do a great deal more than what you've done in previous seasons without a good reason is risky. By forcing yourself to exceed what you are capable of handling, you'll frequently be on the edge of fatigue with fitness going downward. There is nothing to be gained from that. Better to do too few hours with energy to spare than to push beyond your limits and risk not only your performance but also your health.

> **Be realistic. Better to do too few hours with energy to spare than to push beyond your limits.**

After you've found your Base 3 weekly volume in Table 4.2, read the columns to the left and right of that number and you will find what your weekly suggested volumes are for every period of the season. The Preparation period is not included in Table 4.2 as that period is for cross-training and frequency. Duration is not the focus of these periods. The Transition period is also omitted as it is an unstructured time at the end of the season with the focus on R&R.

In Table 4.2 you will also see columns labeled "Base 4" and "Build 3." These are unique periods that have to do with a rider's capacity for recovery from hard training weeks. Typically, they are used by riders over 50, those who recover slowly, and cyclists who are new to the sport. This will be explained in greater detail in Chapter 6, which addresses the issue of R&R, including when those weeks will be scheduled. For now, don't be concerned with this.

Table 4.2 Suggested weekly riding hours for the Base, Build, Peak, and Race periods
Gym time is not included.

Base 1	Base 2	Base 3	Base 4*	Build 1	Build 2	Build 3*	Peak 1	Peak 2	Race**
20	27	30	30	27	27	27	24	18	18
19	25	28	28	26	26	26	21	14	14
17	23	26	26	23	23	23	20	13	13
16	22	24	24	22	22	22	18	12	12
15	20	22	22	20	20	20	17	11	11
14	18	20	20	18	18	18	15	10	10
12	16	18	18	16	16	16	14	9	9
11	14	16	16	14	14	14	12	8	8
10	12	14	14	12	12	12	11	7	7
8	10	12	12	10	10	10	9	6	6
7	9	10	10	9	9	9	8	5	5

*Note that Base 4 and Build 3 are used only by athletes whose training requires short (three-week) periods (see Chapter 6).
**Hours in the Race period include race time, warm-up, and cool down.

How to distribute the weekly hours from Table 4.2 to your custom training plan in Table 4.3, so that you know how long each workout will be is a challenge as there are so many variables. Other than a few that are somewhat easy to estimate, such as gym sessions and your standard group ride durations, workout times are difficult to predict. There are simply too many variables. Since you know the race for which you are preparing and other factors, such as how long it takes to get to a course where you can do, for example, intervals, I'm leaving it up to you to decide daily workout durations. I'd only be guessing. Just make sure the daily hours add up to the suggested weekly volumes in Table 4.2.

Using the discussions above of the types of workout to include in each period, your selected weekly volume data from Table 4.2, and your experience with daily workout durations, you should be able to fill in much of your annual training plan in Table 4.3. Pencil in the types of workouts you will do and their approximate durations. Leave the row titled "Period Length in Weeks" vacant until after reading Chapter 6. There's one more piece of the puzzle that has to do with R&R weeks and this will also be explained in Chapter 6.

Record your weekly volume for each period at the top of each column, pencil in your workouts for each day so that they fit your lifestyle, and record the estimated "Duration" for each daily workout.

Table 4.3 Your annual training plan by periods

Record the types of daily workouts you will do in each period of the season.

"A" Race: _____

Goal: _____

Limiter: _____

	Preparation	Base 1	Base 2	Base 3	Build 1 and 2	Peak 1	Peak 2	Race	Transition
Period Length in Weeks (Table 4.1)									
Weekly Volume (Table 4.2)									
Monday Duration:									
Tuesday Duration:									
Wednesday Duration:									
Thursday Duration:									
Friday Duration:									
Saturday Duration:									
Sunday Duration:									

*Note that some riders will include Base 4 and Build 3 in their training plans. This has to do with rest and recovery weeks and is addressed in Chapter 6.

KEY TAKEAWAYS

- Create a custom weekly training routine, friendly to your lifestyle, that you can use year-round.
- Always keep your limiter in mind—it is the emphasis of your training.
- When you aren't focused on your limiter, which is a significant part of your training time, maintain your strengths.
- Start the Preparation period no later than 26 weeks prior to your A race—even earlier is better.
- The Preparation period is your time of unstructured training with an emphasis on frequency and cross-training.
- Start the Base period no less than 23 weeks before race day—making it longer than that would significantly improve your race-day fitness.
- The early Base period is an in-between blend of what you did in the Preparation period and will do in the late Base period with an emphasis shifting from frequency to duration.
- In the Build period you will do two race-like workouts weekly, with occasional B and C races.
- The Peak period is marked by a gradually reduced training volume while intensity remains race-like.
- Your purpose in the Peak period is to slowly come into form (freshness) by greatly reducing fatigue.
- In the week of your A race, training volume remains low as high-intensity workouts are done to maintain race readiness.
- The Transition period is an "off season" for restoring your body's vigor by mostly resting.
- After an A race, start an off season by fully dedicating your time to rest, recovery, and renewal.

WHAT IF YOU HAVE ANOTHER A RACE?

I mentioned earlier that you must give up some of your fitness after the first race of the season by taking a Transition period break from training. That's why earlier in this chapter I said that if you have a second A race in a season it needs to be several weeks after the first one. The reason for that is to give you adequate time to unload the stress and then re-establish race readiness. Having important races with only a few weeks' separation gives you little time to prepare and almost assures you of a poor performance in the second event. How many weeks until the next A race are needed to perform at a high level? That is a very difficult question to answer as it depends on who you are, physically and mentally. Base fitness needs to be rebuilt, followed by more periods of Build, Peak, and Race. Some riders could be ready to go, perhaps, in as few as 10 to 12 weeks. Those riders are few and far between. Others may need twice that. That's why I only recommend one A race in a season, along with other B and C races.

THE REST OF TOM'S STORY

Following graduation that spring Tom was offered a teaching position at a high school in the same county as his university. That was good as I was afraid a long-distance move would mean leaving the team that had supported him so well. With everything falling into place so nicely for Tom, it was no wonder that he had a great season, including a couple of wins—with one being his A race. Goal achieved! He and I were both very happy with how training had progressed. But all of that was about to change.

His first semester of teaching that fall proved to be even more difficult and time-consuming than the schoolwork in his senior year in college. He didn't train much as there were just too many demands on his time. In that first year of teaching, he also fell in love and got married. The winter was a pivotal time for Tom and cycling. He tried to make a comeback the following spring, but there was too much going on in his life, so he decided to put racing on the backburner until he got everything under control. That was a wise decision. I heard that after his first year of teaching, he and his new wife decided to move to another state. Unfortunately, I lost contact with him, but he had a lot of talent and was a good guy to coach.

5. TRAINING DETAILS

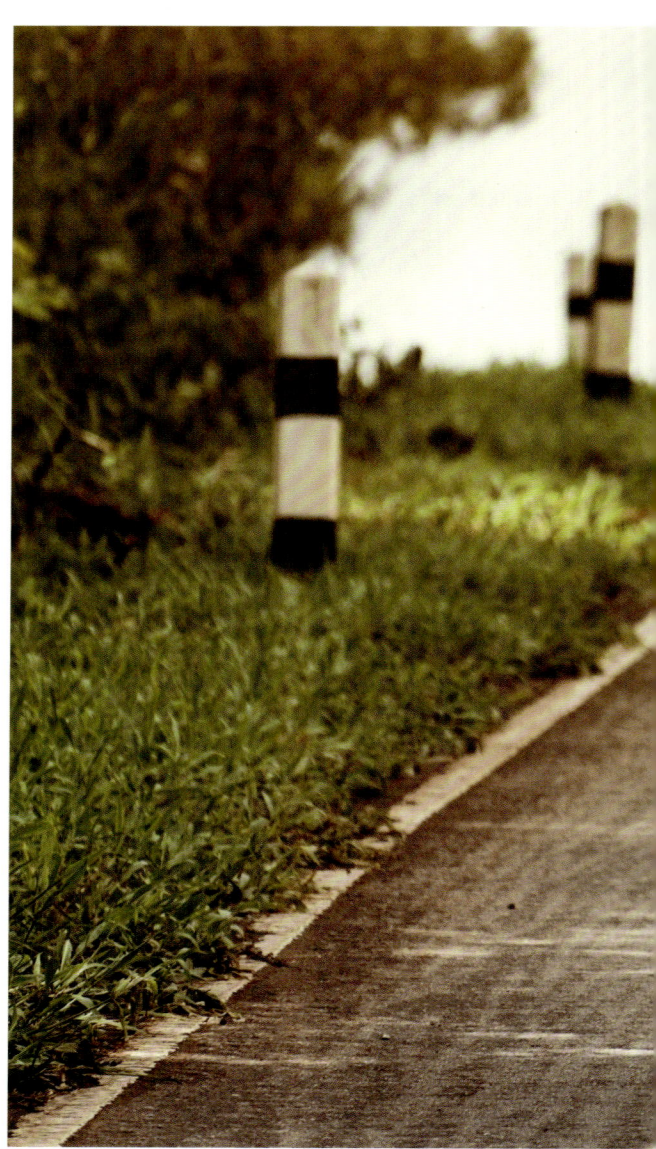

In Chapter 4 you created most of the plan that will be the foundation of your training for the coming season. From that you should now have an idea of how your weekly training will look regarding daily workouts and their durations. That's a good start but it's just the easy part of designing a training plan. In this chapter we will take it up a few more levels by probing a bit deeper into the details of periodized training. By the end of this chapter, you will have almost all your annual training plan set for the coming season. There will be one more small piece that we will cover in Chapter 6.

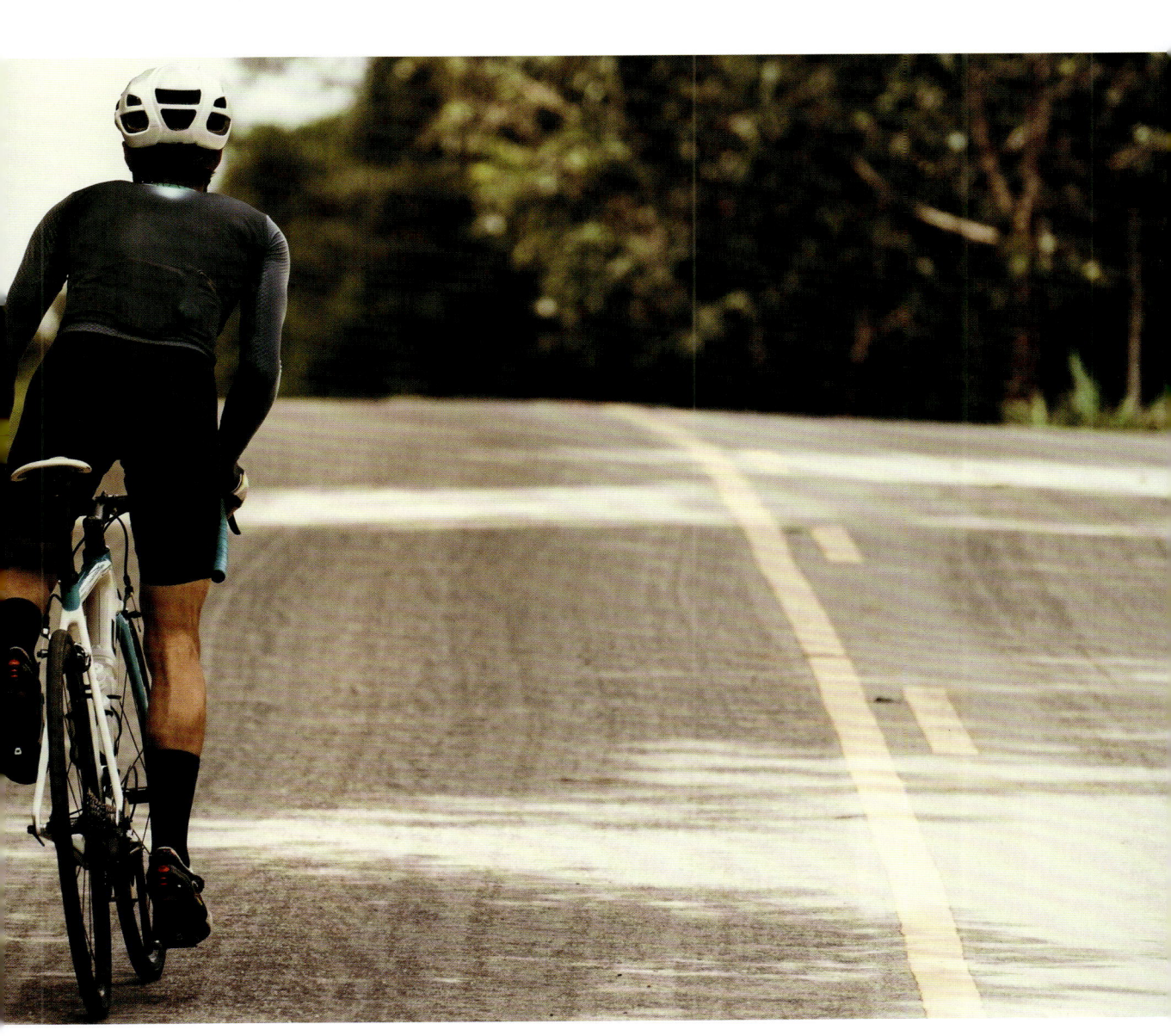

LAURIE'S STORY

I had never heard her so excited in nearly a year of working together. She was always a pleasure to coach but somewhat reserved. On the phone, however, she was telling me, as near as I could tell through all the background noise, excitement, and chuckling, that she had just won the women's division of the Leadville Trail 100 MTB. That was her A race for the year. It was a new challenge, not only for her, but also for the sport of mountain bike racing.

Laurie was one of the earliest mountain bikers, having started racing just a few years before we met. She was a ground-breaker for female athletes as off-road racing was less than a decade old when she won in Leadville. She had been a road racer who switched over to the new sport while it was still in its infancy. And she loved it.

This win was a first for both Laurie and for the sport. The Leadville event was the second-ever mountain bike ultra-distance race in the USA (the first was the Wilderness 101 in Pennsylvania, three years earlier). In its first year, the Leadville race attracted riders mostly from the western states, but would soon welcome athletes from around the world.

To say that Laurie and I were a little concerned in preparing for it would be an understatement. The Leadville Trail 100 is not a race for the faint-hearted. It's an out-and-back course of about 105 miles (169 kilometers) including five serious climbs. It starts in the small town of Leadville in Colorado's Rocky Mountains at 10,200 feet (3,109 meters) and tops out at 12,600 feet (3,840 meters) with an overall gain of about 12,000 feet (3,650 meters). Altitude is certainly a serious concern. Fortunately, Laurie was from Colorado, although she did not live nearly as high as Leadville. She was somewhat adapted to altitude. Elevation was obviously one of our primary concerns going into the race. Given her lifestyle she wasn't going to be able to get in enough time at higher altitude to fully adapt. That could take weeks. The key was to give a high level of effort, but always race within her limits. Breathing and exertion had to be always under control. We talked about this a lot. You must be friendly with altitude. Don't try to beat it. Altitude will always win.

If extreme altitude wasn't enough, there was more. The weather at that extreme mountain elevation can be vicious. Although the race is in August, the rider may be walloped with freezing temperatures, rain, hail, and possibly snow. It wasn't going to be easy. And we knew it. But there was nothing we could do about the altitude or the weather, except keep our fingers crossed.

At 32, Laurie was no spring chicken. She

had been racing for several years, mostly as a roadie, and had maintained an extremely high level of fitness with lots of saddle time. But it's usually in their early 30s that riders begin to see a slight downward swing in performance as the body changes. This could possibly be another challenge. We simply had to accept all these challenges and get on with training.

In deciding how to prepare Laurie for such an extreme event I wasn't worried about her aerobic endurance or off-road, bike-handling skills. Those were her strengths. With all the hilly off-road riding and climbing she did her muscular force was also quite well developed. My biggest concern was stamina. But unlike altitude, weather, and age, this was something we had some control over. Not only did she need the endurance to last up to, perhaps, 10 hours if the weather was nasty, but, given the altitude, she would also have to stay near her physical limit for hour after hour. It would be a grueling day. I wasn't sure she could do it. She never expressed a doubt.

The winter before the race she had to spend quite a bit of time on an indoor trainer due to the fickle Colorado weather. But when she was able to get outside it was the road bike we focused on in the Base period. That made it easier to get in enough ride time to boost aerobic endurance fitness to prepare for what could be a 10-hour race. Then in the late Base and Build periods she did lots of stamina rides on the road and, later, on trails in the mountains. I could tell by the testing we did that she was coming along quite well. And her spring and early summer races were also quite encouraging.

Laurie had a packed racing schedule in 1994, including North American World Cup MTB races, the National Off-Road Bicycle Association (NORBA) series, and the Colorado Off-Road Points Series (CORPS). But Leadville was a different kind of animal. Since the mountain bike race had never been held before, there were no time splits for men or women between aid stations or segments of the course. Since most of her mountain bike races were well under than 30 miles, usually less than 20 miles, Laurie's strategy was to think of this as four 25-mile races, so that she could have mini-goals to measure her progress and sense of accomplishment throughout the day.

Talking on the phone over the loud background noise I could tell that, although tired, she was excited to have won. And her time was just a couple of minutes over nine hours. Not only did she win for the women, but also finished 19th overall among the men. We went through some of the details from her day—the ups and downs, literally, of a nine-hour race. She was already talking about next year in Leadville and how she could be faster from knowing the course, and how to better fuel and stay hydrated. Looking ahead positively is always a good sign.

Laurie was a pleasure to coach. She trained consistently, seldom missing a workout. And, just as important, she kept me informed of how her training was going. My only concern was that I had to hold her back. It was nothing for her to throw in an extra hour on the bike a couple of times weekly. She was also a bit hesitant when I scheduled R&R weeks. I often ran into this burning desire to excel with other highly dedicated riders. It can be dangerous. Unrestrained motivation can easily lead to injury, illness, and overtraining. I had seen this in other riders before and expressed my concerns to Laurie. She always heard me out, but holding her back continued to be a coaching challenge.

But that was all behind us. Now it was time to celebrate. Unfortunately, I was half a state away. Our celebration was confined to a very happy phone call.

While you are drawing up a plan that guides you to a high-performance race, you must always have one question in the back of your mind: "Is this really what I want to do?"

THE PLANNING PROCESS

I don't take your planning process lightly. I understand that it's a lot of work, but necessary if you really do want to excel. This is just one piece of high-performance racing. I must admit, however, there is a bit of hesitation for me in taking you through this planning process. My concern in writing these periodization chapters with all their *whys* and *hows* is that you begin to feel that the fun is being taken out of riding a bike. That's always a concern of mine at this stage of the coach-athlete relationship. Why? Plan-building is so mechanical that you may feel like a robot that simply follows a master plan. The fun part of cycling is missing in the planning. Once the fun is gone, riding eventually loses its appeal. That is certainly something you should never lose. You must realize that while you are in the process of drawing up a plan that guides you to a high-performance race, you must always have one question in the back of your mind: "Is this really what I want to do?" If the answer is "no," then the only avenue forward is to stop planning and ride when you want to and how you want to. That is the epitome of fun. The downside, of course, is the high possibility of a poor race performance when you most want it. If you are truly focused on racing better, and can physically and mentally manage all the structure I'm introducing to you here, then I feel certain you will race at a high level. But you must keep in mind that what's ahead is a nose-to-the-grindstone season as it takes patience and persistence to achieve at a high level in this sport.

TRAINING BASICS

In Chapter 4 I told you about the seasonal training progression, starting with workout frequency, then gradually transitioning to duration, and finally becoming more focused on race-like intensity in the last few weeks before your A race. This is the sequence you should go through every season from its beginning to race day. But I didn't say much there about *how* these progressions should blend into your training. "Blend" is the key word here. In the Preparation and early Base periods the challenge is to smoothly mix aerobic endurance time on the bike and cross-training with gym workouts, while also improving your bike-handling skills. All of this should fit together like the pieces of a puzzle. The Build period workouts with their emphasis on advanced abilities should also be gradually blended into your training as the basic abilities go into a maintenance mode. These changes to your weekly plans should be gradually applied, not suddenly inserted.

PROGRESSION TRANSITION 1: FREQUENCY

Let's do a quick review of seasonal training. In the Preparation and early Base periods there are two key factors at play. One is cross-training, and the other is the frequency of training. I mentioned in Chapter 4 that there are several non-cycling, endurance sports I'd suggest you choose from in this period, such as running, hiking, walking, rowing, Nordic skiing, and snowshoeing. There could be other options so long as they are aerobic. Frequency, as I'm using the word here, refers to doing two, somewhat brief workouts daily, early in the season. That could include doing only cross-training sports twice daily, or it might be a combination of cross-training and cycling—one of each daily. And two times per week one of your two-a-day workouts is a gym session. By "brief workouts" I mean each is less than half of what your single, daily workout durations are on the bike at the height of your seasonal training volume. For example, let's assume your *average* daily ride duration in the Base 3 period is two hours. That would indicate that you should do two workouts daily in the Preparation and early Base periods that are each less than an hour. There's a lot of latitude for exactly how long those workouts should be. Since the frequency stage of training is somewhat of an in-between period, it's more a matter of staying aerobically active than of building great fitness. But you are indeed developing the early stages of your aerobic endurance, which will eventually result in a higher aerobic capacity. In Base 1 of this frequency stage of training you begin to replace cross-training sessions with increased time on the bike. That brings us to the second progression stage.

TRAINING DATA ANALYSIS: DIRK FRIEL

Franz Stampfl, the coach of the first runner to break the four-minute-mile barrier, Roger Bannister, once said, "Training is an act of faith." By that, he meant that the coach and the athlete can never be sure that what they are doing in preparation for competition is working. You find out on race day. One must simply come up with the best plan possible, follow it closely, and hope for the best. In many ways he was right. But now, some 70-plus years later, there are some indicators we can look for along the way that provide feedback on how the athlete is progressing. But this doesn't eliminate the act of having faith in your training. However, measuring the right data at the right times makes the process of training much more predictable.

Making Sense of Metrics

There is an ever-growing choice of metrics an athlete could track with the advent of modern wearables. Yet as the landscape of self-quantification advances, I seem to find more value in the basics as they relate to each other. Reading training data is in many ways pointless without context. Knowing the goal date and event limiters along with the prescribed training add much more clarity to training data, but what I keep coming back to the most as a cyclist are the tried-and-true data channels of time, power, and heart rate, and how they relate to each other.

Time

Training volume expressed as daily and weekly hours says a lot. Time is also more relevant than distance when it comes to training adaptations.

Normalized Power (NP)™

The training software TrainingPeaks brought the concept of normalized power to the cycling market to better express the physiological demands of a ride versus average power. The downside of tracking average power is when a ride is very stochastic or variable, such as in a criterium or mountain bike race, where there may be a lot of short time periods coasting at 0 watts due to cornering or descending. The addition of zero output will drag the average watts down, yet physiologically, the heart rate and lactate levels may still be very elevated. Normalized power expresses the intensity that the body would feel if the ride were conducted at a constant power output. Conversely, Average Power within a steady state time trial will be very close or equal to NP (aka Variability Index, also shown in TrainingPeaks).

Training Stress Score™

Once we know NP and the duration of the workout, TrainingPeaks will calculate the Training Stress Score (TSS), which in effect is assigning a workload value to the session. The only remaining value to know is the threshold for the athlete, so an Intensity Factor (IF)™ can be calculated and used within the calculation. The IF is therefore a percentage of the threshold, which is combined with duration to determine the TSS.

Average Heart Rate

The average heart rate of a workout can be a good indication of aerobic fitness, but it becomes even more valuable when looking at average heart rate within intervals. A word of caution, however, is warranted when looking at short intervals of less than five or so minutes as short intervals are not long enough for the heart rate to respond to the actual work being performed.

Decoupling (PW/HR)

The purpose of training is to go faster on race day and ideally as an athlete improves you will see more output (watts and speed) for the same input (heart rate). Another concept that relates to decoupling is heart rate drift. Decoupling is a metric that reflects the amount of change over time between heart rate and power within a session or interval. The aim is to lower the decoupling value as fitness improves, which reflects aerobic fitness. The greater the value the larger the spread is within a given segment between heart rate and power.

Efficiency Factor (EF)

Efficiency factor is yet another way to view the relationship between heart rate and power. Efficiency factor could be compared to miles per gallon in a car. To calculate EF, you divide the normalized power of a steady state segment by the average heart rate of the same segment. Unlike decoupling, EF does not measure the rate of change over time between heart rate and power.

Dirk Friel, a former professional road cyclist and cycling coach, is the Co-Founder and Chief Evangelist of Peakware Holdings and TrainingPeaks. In 2023, the Escape Collective named Dirk one of the Top 50 Most Influential People in American Cycling.

PROGRESSION TRANSITION 2: DURATION

The second transition of the season begins in the Base 2 period—no less than eight weeks before starting your Build period. Now your training focus shifts from frequency to duration. This is when you transition from the cross-training workouts to only riding a bike. This transition should be done by gradually replacing cross-training with riding. It may take a week or two to fully complete this transition. Winter weather at this time in the season could also play a role, so you may want to cross-train more and ride only when the weather permits.

In the Base 3 period the single daily rides should be about as long as, or even perhaps longer than, the combined times of the previous cross-training days in Preparation and Base 1. The durations of your weekly long rides are roughly based on the expected duration (not distance) of your A race and the history of your typical training loads. This stage of training is also when you cut back to one gym session a week (more on this shortly). The ride durations now begin to get longer than the combined times during the previous cross-training stage.

In this second progression stage you may also include group rides, *but only if they are aerobic*. In my years of cycling experience, I've found very few groups that ride easy and aerobically at this time of year. It seems that whenever you find a group to ride with, even if it's billed as being "easy," it is usually an unsanctioned race. These types of group rides are best avoided in the Base period. Such rides at this time in the season will *not* help you race faster when the serious racing begins. It comes down to whether you want to ride for fun or for Base fitness. If you choose the former, you are likely to be lacking in aerobic fitness as you move into the Build period. Disorganized group "races" in the Base period essentially mean that there is no longer a good reason to follow your training plan. You're now riding strictly for fun. Again, there's nothing wrong with that, except for what it means when it's time to *really* race.

PROGRESSION TRANSITION 3: INTENSITY

The final training transition begins when you move up to the Build period. This should start 11 or 12 weeks before your A race (see Table 4.1). Now the ride durations should become a bit shorter than in the late Base period as you begin to shift your energy from long duration rides to race-like workout intensities. This is the time to ride with those groups that are unable to limit intensity to anything other than "race-like" in the Base period. In fact, such rides may now become a central focus of your weekly workouts. With a few weeks to go until your race, they can be beneficial. It's also a good idea to include some C races and occasional B races in this period. But go easy on the latter since you need to reduce the training load for three days prior to the race, which takes us back to losing fitness due to decreasing saddle time, as explained in Chapter 4. The best time to do a B race is at the end of an R&R week, which we'll get to in Chapter 6. Limiting these races to R&R weeks implies you could do two or three B races, at most, in the Build and Peak periods. These will serve as good tests of what you've accomplished so far this season by sticking to the plan.

KEY TAKEAWAYS

- The seasonal transitions from frequency to duration to intensity are important episodes in your quest for race fitness.
- Your first two periods of the season are unique in that frequent aerobic workouts may include both cycling and cross-training.
- In Base 2 and 3 your training focus must shift to bike-only with an emphasis on increasing workout durations at an easy intensity.
- As you start the Build 1 period some workouts are shorter but with greater intensity than in the Base period.

THE BASIC ABILITIES

In Chapter 3 I introduced you to the Training Triad with its basic and advanced abilities (see Figure 3.1). You may recall that these are the categories for the workouts you will be doing throughout the season. To refresh your memory, the basic abilities are aerobic endurance, muscular force, and speed skills. These are the primary workout types you do in the Preparation and Base periods.

But before we get into the details of this let me say once more that your fitness on race day is, for the most part, determined by how well you trained in the Base period. The basic abilities play a very important role in how well you train in the last several weeks before your A race. This is much like laying the foundation before framing a house. A rock-solid foundation means a sturdy building. But if your version of a foundational Base period is doing fast group rides and intervals, don't expect a great race. You could be a lot faster if you follow the plan. Riding hard in the Base period is more than a waste of time. Your body can only handle so much race-like training before things start to falter with fitness going the wrong direction.

Okay, now that I've got that off my chest, let's move on to the details of training in the basic abilities.

AEROBIC ENDURANCE

In previous chapters I've said quite a bit about the importance of the basic ability, aerobic endurance, how to do these workouts, and their importance to your race preparation. Even though it's basic and done at an easy intensity, I consider it the single most important ability of the six listed above, and it's the only one you do weekly for the entire season. In previous chapters I've said quite a bit about this ability, so I won't go back through all that again. Instead, I would like to tell you about the details of the two other basic abilities you must work on in the Base periods—muscular force and speed skills.

MUSCULAR FORCE TRAINING

In Chapter 4 I proposed that you lift weights throughout the season. You may recall that in the Preparation and early Base periods I recommended you work on strength twice weekly. And in the late Base period I advised that you cut back to one session weekly. This single session also extends into the Build and Peak periods. But I didn't provide any details on what to do. Let's address that now. But before getting into the *what* of weightlifting, let's first talk about a closely related, more important topic—*why*.

Why do I recommend lifting weights? There are a few reasons. The overarching reason is that research has shown that weightlifting improves cycling performance. You become more powerful, especially in the legs, which we will focus on. It has also been shown to significantly improve power for time trialing and sprinting. And while I've not seen any research on this, I suspect it is likely to benefit your climbing, also. Not only do you become more powerful, according to this research, but several studies also found an improvement in aerobic capacity and stamina, two of the three advanced abilities you read about in Chapter 2. Another closely related topic we haven't talked about is economy—how much energy you expend when riding at any given power output. Studies have shown that strength training also makes you more economical. Basically, that means it takes less effort and fuel to drive the pedals at a wide range of intensities.

> **Weightlifting can enhance cycling performance and significantly improve power for time trialing and sprinting.**

There's another reason for weightlifting which is even more important for cyclists—health. For runners a common health benefit of their sport is bone density, especially in the feet, legs, hips, and lower spine. That's because of the impact the runner (and walker) experience with every workout. That pounding stress gives the runner a stronger lower-body frame and, hence, helps avoid broken bones. Pedaling a bicycle offers no such benefits, no matter how hard you push the pedals. Many young, serious riders in their 30s have been found to have the early stages of osteoporosis—weakened bones more common in the elderly. And the older you are, the greater the risk. The weightlifting exercises I'll soon recommend you do will strengthen your bones and help you maintain their health. And of course, cross-training sports, such as running, hiking, and walking, are also beneficial to bone health. The bottom line here is that weightlifting has the potential to boost your cycling performance while also keeping you free of major bone injuries.

There are a couple of options for where you do the weightlifting sessions in your training plan. The most common place for lifting is at a health club or gym. Such facilities typically have everything you need to get started. A better option is to have a "gym" in your home. Several years ago I decided to go this route to save travel time to and from the gym, and to also make it harder to have an excuse for not lifting. I turned the third bay in our garage into a gym and began to slowly outfit it with the equipment I needed for weightlifting—a rubberized floor cover, free weights, a bench, a leg-press machine, and other odds and ends, such as heavy-duty elastic bands and step stools. Now I have no excuses for not lifting and the commute takes only seconds. I've known of several athletes who have done this. Yes, there is a cost for this, but take a multiyear approach to stocking your home gym and it isn't so bad, especially when compared with a monthly gym membership. The biggest challenge is, undoubtedly, where in your home to locate it. I can't offer much guidance there, except to be creative—garage, spare room, basement, patio, or wherever you have some unused space.

Now let's get to the details of weightlifting and gym training for cycling. The starting place is exercises that develop leg extension strength— the key to high performance in cycling. As you will see in the list below, your legs are the focus of the weightlifting sessions. The reason for that is obvious since you're building strength to drive the pedals on a bike. It's also important that the leg exercises focus on extension and are multi-joint. Multi-joint means extending the hip, knee, and ankle. None are single-joint exercises. Multi-joint exercises simulate pedaling a bike.

Before you begin to decide which weightlifting exercises you'll do, along with the core strength and hip mobility exercises to be introduced next, I want to make a point for keeping gym sessions brief. You're a cyclist, not a gym-goer. I understand that and don't want to suggest an exercise plan that keeps you in the gym for long sessions. I believe in keeping these short and to the point (which makes a home gym optimal). So, with this in mind, I'm going to lay out a standard gym session that will give you the strength you need without taking a big bite out of your daily routine. Of course, if you enjoy being in the gym and believe you can do more, certainly feel free to do so. Let's get started with your gym workouts.

From the following drawings, select two leg exercises you will do in each weightlifting session twice each week in the Prep and Base 1 periods. Do *not* do all these exercises in each session. You may periodically change your two choices in each gym workout for variety. See Figures 5.1 through 5.6 for how to do each one. All the following are done with free weights, either barbell or dumbbells, except for the leg press (Figure 5.6), which is on a machine.

Figure 5.1 Two-leg squat

Feet pedal-width apart—about 7-8 inches/18-20 centimeters. Squat until the knees are at about a 90-degree angle.

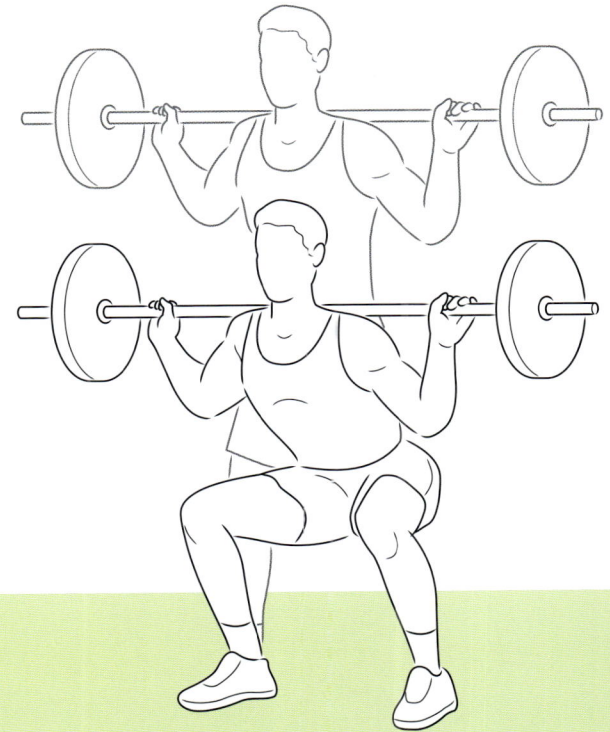

Figure 5.2 One-leg squat ("Bulgarian split squat")
Squat until the forward knee is at about a 90-degree angle.

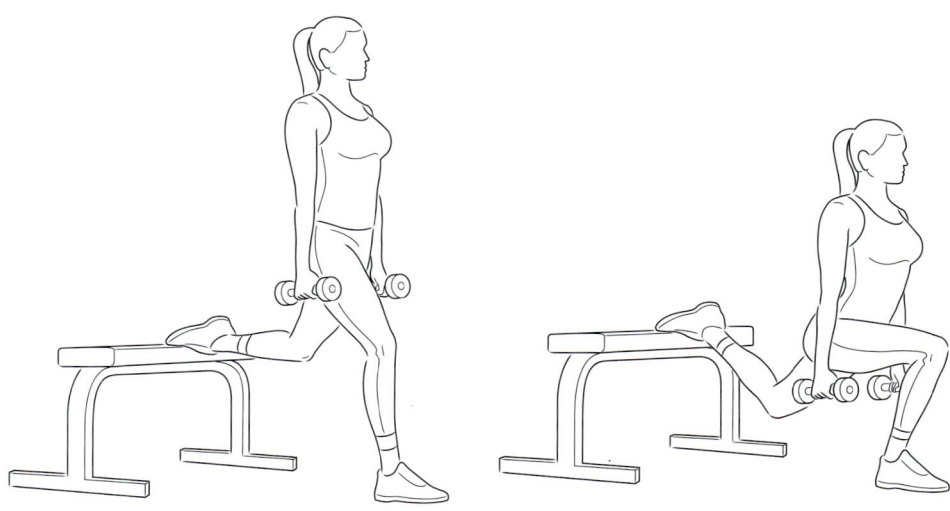

Figure 5.3 Deadlift
Feet pedal-width apart—about 7-8 inches/18-20 centimeters. Keep the head up and back straight. Lift with the legs, not the back.

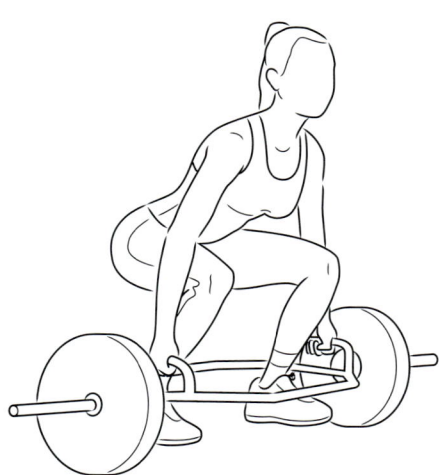
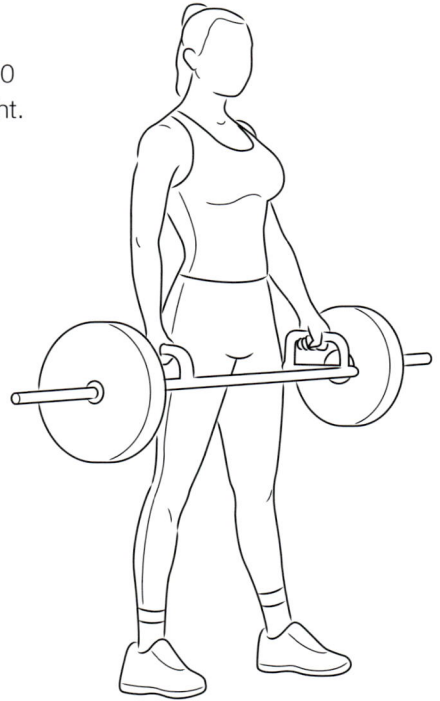

TRAINING DETAILS

Figure 5.4 Step-ups
Platform height is 13-15 inches/33-38 centimeters. Use dumbbells.

Figure 5.5 Lunges
Done with dumbbells. Forward knee at about a 90-degree angle.

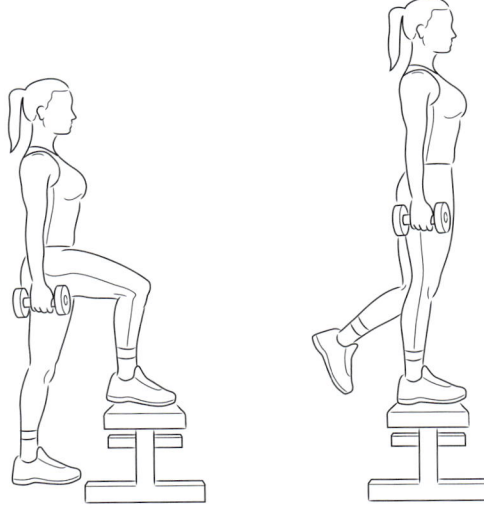

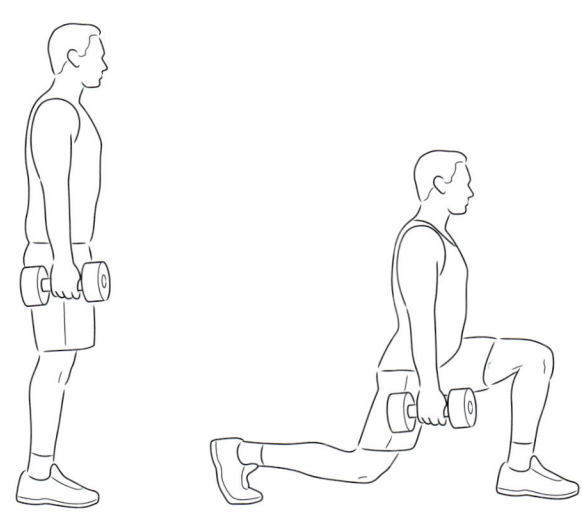

Figure 5.6 Leg press
Feet about pedal-width apart. Knees at about a 90-degree angle.

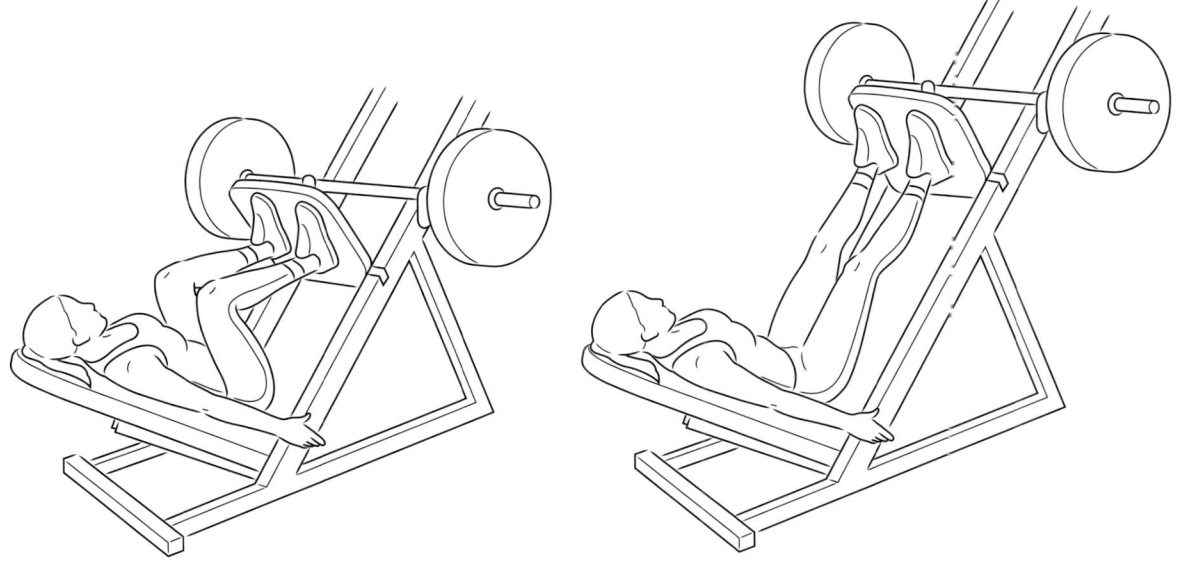

Be patient. Those new to weightlifting should progress slowly to avoid injury.

My main concern for athletes doing these exercises is injury to the knees and back. The weight loads you select every day should be easily managed (more on this shortly). The "depth" of these exercises is determined by the knees being at about a 90-degree angle when bent. Making the knee angle more acute than a right angle increases the risk of injury. Such an acute angle is also not what you do when driving the pedal down. I also strongly recommend wearing a weightlifting belt for these exercises to provide support for the back. If you are concerned about your back, be very conservative with weight loads for free weight exercises while being sure to use excellent posture. That means a straight back, tall pose, and head balanced directly above your torso. Also, look only forward; do not look down. The exercises that are most "back friendly" are single-leg squats, lunges, step ups, and leg presses. The riskiest lift if you are prone to back troubles is the dead lift. Always select exercises that are low risk relative to your known knee, hip, and back limitations.

For junior riders (under age 16) I recommend staying in the Anatomical Adaptation phase (see Table 5.1 below) with relatively light loads and high reps. Other athletes who are new to weightlifting should avoid the Max Strength phase for the first season. My reason for setting such limits for these two groups is to reduce the risk of injury, which is relatively high for young or inexperienced athletes who lift heavy loads. Be patient. Give this until you are 16, or have been in the sport for at least one season before going to heavier loads. If you are unsure if you should lift heavy weights (Max Strength phase) for whatever reason, I'd strongly suggest following your inclinations and using only lighter loads with more reps, such as in the Max Transition phase. On the positive side, the riders who stand to make the greatest improvements from weightlifting are those over 50. The riders who will likely see the smallest performance gains are those in their 20s.

The next topic we need to address is how many sets and repetitions to do in a session and the weight loads. These two variables define the phases of muscular force training. There are four weightlifting phases during the season, as follows:

- Anatomical Adaptation (AA): refine weightlifting skills with light loads and high reps.
- Max Transition (MT): with skills improved, gradually increase loads as reps are decreased.
- Max Strength (MS): maximize strength with heavier loads and greatly reduced reps.
- Strength Maintenance: do one light set (AA) for warm-up and one heavy set (MS) for strength maintenance.

Table 5.1 The details of seasonal weightlifting

Weightlifting Phase	Training Period	Total Sessions	Sessions per Week	Sets per Exercise	Reps per Set
Anatomical Adaptation (AA)	Preparation	3-6	2	3	15-20
Max Transition (MT)	Preparation	3-6	2	3	8-12
Max Strength (MS)	Base 1	6-8	2	3	4-6
Strength Maintenance (SM)	Base 2, 3 Build Peak	13-19	1	2	Set 1: 15-20 and Set 2: 4-6

Table 5.1 provides the details of your seasonal weightlifting sessions with the weight loads determined by how many reps you can do. The most important point here is to stop when you sense that you can only do one or two more in a set. For example, the Max Transition phase calls for 8 to 12 repetitions in each of three sets. When you are in this phase, if you do 10 reps and you feel like you could probably do one or two more, stop the set. *Do not lift to failure.* That greatly increases your risk of injury and does nothing for cycling performance.

Besides building strength primarily in the legs using weights, I'd also suggest working on your core strength and hip mobility. Core strength is necessary to maintain posture on the bike so that your legs can drive the pedals without a "leak" in the power output. This has to do with the muscles of your torso that form the foundation for the movement of your limbs, especially the legs in cycling. If the core muscles are weak, you will not be able to fully deliver force to the pedals. Core muscles primarily support the spine and pelvis, and help to stabilize the body while pedaling at a high power output. They also improve economy by ensuring that the force of driving the pedal down is not compromised. Instead, the energy is delivered to the pedals. Common signs of core weakness in cyclists are lower back discomfort on or off the bike, and shifting your butt toward the nose of the saddle when working hard.

See Figures 5.7 through 5.9 for core strengthening exercises. There are several other core strength exercises besides these three that could be included, such as bridge, bicycle crunch and bug (you can find more online). Do all these core strength exercises in each gym session. Feel free to do more or to do others that you know work well for you.

Figure 5.7 Front plank
Hold this position for 20 to 30 seconds for each of three sets.

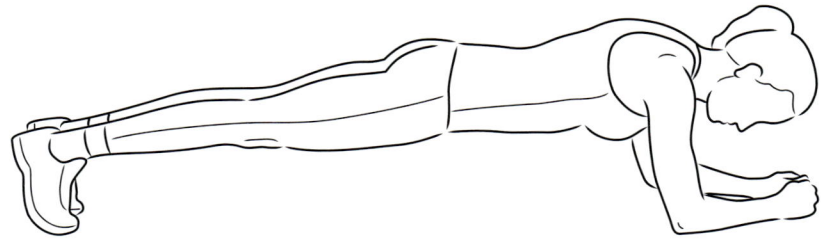

Figure 5.8 Side planks
Hold this position for 20 to 30 seconds for each of three sets, both left and right sides.

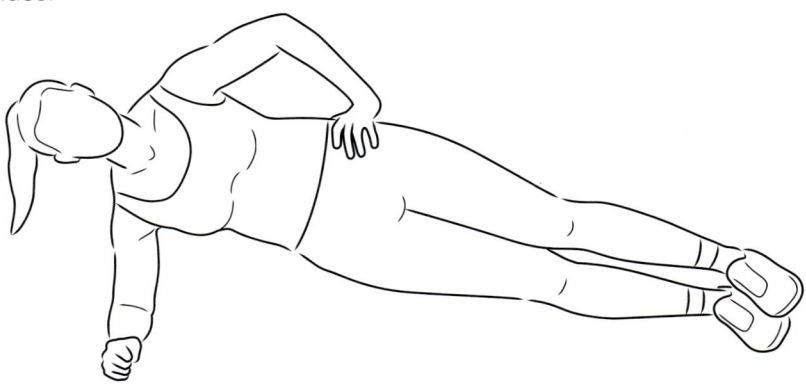

Figure 5.9 Reverse plank
Hold this position for 20 to 30 seconds for each of three sets.

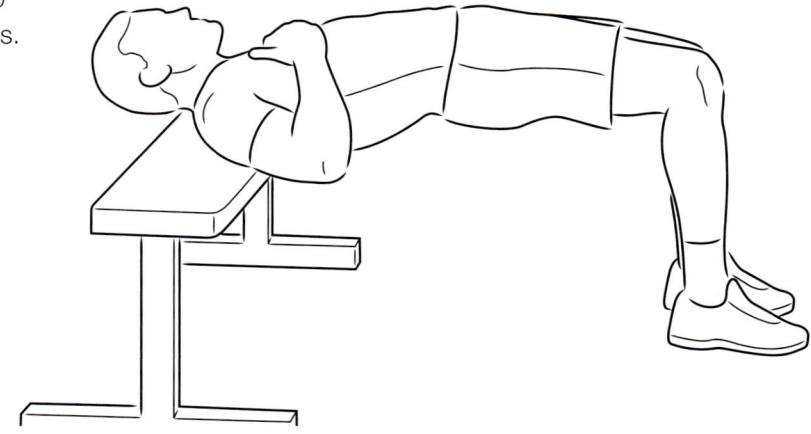

As with most endurance sports, riding a bike is done in a sagittal plane—straight ahead. The hips, especially, become rather weak and tight in the other planes, as when moving side to side and rotationally. And since the hip flexors also play a role in pedaling, weakness here may limit performance or lead to tightness and possible injury. This is likely to show up in one leg more than the other and lead to an imbalance in your left-right pedaling force. To reduce the likelihood of injury and to maintain a healthy range of motion, include hip mobility exercises along with your weightlifting and core strength. The hip mobility exercises I suggest using are shown in figures 5.10, 5.11, and 5.12. Include these three exercises in each gym session. If you would prefer to do different hip mobility exercises that you are used to and that work for you, feel free to do so.

Figure 5.10 90-90 rotations
Complete 10 to 20 repetitions of this movement in each of three total sets.

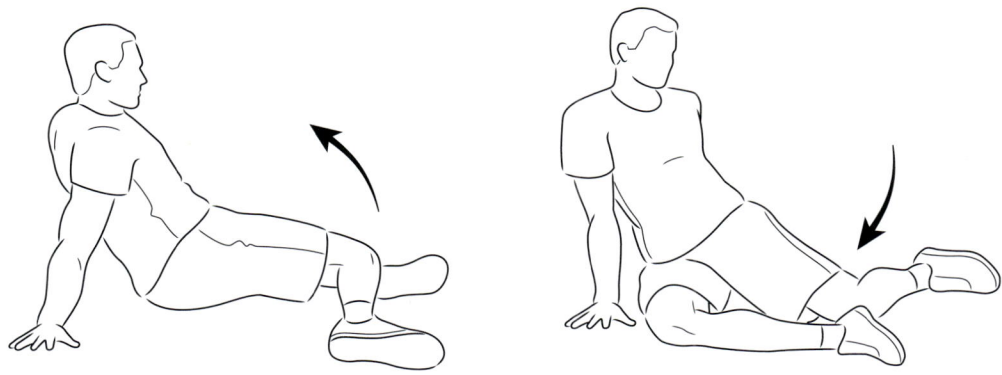

Figure 5.11 Windshield wipers
Complete three total sets with 10 to 20 repetitions for each set.

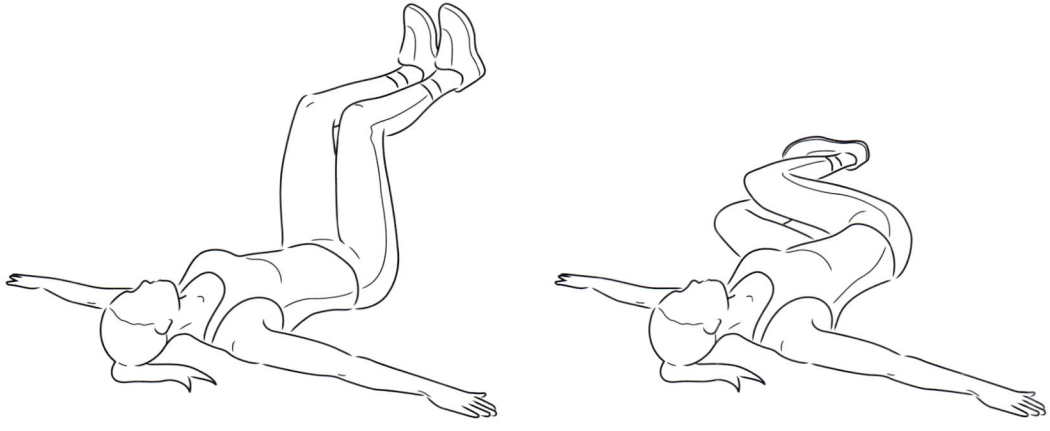

Figure 5.12 Cossack squats

Complete three total sets of this exercise with 10 to 20 repetitions for each set. Keep the head high and the butt low. You may use a light weight. This is done as a warm-up before weightlifting.

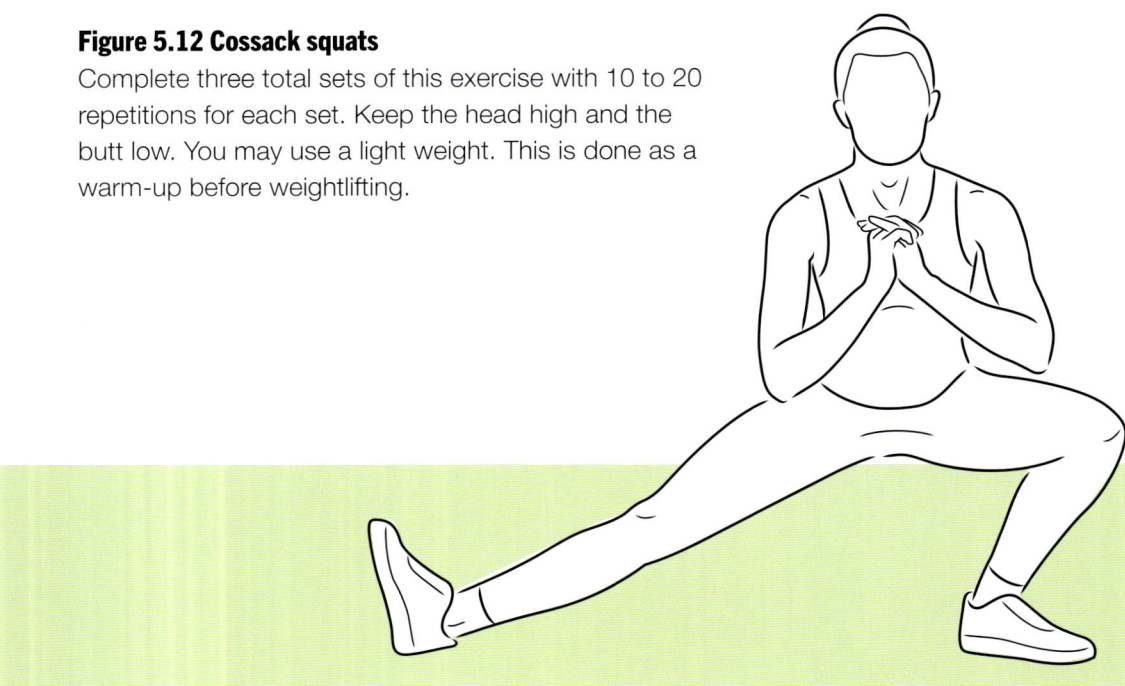

The gym workout including all these exercises can be done in whatever order works best for you at the time. Besides warming up with Cossack squats, the only other workout recommendation I suggest is to separate the two leg weightlifting exercises by a few minutes, during which you can do planks and mobility exercises. Otherwise, how you organize the session is up to you. In a gym it often comes down to which exercise stations are open, but be cautious not to do so much that you cause excessive fatigue, which will impact your next bike or cross-training workout. You're not lifting to become a body-builder. A suggested routine follows:

- Warm-up: Cossack squats.
- Weightlifting.
- Core strength.
- Weightlifting.
- Hip mobility.
- Repeat.

Now that we've got all the gym workouts determined, let's insert them into your early season periodization plan. In the previous chapter I proposed

Table 5.2 A suggested weekly training plan for the Preparation and Base 1 periods with an emphasis on gym sessions

Monday	Tuesday	Wednesday	Thursday	Friday	Saturday	Sunday
Gym session. Day off from bike and cross-training.	Easy ride and cross-training (or two cross-training sessions).	Easy ride and cross-training (or two cross training sessions).	Easy ride or cross-training. Gym session after.	Easy ride and cross-training (or two cross-training sessions).	Easy ride and cross-training (or two cross-training sessions).	Easy ride and cross-training (or two cross-training sessions).

a plan for a 4+3 training week in the Base periods and suggested that you redesign it to better fit your lifestyle, being sure to separate the gym sessions by two or three days. This latter point is very important. Scheduling weightlifting sessions too closely—only one day of separation—increases your risk of injury and reduces the benefits of strength training. Table 5.2 shows what that suggested week might look like in the Preparation and Base 1 periods when most of the gym work is done. As for weightlifting, these periods include the Anatomical Adaptation, Max Transition, and Max Strength phases of weightlifting. When you start Strength Maintenance in the Base 2 period you will only be lifting once each week. Again, adjust the days of the various workouts to match the personal training weeks you created in Chapter 4. This weekly program will take you through the Preparation and Base 1 periods. Also, note that in Base 1 you begin to phase out cross-training and gradually get more time on the bike.

There are going to be days when you just don't feel like doing a gym workout or you don't have much time. Those days happen to all of us, including me. Make a promise to yourself that on such days when motivation is low, or you are pressed for time, that you'll accept the situation by only doing one set of each of the exercises, if possible. There are eight exercises in total that I suggested above for weightlifting, core strength, and mobility. Each set will take one to two minutes. That's about 15 minutes. If even that feels like more than you want to or can do, cut back to only one of the weightlifting exercises after warming up. At home you may even do one set of one-leg squats with bodyweight only. Just do something. This will maintain your streak of consistent training and retain your fitness until you get back to a full session—soon, I hope. Less is better than not at all.

SPEED SKILLS TRAINING

Besides aerobic endurance and muscular force workouts, the other basic ability workouts I want to describe have to do with your bike skills, especially pedaling, sprinting, cornering, group riding, and descending. The detailed descriptions for most of these workouts may be found in the Appendix under the heading Speed Skills Workouts. If you've been around the sport and training seriously for several years, your skills are probably well honed. But if you're new to cycling, meaning in the first three years of racing, you may have a lot of room for skill improvement. In either regard, skills should never be taken for granted. Even the top pro riders work on their weak bike-handling skills.

I won't go into details here as the workouts in the Appendix speak for themselves. I have only a couple of comments. The first is that the purpose of such training is to hone skills so that you conserve energy and increase speed. Riding with poor skills not only slows you down, but also increases the energy cost of riding a bike. My second comment is that improving your skills makes riding a bike a lot safer for you. Descending, cornering, and riding in a tight group at high speeds are all risky, especially if your talents have room for improvement. The more skilled you are at riding a bike in various situations, the safer you and the others around you will be. On the other side of this, if you have good bike-handling skills and you are aware of another rider in your group ride who lacks such skills, maintain some distance for safety—yours and the other rider's.

The time to focus on skills is in the Base period. Work on your skills, especially for sprinting, cornering, and descending, every week. These can be built into your daily workouts regardless of what the primary purpose of the ride is. The best time to work on bike-handling skills is at the start of a ride when you are fresh. In the Base period pick a skill from the Appendix daily that will fit in with your day's workout. Be very aware of your bike-handling for that skill. Refining your movement often involves relaxing. Eventually, you'll be able to ride more skillfully at any time, even when tired. Just be aware that when you are in a risky situation, such as high-speed descending, that you must stay focused on safe technique and stay within your skill limits.

KEY TAKEAWAYS

- Twice-weekly gym workouts are important for your performance and health and are done in the Preparation and Base 1 periods.
- In the Base 2 period phase out cross-training and focus on the bike with increasing workout durations as you also transition to one gym session a week.
- Why lift weights? Research has shown that weightlifting is beneficial to cycling performance.
- Weightlifting will not only improve your performance, but also build stronger bones that are essential to your health and well-being.
- Do two hip-knee-ankle extension exercises each time you lift, along with core strength and hip mobility exercises.
- The best time to work on your bike-handling skills is in the Base period.

THE ADVANCED ABILITIES

In the Base period you focused on the basic abilities: aerobic endurance, muscular force, and speed skills. I've described in the last three chapters how to do these workouts and their performance benefits. Now it's time to move on to the more advanced training of the Build period. This is when you greatly boost race preparation by doing race-like workouts, along with B and C races. Training the advanced abilities is the icing on the "cake" that you baked in the Base period.

AEROBIC CAPACITY

Aerobic capacity has to do with the shuttling of oxygen from the lungs to the muscles. It is largely a product of your ancestry. There are several "fitness" genes that have been passed down to you by your parents, which they also inherited. But aerobic capacity, also known as VO_2 max, is not entirely an inherited marker of fitness. While close to half of your potential for aerobic capacity results from genetics, the largest portion is strictly a result of training. And VO_2 max is highly trainable. It is also one of the best indicators of your race readiness, especially for shorter races.

As I mentioned earlier, aerobic capacity is somewhat lower in women than men. The reason for this is that VO_2 max is based on oxygen consumption and body weight. And since women, on average, have more body fat than men, their aerobic capacity is lower even if their oxygen uptake is the same as a man's. Another reason for this difference is that women have somewhat less hemoglobin, the blood cell which transports oxygen from the lungs to the muscle mitochondria where energy is produced. Generally women's aerobic capacities are about 10 percent lower than men's.

Regardless of genetics and gender, a key purpose in your training is to increase your aerobic capacity, but before looking at how we are going to improve it, let's step back into the Base period first to recall how VO_2 max was initially improved. Your aerobic capacity progressed significantly in the Base period due to all the aerobic endurance workouts (AE1 and AE2) you did. Its current high level is also a product of heredity and your training done over many years. Early in the current season, some of those gains were made both on the bike and with cross-training sessions done consistently. In the Build period all we are doing is putting icing on the cake. We're going to raise your aerobic capacity by only a few percentage points with high-intensity training—10 percent would be a lot. In other words, the greatest improvements in your aerobic capacity were made before you even started the Build period. The improvements to be made now are comparatively small (see Figure 2.1). But they are still significant when a race calls for pushing yourself to the limit. That last 1 or 2 percent may be just what it takes to hang on climbing a steep hill, closing a gap, or riding hard into a cross wind.

The science of physiology tells us that the primary determiner of aerobic capacity is how much blood the heart pumps with each beat. This comes down to the heart's left ventricle, which is the primary pump for getting blood, along with oxygen, to the muscles. Your left ventricle doesn't know whether you are riding a bike, running, walking, Nordic skiing, or doing any other endurance activity. It only knows that you have a demand for oxygen. That's one of the reasons I recommend cross-training in the Preparation and early Base periods. By doing something other than riding you are still building fitness while taking a break from endless hours on the bike, which you will do throughout the season.

The next significant determiner of your aerobic capacity is how dense your capillaries are in the working muscles. This requires riding a bike. Cross-training won't do. In the Base period when riding easy, as in zone 2, you are slowly building large capillary beds in the active muscles and thus increasing your aerobic capacity.

A primary focus of the Build period is doing hard group rides and high-intensity intervals (see Appendix, Aerobic Capacity Workouts). These workouts will challenge your aerobic system to boost its delivery of oxygen to the muscles. We'll test it every few weeks to measure progress (more on testing below).

Is there anything else you can do in the Build period besides traditional high-intensity rides and aerobic endurance workouts to maintain or even boost aerobic capacity? The first option is probably obvious. You must have energy available, mostly from carbohydrate, to produce energy at all levels of intensity, but especially when you are riding at a high intensity, as in a race. The key here is to come into your long races, especially those beyond two hours, well-nourished. Then during such long races, you must replenish your carbohydrate stores (more on this in Chapter 8).

Another simple way to at least help maintain your aerobic capacity when training or in a race is to stay well hydrated. When hydration levels are low and blood volume is reduced, aerobic capacity is also reduced. Thick, dehydrated blood doesn't transport oxygen very well. Avoid dehydration. That's simple.

Here's another unique way of improving your aerobic capacity, which is relatively new in sport science. Train in the heat—sometimes. This has been shown to increase aerobic capacities in well-trained cyclists by 5 to 8 percent when done persistently for several weeks. That may not sound like much, but it is quite a bit. The resulting VO_2 max benefits in these studies were like those found in training at altitude. In the small number of research studies that have been done on this so far, riders spent 30 to 60 minutes in temperatures of 90 to 100 Fahrenheit (32 to 38 Celsius). These subjects rode indoors on trainers.

There may be several ways you could incorporate this into your training. It could be as simple as finishing your ride in the hottest time of day two times per week for eight weeks before your A race, if the temperature gets that high where you live. Or you might do that for eight weeks and then do such rides once weekly for a few weeks for maintenance. If your daily temperatures aren't that high, another option is to finish your ride by going indoors to ride in a warm room on a trainer in zone 1, without fans or other cooling devices. I've even known athletes to use a portable heater to raise the temperature when riding indoors in a rather cool environment. All such hot rides should be done in zone 1 as the subjects in these studies did. Going harder will not increase the benefit and may put you at risk of heat exhaustion or worse. And, of course, you must stay well-hydrated when doing such rides.

Be aware that doing a hot ride, even at low intensity, after a hard workout could be dangerous (I've experienced heat exhaustion on a ride followed by a trip to the emergency room after a hot ride—it's not fun). You are better off doing these rides only after low-intensity rides, such as AE1 and AE2. Short, hot rides are another painless way of raising your aerobic capacity. See Chapter 9 for more on heat adaptation.

STAMINA

In Chapter 4 I made the point that stamina is very important to high performance in cycling, especially for long races. You may come across it in your reading as "durability." They are the same thing. Learn as much about it as you can. It's critical to high performance in long races. Let's look at this a little more closely.

Stamina has to do with maintaining a high percentage of your aerobic capacity for more than an hour. But since you probably don't know your VO_2 max, and certainly don't know it while you're riding, we'll use your current FTP instead, since it's closely related to stamina. Of course, to do this it's imperative that you have a known and accurate FTP. The Appendix tells you how to determine it with a field test (see Field Tests, and T1 Functional Threshold Power (FTP) and Heart Rate (FTHR)).

Your stamina is highly trainable, even more so than your aerobic capacity. If you do long races and have developed a solid aerobic capacity, then the next critical step is being able to ride at a high percentage of it for more than an hour. If both aerobic capacity and stamina are well developed, then you are certainly a high-performance rider. This should be the goal of all serious cyclists.

While aerobic capacity is often considered the most important marker of endurance fitness, it does not always decide the outcome of a race. In a very long race a rider with a very high aerobic capacity may not be able to hold the wheel of a rider with a lower VO_2 max who has great stamina. This difference has to do with the unique physiologies of the two riders. It could be a result of different muscle types, the density of mitochondria which produce energy, how large the muscles' capillary beds are, and the availability of aerobic enzymes. Stamina is one of the best indicators of performance in long cycling events. In fact, the longer the race, the more important stamina is when compared with aerobic capacity. But there are limitations to stamina, of which you should be aware.

For the athlete with excellent stamina, race outcomes often come down to "matches burned." A match is a brief but extremely high-power output, almost like a sprint. Every rider has a limited number of matches at their disposal on a given day—some have more than others. When the matches are gone, stamina is also gone. This usually becomes apparent late in a long race when riders, often in a break, challenge each other with accelerations. If you have

JOE FRIEL'S HIGH-PERFORMANCE CYCLIST

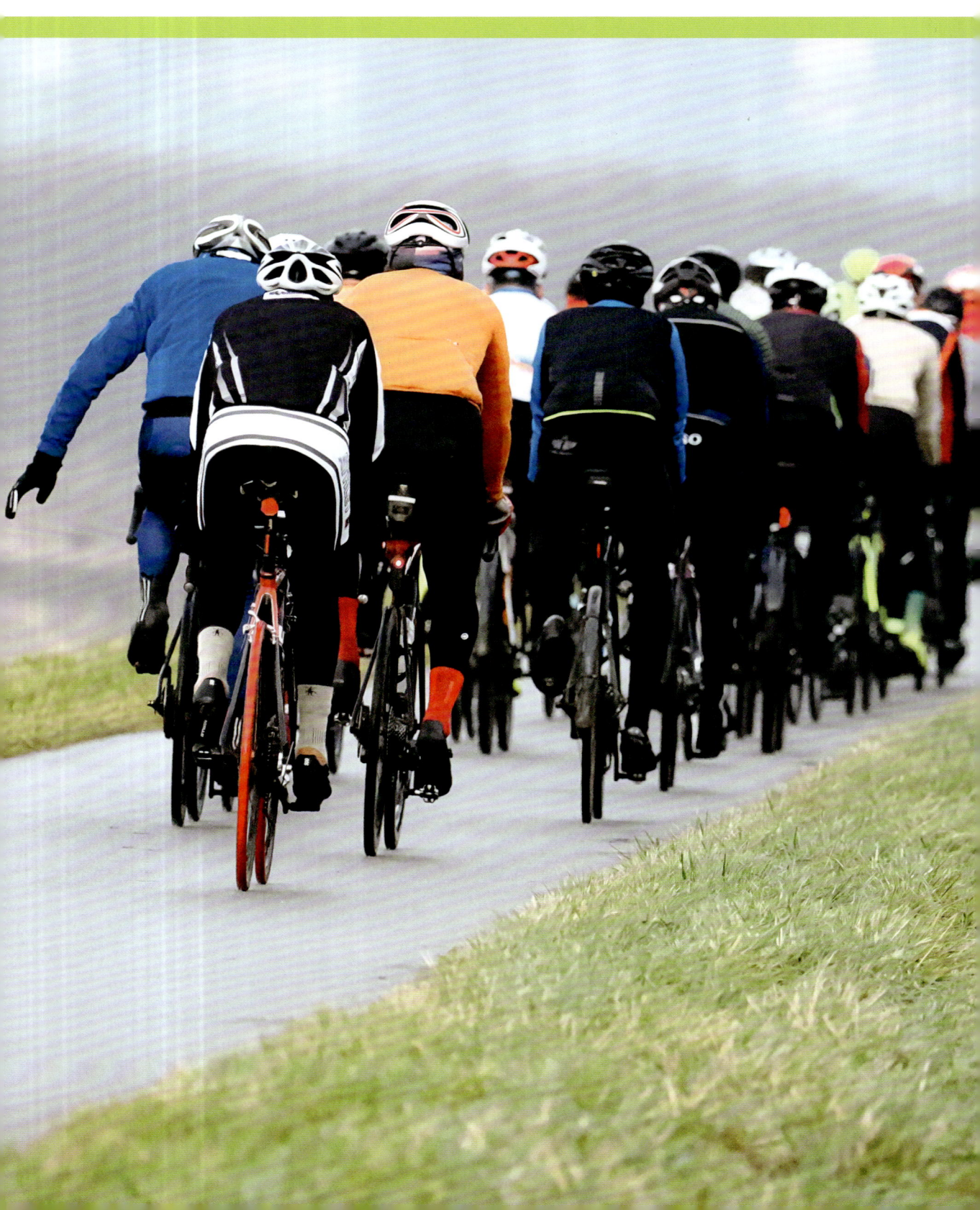

been "wasting" matches throughout the race by greatly accelerating at times when there was no clear advantage to come from it, then you are in danger of burning all your matches before the finish and getting left behind. You must be careful not to waste matches, especially early in the race. This is why you often see a rider who was dropped from the breakaway late in a race working to gradually return to the group without fast accelerations. The rider is saving matches and maintaining stamina.

Matches burned are much less of a concern for riders in short races, such as one-hour or shorter events. In such races aerobic capacity plays a greater role than stamina in the outcome. However, burning matches can still be an issue, especially for riders whose general fitness is poor. Match consumption in a short race is usually highest in two groups of riders—those who are new to the sport and excited about the race, and those who have excellent fitness, especially aerobic capacity, and have done many races. Only the latter will benefit from burning matches in such races.

What makes it possible for a rider with great stamina to also be able to burn a lot of matches? The key is, once again, a high capillary density. In other words, this rider can repeatedly call on lots of energy, while also removing waste products that may inhibit muscle contractions. How do you develop large muscle capillary beds? By doing lots of riding at intensities just below two millimoles per liter of blood lactate (LT1 in Table 3.1). In other words, large capillary beds are largely a result of easy riding in zones 1 and 2. This is another of the reasons I've put so much emphasis on the importance of "easy" rides, especially in the Base period. There is a great deal to be gained by doing this—and when it comes to building fitness, this is "low-hanging fruit." But it is unfortunately often pushed aside by self-coached riders intent on fatiguing themselves with somewhat higher intensities that do little, if anything, to boost high-performance racing. I call them "intensity addicts."

We will build your stamina starting in the Base period with increasingly long workout durations done in zones 1 and 2. And in the late Base and Build periods we'll add in zone 3 stamina workouts. This will begin to develop your stamina, which will be field-tested at the end of the Base period. If you meet the "excellent" standards described in the Appendix (see Field Tests and T3 Stamina Test), you should consider stamina a strength and not a limiter. Maintenance in the Build period is then all that's needed. But if it continues to be a limiter for you, in the Build period you will do stamina rides such as St3 Cruise Intervals (see Appendix, Stamina Workouts), fast group rides, and B and C races.

The perfect time to do a stamina ride in the Build period is at the end of a workout that started out with another purpose, such as aerobic capacity development or a long aerobic endurance ride. Since the purpose of stamina is to maintain a relatively high and long power output late in a race, doing such an effort in the latter part of a ride is a great way to simulate race conditions. It also serves as a marker of how sustainable your power is when fatigue is setting in. Here's another way to incorporate race-like stamina workouts in your training. In the Build period "sit in" on a group ride or C race until late in the ride or race, and then move to the front or break away and ride hard, albeit within your stamina limits. Not only will this be a good stimulus for stamina development, but also a good rehearsal for your A race.

Just as with aerobic capacity, when calling on late-race stamina it's very important that you refuel and stay well hydrated. Disregarding either will significantly slow you down. The time to figure out how much fuel and fluids you typically need is in workouts with late stamina sessions. Riding hard for a long time when fatigue is setting in is a great indicator of your stamina. Pay close attention to how you are feeling as the late-ride effort progresses. When heart rate begins to rapidly rise even though power is steady, you are approaching your limit for stamina. This could be due to the need for fuel or hydration, your general training fatigue, or it may simply be an indicator of your current stamina status. Make note of this for comparison with similar rides in the future. And give a lot of thought to what you can do to improve your stamina with training in the coming weeks.

Doing combined workouts, such as aerobic capacity and stamina, in the Build period is a very smart way to train in that period as it closely simulates what you can expect in a race. Making workouts like portions of the race is the fundamental purpose of the Build period. To carry this race-like training concept a bit further, you could finish such a long and hard aerobic capacity-stamina ride with a sprint or series of sprints. Hard group rides in the Build period are an excellent time to mimic such race-like workouts. When doing a group workout, it's good to have a plan for what you want to accomplish. Ride with a purpose. I suggest that your limiter should usually be the purpose of such workouts. The above multifaceted aerobic capacity-stamina-sprint combination workout is a great option, especially as you're getting closer to race day.

SPRINT POWER

If sprint power is your limiter, you need to focus on it throughout the Build period. When doing races shorter than an hour, it would be wise to combine aerobic capacity and sprint power workouts in your two weekly hard rides. But if your A race will be longer than an hour it's probably better to combine stamina and sprint power training. Again, in the Build period make this combination as similar as you can to what is anticipated in your race.

By the time you get to the Build period you should have developed strength in the gym, refined your sprint technique, and built muscular force on the bike with big-gear sessions (see Appendix, Muscular Force Workouts). Of course, aerobic endurance workouts, including long, easy rides, should also have prepared you for the demands of training in the Build period. Now the focus shifts to your limiter.

If sprint power is your primary limiter, I'd suggest doing two workouts weekly that include sprint training along with either aerobic capacity, stamina, or aerobic endurance. Be sure to work on your sprint in a variety of situations such as uphill, downhill, straightaways, out of corners, alone, and with other riders. The latter is certainly something you should focus on late in the Build period.

It may also be that sprinting is a limiter, but you are not a pure sprinter but rather better at climbing or at time trialing. Your sprint weakness shows up when short accelerations are needed in a race—a gap opens, or you must come out of a corner and quickly accelerate to stay with the group. In this case you will train somewhat differently than how a pure sprinter does. It will be more beneficial for you in the Build period to include random sprints in workouts and, especially, in group rides. It's important, also, that you do the related, preliminary sprint power workouts in the Base period described above.

KEY TAKEAWAYS

- High-intensity training in the Base period will negatively impact your race preparation—save it for the Build period.
- Your aerobic capacity is mostly a product of Base period training, and in the Build period the increase is comparatively small, but necessary.
- Cross-training in the Preparation and Base 1 periods boosts your aerobic capacity by enlarging your heart's left ventricle.
- Carbohydrate stores and hydration status have a lot to do with your aerobic capacity on race day.
- Frequent heat training has been shown to increase aerobic capacity.
- Your stamina has to do with riding for a long time—more than one hour—at a high percentage of your FTP.
- A high aerobic capacity and great stamina are what defines the best endurance cyclists and should be your goal.
- Limit your matches burned in races to maintain stamina for when it's needed.
- Riding at a high percentage of FTP in the last hour and longer of a Build period workout is the perfect time to train stamina.
- Your heart rate rising late in a stamina workout, even though your power remains constant, is possibly a sign of the need for more endurance training.
- Your hard rides in the Build period should imitate the demands of your upcoming race.
- Combining sprint power training following either aerobic capacity or stamina training is a good way to prepare for your race.
- Sprint power training in the Base period involves weightlifting, skill development, and muscular force workouts on the bike.

PREPARING TO RACE

I've said quite a bit about the Preparation and Base periods, and how improving your aerobic endurance, muscular force, and speed skills are your primary goals for that time of the season. Let's shift the focus now to the Build, Peak, and Race periods when your race readiness is realized.

THE BUILD PERIOD

In the Build period you have four goals: increase aerobic capacity, improve stamina, and boost sprint power. But that's only three. The fourth is a bit different in that you must maintain the gains made in the Base period for your aerobic endurance, muscular force, and speed skills. If you now ignore these abilities after weeks of improving them, they will erode. Use it or lose it! But note that it doesn't take as much time to maintain an ability as it does to develop it in the first place. That means you'll devote much less time to those abilities after the Base period.

In the Base period it really didn't matter how you weighed the importance of the basic abilities as, at the time, they were nearly of equal value. Each was essential in its own way, and you worked on all three of them. But now in the Build period you must prioritize the three advanced abilities. The key questions are: of the advanced abilities, which is my strongest, and which is my weakest? The answer to this question requires a comparison of the demands of the race you are preparing for and your known weaknesses.

For example, if the course is hilly and the race usually comes down to high-intensity climbs lasting several minutes and that is a weakness, then the Build period emphasis must be on your limiter—aerobic capacity. But if the course is relatively flat or has long gradual climbs and the outcome often comes down to long breakaways, or the race is a long time trial or off-road race, then stamina is the likely limiter if this is a weakness. If aerobic capacity and stamina are good but the race is likely to come down to a sprint, but that is a weakness, then sprint power is your limiter.

These examples are easy calls. Yours may be much more intricate. Your limiter decision could also be some combination of the three advanced abilities. What it always comes down to is how much training time you will need to concentrate on each ability. The more important an ability is in contributing to your goal success, yet it is a limiter, the more time you must devote to it in the Build period. This is without doubt the most difficult decision you will make in planning your season. But it's critical to your race-day success so give it lots of thought before starting to make decisions about your Build period training plan.

Of course, one or two of the three advanced abilities are probably strengths. We will treat a strength as if it's a basic ability and just train to maintain it for the entire Build period. That means devoting much less time for such workouts. A good time to work on maintaining a strength in the Build period is during a ride that is focused on a limiter. For example, if stamina is a limiter but sprint power or aerobic capacity is a strength, within a ride mostly devoted to stamina, include some sprints or aerobic capacity intervals. A once-weekly focus on a strong ability is usually enough to maintain it.

There's no reason why, however, you can't do it twice in a week on the days you do your hard rides. Table 5.3 offers a suggested weekly routine for the Build period and may help with your Table 4.3 planning.

Table 5.3 A suggested weekly bike and gym training plan for the Build period with an emphasis on your limiter, strengths, and maintaining basic abilities

Monday	Tuesday	Wednesday	Thursday	Friday	Saturday	Sunday
Gym session (SM)	Long, easy ride (AE1 or AE2)	Your strength (Aerobic Capacity, Stamina, and/or Sprint Power workout)	Very easy ride (AE1)	Easy (maintain basic abilities)	Long, easy ride (AE1 or AE2)	Your limiter (Aerobic Capacity, Stamina, and/or Sprint Power workout)

THE PEAK AND RACE PERIODS

Following the Build period, you will start the relatively short Peak period (see Table 4.1). This is when you begin to gradually reduce workout durations to taper your volume, thus improving form. While you will be training less, you will still include race-intensity workouts that are focused on your limiter. They just won't be as long as they were in the Build period. All workouts are gradually shortened to allow you to begin developing "freshness" in your readiness for race day. If you do a 10-day to two-week taper as suggested in Table 4.1, reduce the duration of your workouts by 10 to 20 percent each day compared with what you were doing in the Build period for similar workouts. The idea is that your rides will gradually get shorter over the period of several days. By the end of the second week your ride durations should be about 50 percent of what they were in the Build period. This tapering in the Peak period should be accompanied by gradually increasing feelings of impatience and readiness to race. That means you are coming into "form." You may find it difficult to keep the intensities of the easy workouts under control, but you must. Table 5.4 offers a suggested Peak period week.

Table 5.4. A suggested weekly training plan for the Peak period Workout durations in the second week of a two-week Peak period taper are shorter than those of the previous week.

Monday	Tuesday	Wednesday	Thursday	Friday	Saturday	Sunday
Gym session (SM)	Easy ride (AE2)	Your strength (Aerobic Capacity, Stamina, and/or Sprint Power workout)	Very easy ride (AE1)	Easy ride (AE2)	Group ride or B, C race, or your limiter (if race tomorrow do AE1 today)	Group ride or B, C race, or your limiter (if race yesterday do AE1 today)

By Race week, if all has gone well, you will feel exceptionally fresh, fit, and eager to race. Now you can do several race-like rides with a focus on aerobic capacity and/or sprint power, depending on your limiter, but they *must* be quite short—less than half of what you did in the Build period for similar rides. Warm up and then do a few high-intensity efforts followed by a cool-down. You must now avoid using up your stamina until race day as it requires long efforts and produces a great deal of fatigue. A week without stamina training will not present any problems on race day, so long as you maintain aerobic endurance. Also, by Race week, the basic abilities will remain strong and so won't require maintenance, as long as you've been refreshing them weekly in the Build and Peak periods. Table 5.5 provides an example of what a Race period week may look like.

Table 5.5 A suggested weekly training plan for the Race period with an emphasis on short, intense rides

Monday	Tuesday	Wednesday	Thursday	Friday	Saturday	Sunday
Day off	Short ride with 4–5 Aerobic Capacity Intervals and/or several Power Sprints with long recoveries	Short and very easy ride (AE1)	Short ride with 3–4 Aerobic Capacity Intervals and/or several Power Sprints with long recoveries	Short ride with 2–3 Aerobic Capacity Intervals and/or several Power Sprints (or very easy ride if any fatigue)	Race (or, if Sunday race, same as Friday)	Race (or very easy ride if you raced yesterday)

KEY TAKEAWAYS

- In the Build period do more high-intensity group rides, long and steady stamina rides, intervals, and B and C races while maintaining the basic abilities.
- Easy riding is a key part of your race preparation year-round to develop (Base) and then maintain (Build) aerobic endurance.
- Determine your limiter—aerobic capacity, stamina, or sprint power—and focus your training on it in the Build and Peak periods.
- Maintain your strengths, along with the basic abilities, throughout the Build period.
- Maintain your gym strength with one strength maintenance workout weekly, done after a hard workout.
- Taper your volume by gradually reducing workout durations in the Peak period.
- In the Race period keep the workouts short and with race-like intensities.

FILLING IN THE GAPS

In this and the previous chapter I've tried to cover all the bases for training throughout the season, but there are three gaps. The first has to do with testing. The second is an overview of all the details I've thrown at you so far. Both are addressed below. The third has to do with R&R breaks throughout the season. This is so critical to your training and eventual performance that I've set aside Chapter 6 for it.

FITNESS TESTING

I've mentioned testing several times in this chapter. By now you may be wondering what sort of testing and when will you be doing it. In the Base period testing is primarily to determine and update your functional threshold power and heart rate zones (see T1 Functional Threshold Power (FTP) and Heart Rate (FTHR) in the Appendix under Field Tests). But you should also be measuring your efficiency factor on a daily basis when doing AE1 and AE2 rides throughout the Base period (memory refresher: efficiency factor is normalized power divided by average heart rate for a ride). Your efficiency factor should slowly ratchet up over the course of a few weeks indicating that you are producing more power per heartbeat. That's great feedback on how your aerobic endurance is coming along.

In the last week of the Base period, you will test your stamina to determine if this is a limiter and to establish a baseline. If the test results meet the "excellent" stamina standards listed in the Appendix Field Test section, that indicates stamina is not a limiter for you. Functional aerobic capacity and sprint power testing will also be done in the Build period. The timing of tests is explained in Table 5.6.

SEASONAL TRAINING DETAILS

In this and the previous chapter I frequently referred to when different types of workouts should be done relative to race day, along with comments about the periods, such as "early Base" and "late Base." It's time to put all of this into one chart that helps you see the big picture of your season more clearly. Table 5.6 brings much of what you've read about so far together.

Table 5.6 An overview of the season's training details

Period	Preparation	Base 1 ("early")	Base 2 ("late")	Base 3 ("late")	Build 1	Build 2	Peak	Race	Transition
Length	3–6 weeks	3 or 4 weeks	3 or 4 weeks	3 or 4 weeks	3 or 4 weeks	3 or 4 weeks	10 days–2 weeks	5–7 days	1–4 weeks
Daily Workout Type	XTrain x 2 or XT+bike	XTrain x 2 or XT+bike	Bike	Bike	Bike	Bike	Bike	Bike	Limited aerobic exercise
Progression	Frequency	Frequency and Duration	Duration	Duration and Intensity	Intensity	Intensity	Intensity	Intensity	Greatly reduced training
Training Triad Abilities	Basic	Basic	Basic	Basic	Advanced (maintain Basic)	Advanced (maintain Basic)	Advanced (maintain Basic)	Advanced	Aerobic endurance only
Weightlifting	AA-MT (2/week)	MS (2/week)	SM (1/week)	SM (1/week)	SM (1/week)	SM (1/week)	SM (1/week)	None	None
Field Testing* (in last week of each period) and weekly measurement of Efficiency Factor (EF) following AE1 and AE2 rides	Daily: Efficiency Factor (EF)	Last Week: T1 FTP/FTHR Daily: EF	Last Week: T1 FTP/FTHR Daily: EF	Last Week: T3 Stamina Daily: EF	Last Week: T2 Aerobic Capacity and T4 Sprint Power and T1 FTP/FTHR	Last Week: T2 Aerobic Capacity and T3 Stamina and T4 Sprint Power	None	None Your race is the ultimate test	None

*See Appendix "Field Tests" for details

Note that the length of the Base and Build periods is three or four weeks. Why three or four? This has to do with your typical rate of recovery, which may be age-related. I'll explain this in Chapter 6. Note also that Table 5.6 lists both field tests and "measurements" in the last row. The latter refers to the efficiency factor (EF), which is explained above and is a great indicator of your aerobic endurance.

> ### KEY TAKEAWAYS
>
> - Throughout the Base period measure your efficiency factor after every AE1 or AE2 ride—it should ratchet up over time.
> - The advanced abilities—aerobic capacity, stamina, and sprint power—will be tested in the late Base and Build periods.
> - Test functional threshold power and functional threshold heart rate in Base 1, Base 2, and Build 1.

THE REST OF LAURIE'S STORY

Laurie did the Leadville Trail 100 MTB race three more times as a pro—and returned to the top step of the podium each time. Three years later (1997), she would have the ride of her life and finish in under eight hours—7:58:52—taking more than an hour off her first race and taking seventh overall among the men. No woman had ever even come close to eight hours in the 1990s, and since then only two other women have finished in the top 20, which she did all four years in the race. That record of under eight hours would stand for the next 14 years. Keep in mind that in the 1990s, mountain bikes had small 26-inch wheels with narrow tires, triple chainrings, rim brakes, primitive suspension forks, and little-to-no rear suspension. With the advent of 29-inch wheels with wider tires, single chainrings, disc brakes, and full suspension carbon fiber bikes in the mid-2000s, course times dropped significantly for men and women. Laurie went on to be ranked in the top 10 women riders in the world and nationally. She won the Colorado State Championship three times, and was truly a high-performance athlete.

After leaving the sport's pro ranks, she went back to being a geologist, for which she has Bachelor's and Master's degrees. That didn't mean the end of her racing career, however. She continued to train and race well, becoming a USA Master's National Champion twice for women 55-59 and once for women 60-64. Reflecting a strong commitment to both her hometown of Montrose, Colorado, and the sport of off-road racing, she helped start, and was the team director and coach, for a mountain bike team at the local high school. Both of her daughters, Paige and Abby, raced all four years on the school's team. Laurie also continues to teach mountain bike skills clinics through the Montrose Recreation District, sharing her knowledge of skills and her passion for the sport. I'm proud to say I coached her.

6. STRESS AND REST

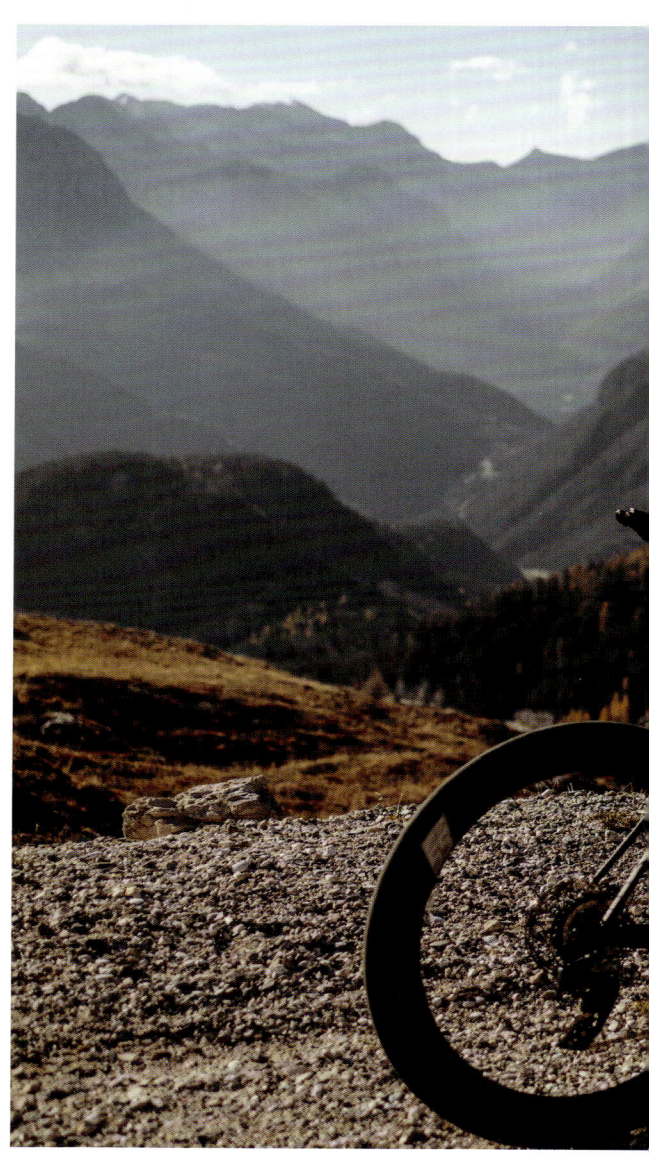

Training for a high-performance race is a complex undertaking, especially for the self-coached rider. As you've probably come to realize in previous chapters, there are a lot of details to consider and decisions to be made. It's not just throwing your leg over a bike and riding however you feel with your buddies. This is probably why the most successful athletes have coaches. Someone with the experience and know-how to make the many critical decisions. It's certainly possible to coach yourself well. I've known many riders who have done a great job of it. But it's not easy and there are a lot of details to understand and get right. In this chapter I'll address what is undoubtedly the hardest part of self-coaching: balancing stress and rest.

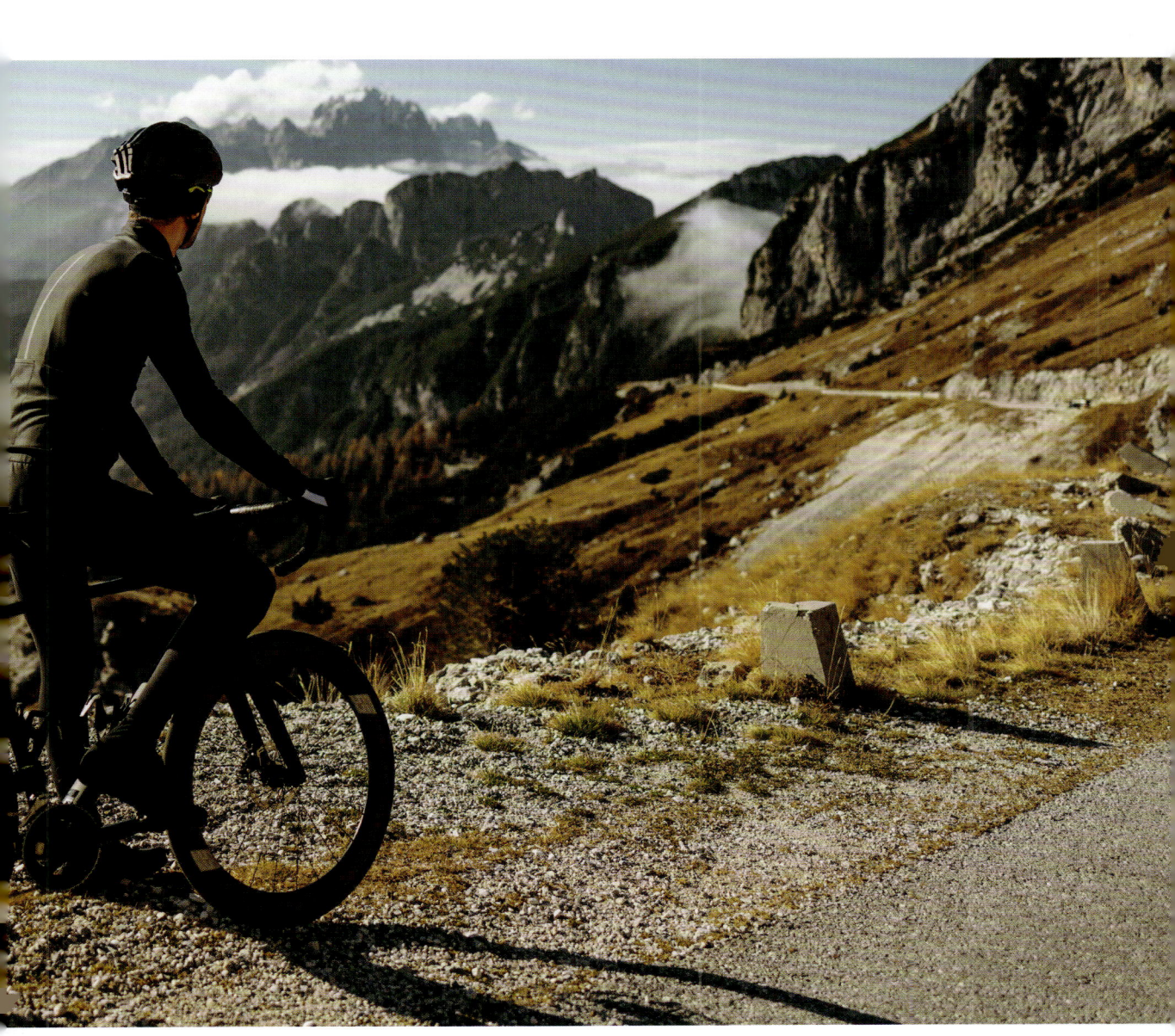

WES'S STORY

We met at a coffee shop near my home. It was late winter. I arrived first and was at a table warming my hands with a cup when he walked in. I could tell at a glance that he wasn't his usual self. When I had seen him at races, he was the life and soul of the party—always smiling, trading barbs with friends, happy to be there, and full of energy. He wasn't that way today: a forced smile and limited eye contact.

We had never met but I knew quite a bit about Wes. He was an icon in the sport, having raced professionally for several years. The United States Olympic Committee had awarded him the title of "Triathlete of the Year" a few years earlier. He was currently ranked in the top five in the USA at the Olympic distance and had been for several years. He was at the top of his game. I wasn't sure I could help him as he was obviously a world-class athlete already. But then, I didn't know what he wanted to talk about.

Wes got a cup of coffee and sat down at my table. I could tell from the start that something was wrong. We made small talk about how we were looking forward to the end of winter, but we were meeting for a reason. What was it? He pulled out his training diary. That's usually a bad sign. After thumbing back a few weeks in the diary, he took me on a journey through his recent training. A few months prior he had decided to ditch his coach so he was on his own. Despite his amazing level of success over the past several years, he had decided he could still race faster. All he had to do was train harder, he said. If he could do more high-intensity training, he could be faster in the coming season. He just had to commit to working harder and resting less, he told me. My thought was, "Hmmm, that's not a good sign."

Then he got into the details. He told me that a couple of months ago he had started a challenging eight-week plan. No rest. No easy days. Just train long and hard with lots of high-intensity workouts. He'd be unbeatable in the coming season. He told me what he'd been doing for the last seven weeks. It was remarkable. On Tuesday, Thursday, and Saturday he did hard group rides with local cyclists in Boulder, Colorado. Also, on Saturday mornings he met with a group of high-level runners to do a five-kilometer race. Each of the eight weeks also included running intervals on the track, and two long runs to build endurance. Then there were several swim sessions weekly made up of mostly high-intensity interval sessions. He had been putting in up to 24 hours of training with lots of anaerobic work for each of the past seven weeks. He looked tired. And there was no wondering why.

Wes was now in the eighth week of his plan, but he was wasted. He still wanted to complete the eight-week plan but was finding it hard to get out of bed in the mornings, having slept very little for days. He was a wreck. The bottom line was: could I help him get back to his normal training routine again? There was no doubt that he was overtrained. I had seen a few overtrained athletes before, but he had taken it to an even higher level. He was at his physical and mental limit but was looking for a way to soldier on. He wanted me to help him do it.

I knew he wasn't going to like what I had to tell him: he needed to take some time off. "How much?" he asked. I didn't know the answer, but I did know that it would be longer than he could tolerate. I suggested one week of rest with no training of any kind. Then we'd see how he was coming along. We'd talk then and decide what to do next. He reluctantly agreed. It wound up being about three weeks before he was sleeping normally again and sounded like his old self on the phone. So, we tried a short and easy bike ride to see how he'd respond. That went okay, so two days later we tried a longer, yet still easy, ride. Again, the takeaway seemed to be positive. Slowly we began to move his training back toward something normal for him, but not his eight-week plan. That was a disaster. Going forward I included frequent R&R weeks with far fewer hard days separated by quite easy ones. Within two months he was starting to train well again. There was still a long way to go. One of the best signs was he gradually returned to his old chipper self, but he was somewhat scared of what lay ahead for racing in the fast-approaching season.

The extended rest periods followed by easing back into normal training was a very slow process. That brought us to the start of the race season in May. His early races that season, finishing well back of the winners, were nothing like he had done in previous years. He was extremely disappointed with a rather lackluster season in our first year together. He had some decent results, but nothing like before. It was amazing how just a few weeks of chronic fatigue affected his performances for an entire season.

The following season we shifted our attention from the shorter Olympic distance races to something a bit longer. It was his idea and I liked it. This would allow him to focus more on endurance and a bit less on intensity that late winter and spring. We aimed for the Escape from Alcatraz race in early summer, which was a unique distance with a 1.5-mile swim, 18 hilly miles on the bike, and an 8-mile trail run. That turned out to be the best decision we made that season. He won and started to get some of his mojo back. He was positive and happy again, more like the old Wes.

The next challenge he had to take on was qualifying for the USA Olympic team early in the following spring. Despite the win and feeling much better, he was still not the dominant athlete he had been two seasons prior. I hoped that after some downtime at the end of this second season together he would bounce back and be ready to take on the Olympic Trials test. Things seemed to go well throughout his next Base period. Wes was always a very strong cyclist and good swimmer. Those sports progressed quite well in late winter. Running stamina was his limiter. It seemed that nothing we did got him to the level of runner he had to be to make the team. There were some very fast runners in the USA and a new draft-legal rule took away much of Wes's cycling advantage. Neither of us were very positive about what we might expect at the Trials, but we both tried to hide it.

The next spring he raced the USA Olympic Trials race in Dallas, Texas, much better than I thought he might. Fifth place was a very good outcome for him in this new way of triathlon racing and all he'd been through. With the top three going to the Olympics, he was close. We finished the season with some good races, but he was still short of his former self. That was a mix of both the still-lingering effects of overtraining and the sport's very significant changes. Both of us learned an important lesson about the effects of pushing your limits without concern for health.

THE RIGHT BALANCE

Getting this balancing act right, week after week, is often the difference between a good race and poor one. This stress-rest relationship is closely tied to successful training and is the most likely culprit for a lackluster race season. Should you upset the stability of a well-balanced training program for a few weeks, the entire season—and even more—may be lost. If stress and rest aren't carefully balanced, then the athlete is either overtrained or undertrained. Both have dire consequences that must be avoided. More than anything you've read about here so far, this teeter-tottering of stress and rest is the single most important reason for having a training plan. The equilibrium between these two must be reflected in your plan and given a lot of follow-up attention daily. The balancing of stress and rest will seldom be perfect, but there must never be an exceptionally prolonged shift toward either. The key is to find that successful coupling of yin and yang, and stay as close to it as you can: never too much of one or the other, always balanced and steady.

Most athletes have a good understanding of what the word "rest" means, even if they choose to disregard it. Rest is too often considered to be something that must be minimally used in training. And while athletes often try to produce as much physical stress as possible, they don't always understand exactly what that means and how it can be too high. When is stress too high? And when is it too low? I'll try to answer those questions in this chapter.

To finish designing your training plan, you've got to understand how to maintain this fragile relationship. By the end of this chapter, you should have a finished training plan with all the details necessary for producing your best A race. Let's start toward that goal by getting a better understanding of stress and rest, and how can you use both for high-performance racing.

STRESS

Stress can refer to both physical and mental situations. As an athlete, both are important. Let's start with some stress history to get a better understanding of this key term. The word "stress" was not used as it is today until the mid-20th century. Prior to that the common use of the word was in the field of physics, for example, when referring to repeatedly bending a piece of metal until the stress causes it to break. That was how we typically talked about "stress." More than 70 years ago a Hungarian-born, Canadian endocrinologist, Hans Selye, introduced the concept of stress in a biological setting. He is often referred to as "the father of stress research" for all the studies he did using animals to see how they reacted biologically to various traumatic situations. He introduced two variations of the word to better describe the two types of stress he discovered: *eustress* and *distress*. Eustress means "good stress," the kind you experience when training is going well, or you win the lottery. Both are stressful but in positive ways. Distress, however, has a negative connotation—"bad stress." That's what happens when you are so tired from a hard workout that you can't get out of bed the next day. It may also be what you experience when your tax payment becomes due.

Today the word stress has commonly come to mean *distress* in how we use it. We view it as a negative experience. Eustress is seldom used in daily life but is still common in psychology. In cycling we often use the word "stress"—implying distress—in the context of terms such as pain, agony, suffering, or severe discomfort. Using such words to describe a hard workout or race is quite common in our sport.

Eustress is what I want you to focus on this season—the beneficial stress of training. How can stress be beneficial? When it causes your body to adapt, become stronger, and better able to cope with the workload you just placed on it in a ride. That, of course, is what training is all about. The body becomes more fit due to a eustressful workout followed by rest. The ultimate form of rest is sleep, especially deep and prolonged sleep. That's when fitness occurs. The workout didn't make you more fit. It only created the *potential* for fitness. More on this later in the chapter.

I'll often refer to the stress of training in this book. Distress, of course, is experienced in various degrees. But any amount of it can lead to a physical and mental breakdown if it continues long enough. There are only three situations in which you may experience distress. The most usual is in a race in which you are going full gas and pushed to your physical and mental limits. Another common one in cycling is very hard, race-like group rides or very high-intensity intervals. The third is a field test in which you are exploring your limits to measure how fit you currently are, especially by doing the stamina or FTP field tests (see Appendix).

Each of these distressing episodes requires a lot of R&R time, especially sleep, afterward. It will probably take more than one day of easy training or a day off to fully recover from something this challenging. And that's why I will seldom have you do a ride that is truly distressful. While that is obviously necessary on occasion, it must not be common in your training. There must be broad gaps between

USING HEART RATE VARIABILITY (HRV) TO MONITOR STRESS: MARCO ALTINI

HRV, or heart rate variability, quantifies the variation between heartbeats in numerical form. This variability between beats is not random, but when measured under certain circumstances (clarified below) it allows us to capture our body's response to stress. In particular, our body continuously strives to maintain equilibrium, known as homeostasis. Various bodily functions such as heart rate, blood pressure, glucose levels, and hormone secretion respond to challenges, notably stress, with the autonomic nervous system regulating these responses to ensure optimal functioning and prevent the onset of chronic conditions or enhance performance. When we measure HRV following best practices, we get insights into our body's response to physical exertion, lifestyle factors, psychological stress, or other sources. A decline in HRV typically indicates reduced parasympathetic activity, suggesting incomplete recovery or heightened stress on the body, hindering a swift return to baseline levels. Thus, HRV serves as the most convenient, non-invasive, and cost-effective method for assessing how we respond to stressors.

To effectively use HRV, it is crucial to gather data using reliable methods and adhere to best practices. This means using accurate sensors, but also measuring at the right time, and interpreting the data with respect to our own normal range, as there is no universal frame of reference. To measure accurate data, several sensors are available, including chest straps such as the Polar H10, or optical sensors like the Scosche Rhythm24. Accuracy is paramount; hence ensure you use validated apps or sensors, like HRV4Training.

Keep in mind that our primary focus lies in assessing underlying physiological stress levels, resulting from both acute stressors (for example, intense workouts, or long-distance travel) and chronic stressors (for example, work-related concerns). By monitoring how these stressors affect resting physiology, meaningful adjustments can be made to enhance health and performance. Thus, measurements should be taken far away from stressors to determine if our physiology has re-normalized after a few hours. Physiological changes during or immediately after stress are normal, and this is why we should not monitor HRV continuously, but we should assess our body's response after several hours, in a resting state.

Practically speaking, measuring at the right time means using a morning spot check or a full-night measurement. Both these methods are established as reliable once accurate data acquisition is ensured. However, there can be some key differences. For example, stressors (alcohol, but also training, food intake, and so on) impact your resting physiology acutely, and therefore late stressors might impact your night HRV data more, simply because the measurement comes earlier. By the following morning, everything might be perfectly normal (unless the stressor was particularly strong). If you often eat late, drink, or exercise in the evening, morning data might be more helpful, simply because night data is measured too close to the stressor and does not allow for a proper assessment of our response. Finally, measuring in the morning allows us to use orthostatic measurements (this simply means measuring while sitting or standing), resulting in a little challenge for the system and therefore making the measurement more sensitive to stress, and more useful to determine our state. As such, morning measurements are better for capturing your readiness for the day, while night measurements might capture more of your previous evening's behavior.

If you decide to go for a morning measurement, here is a simple protocol: after you wake up, grab your phone, and measure either using the phone camera, a chest strap, or a reliable optical sensor. Your morning measurement can last just one minute. During the measurement, limit movement and breathe naturally, avoiding yawning and swallowing. If you need to go to the bathroom, please do so before your measurement. Finally, my recommendation would be to measure while sitting, especially if your heart rate is particularly low or you are an endurance athlete.

Consistency is paramount in HRV analysis due to the myriad factors influencing it. Whether morning or night measurements are chosen, adherence to a consistent protocol is essential for meaningful interpretation and trend analysis over time.

Once you start collecting some data, the most important thing to remember is that you always need to interpret your HRV data with respect to your historical data. Your normal might be different from your friend's normal (it probably will be). Thus, focusing on changes over time in relation to our own historical data often provides the most meaningful insights for health and performance optimization.

Marco Altini holds a PhD and two MScs, including one in human movement sciences and high-performance coaching. He has published more than 50 papers and patents at the intersection between technology and human performance, and is the co-founder of HRV4Training.

distressful workouts. Unfortunately, some riders are inclined to frequently make it a common part of their training, thinking it will make them "faster" or "tougher." It won't. You'll only become more fatigued. This degree of distress must be rare so that you avoid injury, a weakened immune system, and overtraining. Weariness following a hard ride is to be expected. That's an early stage of eustress. But if you are frequently exhausted from having pushed beyond your limits then it is distress, and not beneficial to your purpose in training. Tiredness after a hard workout should usually be fleeting—totally gone within two days at most, and usually less than that. Twenty-four hours later you should feel recovered. That's eustress and it means you will adapt and become more fit. To experience frequent distressful fatigue sets you up for one of the worst experiences of an athlete—overtraining syndrome. Overtraining is one side of a two-headed coin. On the other side is "under-recovering." That isn't as well understood by most athletes. So, let's start there.

UNDER-RECOVERING

Although among the slowest animals on the planet, humans are some of the very best when it comes to endurance. Our Stone Age ancestors survived in a very challenging world because they could chase any animal until it became tired and they could thereby feed the tribe. We've inherited that quality. We're designed to ride bikes long distances and at easy to high intensities.

Then there's the bicycle. What a gift to humanity! It's the most efficient transportation machine ever invented. Put these two together—great endurance and a highly efficient machine—and we have the modern-day cyclist. But with everything in our favor we still experience temporary setbacks. We call it "fatigue." Without that we'd be like Superman—faster than a speeding bullet. Fatigue is our Kryptonite. And that's a good thing. Occasional weariness is a healthy product of well-managed training. It keeps you from doing too much and sets you up for improved performance once recovered.

Training, as mentioned earlier in the book, is a combination of workouts and lifestyle. Both play a role in how your body relates to the stress you are experiencing throughout the day, whether it is from a hard workout or a stressful ("distressful") lifestyle. A stressful lifestyle could be the result of a hard day at work, a pressing problem that must be dealt with, inadequate sleep, an argument with your partner, or a sore throat. They're all stressful and your capacity for training is reduced because of them. Each is just a different kind of stress, but the result is the same: you're fatigued and unable to work out at your normal levels of duration and intensity. You need to honor that fatigue and not try to train through it. There's nothing to be gained from that.

That reduction in your physical capacity for working out is often referred to as "overtraining"—doing too many hard workouts. But that may not be right. You may *not* have trained too much. Instead, it could be a result of under-recovering since both come from the same two sources—working out and lifestyle. Do you overtrain or under-recover? When I take up this dilemma with an athlete it's often a mix of the two. It's common to do more in a workout than you should. I see that a lot. You push yourself to the limit by increasing the volume or the intensity—or both—just a little too much and too often. You may do hard workouts on subsequent days. Then you follow that with limited R&R on top of a stressful job, too little sleep, and more to do than you can handle. You overtrained a little but under-recovered a lot. Your goal is in jeopardy.

As mentioned in Chapter 2, something I look for in an athlete to reduce the chances of an overtraining breakdown is how much sleep they get. I've found that the more commitments in an athlete's daily life, the less sleep they get, and consequently the lower their workout quality is. Fitness suffers. As mentioned in that chapter, I've told many a prospective athlete-client that for me to coach them they must get more sleep, which means reducing their obligations. If they have a very challenging goal, I tell them they can have only three responsibilities—family, career, and training. Nothing else. If they are unwilling to accept this then we go our separate ways. That may sound mean, but trying to produce a high-performance race with an athlete who is dragging an anchor is pointless. Why do some refuse to cut back? Interestingly, there are folks who actually look forward to and thrive on stress, and feel less important if they don't experience it constantly. That's not a healthy lifestyle and one that is likely to not only diminish performance but also to reduce health and shorten lifespan.

Why do I make such a big deal about limiting stress? As mentioned above, sleep is when fitness happens. Ultimately, inadequate sleep means poor performance. It's during sleep that the body releases anabolic (tissue-building) hormones, such as growth hormone, insulin-like growth factor, androstenedione, testosterone, and more. These hormones are responsible for the growth and repair of tissues throughout the body—the stuff that *makes* you more fit. These They are released in waves of roughly 90-minute durations throughout the night. If you cut your sleep short with an alarm clock, one or more of those waves may be missed and you won't reap the full benefits of the previous day's workout. For this reason, I'm not a big fan of alarm clocks. If you must be someplace early in the day, the solution is not an artificial and stressful awakening from deep sleep but rather going to bed earlier. If you can't do this then you have too much going on in your life.

OVERTRAINING

Many athletes don't realize how serious overtraining is. They seem to think it's normal and means you are simply tired. That is far from what the real problem is. Overtraining is *not* normal and much more serious than most athletes think. Wes's story at the start of this chapter illustrates this dilemma quite well. His season, and eventually his career, was cut short due to one winter of trying to train too hard and too often. He continually pushed himself beyond his limits. That resulted in a sad outcome for what was otherwise an outstanding career.

My point here is that we must keep your training very much on the side of eustress. And we will balance that with a lot of sleep and otherwise do what we can to enhance your post-workout recovery. This is crucial to successful training. We'll get into this topic in greater detail shortly.

Overtraining starts with overreaching, which is a normal result of focused training over several days or a couple of weeks. Overreaching is marked by tiredness. That weariness must be accepted and eventually relieved—sooner rather than later. You may have also noticed in Wes's story that he decided not to take an R&R break following what was a very difficult period of training. He was highly motivated to push himself as much as he could. He both overtrained—the workouts were too hard—and under-recovered—he didn't include any R&R. The result was catastrophic for his season and his career.

How do you know if you are overtraining or under-recovering? Since there are no sure biological indicators of this condition, there is nothing your doctor can test to see if you are truly overtrained. To make it even more of a challenge, there are other conditions that have nearly the same symptoms as overtraining, such as Lyme disease from a tick bite and chronic fatigue syndrome. While your doctor may not be able to diagnose overtraining, it is a good idea to be checked when you have the symptoms of overtraining (unfortunately, chronic fatigue syndrome is also difficult to diagnose). How do you know if you are overtraining or under-recovering? Either or both provide the same signs. Overtraining may be accompanied by a few of the following symptoms, but not all, and the first two in the list below are the most common:

- Unrelenting fatigue.
- Reduced performance in training.
- Moody, grumpy, and emotional.
- Depression.
- High perceived exertion for a common power output.
- Low motivation.
- Colds, flu, and allergies.
- No improvement with a short recovery.
- Low heart rate variability.
- Elevated resting heart rate.
- Unusual changes in appetite.
- Restless sleep, insomnia.
- Menstrual cycle dysfunction.

Of course, fatigue, the single best indicator, is to be expected following very long or highly intense

Overtraining is the product of distress and is commonly tied to excessive workouts—too often, too long, too intense, or all three.

workouts or races, and it's usually accompanied by a sense of "heavy" legs and low motivation for the rest of the day following such a ride. However, if it lingers and refuses to go away despite backing off from training for a few days, then the chances of overtraining are quite high, especially if you've been riding more than usual or not recovering often enough. Of course, it doesn't come on suddenly. It sneaks up on you. A long streak of hard workouts with limited R&R is the culprit. As with Wes, the only cure in such a situation is a prolonged break from training. How long is difficult to say as it depends on how advanced the condition is. You may take a week off and find that you are still experiencing the symptoms. Or it may go away quickly if you caught it early enough. Most riders don't.

The bottom line is that this situation is best avoided by training conservatively and emphasizing regular R&R. This is why I highly recommend a "5+2" training routine when high-intensity training starts (see Chapter 4). If you make a mistake, make it on the side of doing too little hard riding and a little too much easy riding. If you do this your cycling career will be long and rewarding.

UNDERTRAINING

Let's look at the opposite of overtraining. What happens if, for some reason, you take a significant amount of time away from training by reducing your weekly workouts from six to three rides for a few weeks? Here's what the research suggests you might experience from two to four weeks of "detraining."

First, you could expect a loss of fitness of around 10 percent at most, which isn't as bad as it may at first seem. Such undertraining is a reversal of the markers of your aerobic endurance. A reduction in your heart's left ventricle stroke volume would be accompanied by an increased heart rate, the capillary beds in your muscles would become less dense, there would be a reduction of blood volume, fuel for movement would come more from carbohydrate and less from fat—and the list of problems would continue. These changes occur within two to four weeks of greatly reduced training. If your detraining continues beyond four weeks there is a further reduction of performance due largely to a decreased aerobic capacity and lowered lactate thresholds (LT1 and LT2 in Table 3.1). But the good news is that at this stage you are still more aerobically fit than your sedentary next-door neighbor.

If your reduced bike time was due to a temporary setback, such as foul weather for riding, cross-training is a solution. By running, hiking, walking, Nordic skiing, snowshoeing, rowing, or doing any common aerobic activity, the losses are likely to remain rather small. The take-home here is that any aerobic endurance exercise can maintain a fairly high level of aerobic fitness in the absence of riding. That's one of the reasons why I suggest cross-training during the Preparation and Base 1 periods when weather is most likely to be a problem and training can be quite general. Illness as a cause of missed workouts is an altogether different animal. I'll address that in Chapter 8.

KEY TAKEAWAYS

- Stress can be either detrimental (distress) or beneficial (eustress).
- Beneficial stress primarily comes from widely spacing hard rides and separating them with easy ones to allow for recovery while seldom pushing yourself to the limit.
- Overtraining is the product of distress and is commonly tied to excessive workouts—too often, too long, too intense, or all three.
- Instead of overtraining, a distressed athlete may be under-recovering with inadequate R&R.
- Insufficient sleep combined with excessive exercise is a likely contributor to overtraining.
- It's during sleep that the body becomes more fit due to waves of anabolic hormones throughout slumber.
- Your tiredness is normal and to be expected with focused training, but when pushed to deep fatigue can become overtraining.
- There is no sure medical test for diagnosing overtraining, but the many symptoms always include extreme fatigue.
- When experiencing overtraining, a couple of days of rest is not enough to remedy the fatigue and other symptoms—you will likely need weeks.
- Volume and intensity must be cautiously blended into your training plan as large increases over what you have done recently are problematic.
- With a significantly reduced training load for two to four weeks you could expect a loss of fitness of around 10 percent.
- If you aerobically cross-train during extended periods of off-bike time you can maintain much of your endurance cycling fitness.

REST AND RECOVERY

Once you understand the dire consequences of overtraining and under-recovering, the need for frequent R&R breaks in which you can shed accumulated fatigue is obvious. During these R&R breaks your body and mind rebound, allowing you to return to challenging workouts. Without such breaks from serious training, you would soon become a zombie pedaling a bike without purpose or benefit. Such breaks from serious training typically require three to five days of greatly reduced workout durations and intensities. Young athletes who have a great capacity for training loads will often get by with only three or four days away from their normal routines. Older riders are likely to need longer R&R breaks in their training plan. What are "young" and "older" riders? That's difficult to nail down. I've known of riders in their 30s who usually needed long breaks and some 50 or older who could get by quite well on short R&R periods. Age is just a quick, but not always accurate, way of categorizing the R&R needs of riders.

For most riders in the Preparation and Base 1 periods the need for R&R is quite low, if needed at all. But for the Base 2 and 3 and the Build periods it is imperative as the stress load increases. If you can't get through these first two periods of the season without an R&R break, then you are already training much too hard. The first two periods of the season are meant to be very easy, except for weightlifting. The focus is primarily on aerobic endurance and low-intensity workouts. As the volume of training goes up in the late Base and intensity increases in the Build period, the need for R&R rises considerably. This is when you *must* take frequent breaks or risk deep fatigue and possibly overtraining.

I keep using the words "rest" and "recovery." What's the difference between the terms? In the context of this book, rest means a day off from riding. Recovery, on the other hand, means greatly reduced workouts—short durations and low intensities. A period of three to five R&R days is meant to mostly shed your fatigue, and have you physically and mentally ready for the long, serious training period ahead. What does "long" mean? Again, it depends on who we are talking about. A young rider (same definition as above) is likely to train in four-week blocks with *three* weeks of a moderate to high training load and a few days of R&R followed by testing. An older rider may instead do *two* weeks of high-load training followed by an R&R break and then testing. But, again, there are exceptions.

The specifics of R&R—when and how long—are hard to define. It comes down to who we are talking about and what their unique needs are when it comes to R&R. How should you include R&R breaks in your training? There are two common ways to resolve this dilemma—*planned recovery* and *recovery on demand*. Each has its benefits and shortcomings.

PLANNED RECOVERY

The most common way for self-coached riders to recharge during Base 2, Base 3, and the Build periods is to pre-plan their R&R breaks from challenging training weeks by scheduling them in a training calendar. This is the easy way to do it. And it works well, although there is certainly the possibility for error. The biggest mistake is working too hard in the preceding two or three weeks and accumulating significant fatigue long before getting to your planned R&R week. But even then, the likelihood of overtraining is greatly diminished since a few days of much reduced work will soon follow.

Determining when the R&R weeks should occur in your training plan is based on how quickly you usually recover after two or three weeks of serious training. If you commonly experience fatigue and find it hard to shed, it's wise to include a training break every third week. That means two weeks of high-training load followed by a week of rest, recovery, and testing. If you are somewhat resistant to fatigue (or your training load is reduced) then an R&R week would probably be best after three weeks of training. However, that is often hard to judge as many self-coached riders are not fully aware of what borderline excessive fatigue feels like. And, unfortunately, many would deny it's even occurring although it may be obvious to a coach, the rider's spouse, or even training partners. Many serious riders disregard feelings that suggest an R&R break is needed, so what should you do about this?

An easy way to resolve this dilemma, which I've used with athletes when just starting to coach them, is to base the decision on age and experience. In this method riders aged 50 and older are assumed to need a break from training sooner—every third week—than those under age 50 who will take a training-load break every fourth week. The exception is for inexperienced riders under the age of 50. They are encouraged to recover every third week for the first two or three years in the sport. Note that for those following the shorter three-week training periods, the number of periods in Base and Build will change. They will do four Base periods of three weeks each and three Build periods of three weeks each. This means they will have an additional Base period (Base 4) and Build period (Build 3). As a result, older riders (or those who recover slowly) do one more week in the Build period (nine weeks instead of eight). The Base period remains at 12 weeks for both. Tables 6.1 and 6.2 illustrate what a period of training might look like for both three- and four-week training blocks in the Build 1 period.

Table 6.1. A suggested four-week training period for a "young," or quick-to-recover, rider in the Build 1 period*

Monday	Tuesday	Wednesday	Thursday	Friday	Saturday	Sunday
Gym session	Easy ride	Your limiter	Very easy ride	Easy ride	Easy ride	Your limiter
Gym session	Easy ride	Your limiter	Very easy ride	Easy ride	Easy ride	Your limiter
Gym session	Easy ride	Your limiter	Very easy ride	Easy ride	Easy ride	Your limiter
Gym session	Short, very easy ride or day off*	Short, very easy ride or day off*	Short, very easy ride or day off*	Easy ride	Test Sprint Power or Test Aerobic Capacity	Test FTP/FTHR

* Note that the *fourth* week is for rest and recovery. Take only one additional day off the bike in the R&R week on Tuesday, Wednesday, or Thursday.

Table 6.2 A suggested three-week training period for an "older" or novice rider in the Build 1 period

Monday	Tuesday	Wednesday	Thursday	Friday	Saturday	Sunday
Gym session	Easy ride	Your limiter	Very easy ride	Easy ride	Easy ride	Your limiter
Gym session	Easy ride	Your limiter	Very easy ride	Easy ride	Easy ride	Your limiter
Gym session	Short, very easy ride or day off*	Short, very easy ride or day off*	Short, very easy ride or day off*	Short, very easy ride or day off*	Test Sprint Power or Test Aerobic Capacity	Test FTP/FTHR

* Note that the *third* week is for rest and recovery. Take only one additional day off the bike in the R&R week on Tuesday, Wednesday, Thursday, or Friday.

RECOVERY ON DEMAND

The alternative to pre-planned R&R periods is "recovery on demand." This is potentially the more effective of the two options, since assuming that R&R is needed on a fixed schedule may not be realistic. There will be times when a planned recovery period every third or fourth week is either too soon or not soon enough. The degree of fatigue you may experience in a training block is very hard to predict. There will likely be times when you come to a planned R&R break and realize you aren't in need of recovery. There will be other times when you are physically and mentally wasted several days before your scheduled break. Recovery on demand solves this problem, but it's not perfect either. I'll describe what this method entails and then circle back to explain the downside of recovery on demand.

On the surface, recovery on demand looks like the picture-perfect way of taking R&R breaks from high-load training. When you have accumulated enough fatigue, you rest and when freshened, you return to demanding training. I wish it was always that simple. You must pay close attention to how you feel daily, and when the time is right ("on demand") you take a few days of much-needed R&R, test, and then return to normal training again. The periods will be rather fluid, and, in fact, calling them by the common names, such as "Base 3," doesn't make much sense. While there will still be Base, Build, Peak, and Race training, it becomes much more tailored to your exact needs. So, recovery on demand is sometimes "periodization on demand." Train for frequency, duration, and intensity when you sense it's time to do so. If you are self-coached you've got to do a very good job of self-assessment, or things will fall apart badly, and a professional coach will *probably* do a better job of managing your training under such conditions.

Assuming you are self-coached, though, how do you decide when it's time to recover? That's the tricky part. That decision is based on how you rate your current level of readiness to train. Some riders are very good at determining this and others are terrible. You've got to pay very close attention to how you are responding to the current training load, and when it's time for a break you must be willing to back off. Overleaf are some typical indicators that you need an R&R break:

- If tired and leg-weary on the second recovery day after a hard workout, it *may* be time for an R&R break.
- If your efficiency factor (EF) goes down for two back-to-back daily aerobic endurance workouts, it *may* be time for R&R.
- If you are unmotivated to ride two days in a row and must force yourself out of the door, it *may* be time for R&R.
- If you've been training steadily for three weeks or more, it's time for R&R regardless of how good you may feel (a serious downturn is likely just around the corner).
- If your heart rate variability is outside your normal range for two days in a row it *may* be time for R&R.
- If you are unsure if recovery is needed or not, it's time for R&R.

Are these perfect predictors of when you need recovery? No. Most are based on a very prejudicial foundation: your opinion. Many serious riders must be on their death beds before they decide it's time to back off for a few days. That's because most of the above indicators are highly subjective. Only a couple of them are objective. One of these refers to three consecutive weeks of serious training. If that's in the late Base or Build periods I'd strongly suggest you need to take a break regardless of how you feel. Another is if you are debating in your head whether you need a break. Solve the problem by automatically backing off when faced with this conundrum. Whenever you are unsure if you should rest or not, just do it—take a few days away from hard training.

A third objective marker of stress from the above list is heart rate variability, which is an important indicator of how your body is responding to training. But first, a little background on HRV. While HRV was discovered in the 19th century, it wasn't accurately measured until the 1960s. While it's been around for several decades, we are still learning how to effectively use it, especially in sport. What is heart rate variability? It's a measure of the time between heartbeats. They are not steady, and they fluctuate slightly based, to some degree, on your stress status. When variability is low (the times between beats are closer to an even spacing) and within your normal baseline range, it indicates that your sympathetic nervous system is dominant. This system may be thought of as a "fight or flight" response to life. You may be somewhat distressed, perhaps because of recent lifestyle problems or accumulated training fatigue or the early onset of illness. You may not even be aware of this slight sense of distress as HRV is quite sensitive. When HRV is low, your physiological capacity for responding to training is also quite low. To force yourself to ride hard is mostly a waste of time, or worse. You may be on the road to extreme fatigue. This may be a good day for a recovery ride or day off.

When heart rate variability is high (the times between beats vary widely) and above your normal baseline, your parasympathetic nervous system is prevailing. This branch of the autonomic nervous system is often referred to as "rest and digest." You're calm, and perhaps too much so to train well. HRV thus gives you an objective look into your physiological response to training and lifestyle stress.

To gauge HRV, all you need is an app on your phone to help you measure it every morning soon after waking up. If you search the internet, you'll find a few HRV apps. A morning measurement can help you decide if it's time for an R&R break. Please realize, however, that HRV is not a definite marker of your stress status. It's a good one, but it's not perfect. You still must consider several factors, such as those listed above, before deciding if you should take a break. It's just one more indicator of your stress and fatigue status.

Should you decide to use the recovery on demand method of determining an R&R week, you are likely to make mistakes due to the largely subjective indicators of the need for R&R. To be safe, if you make a mistake in the timing of an R&R week, make it on the conservative side—too much recovery. Resting when you don't need it is preferable to the opposite.

When you take an R&R break from training using the recovery-on-demand method, you must also decide when it's time to return to a normal and elevated training load. The following training readiness indicators can help you make that decision. After three days of reduced training in an R&R week, grade your recovery status using the following points. All the indicators you use must be answered "Yes" before returning to your normal training routine. If they aren't, take another day of R&R and then again check your readiness indicators.

- I feel rested and ready to train again.
- My HRV is in the normal baseline range.
- My waking heart rate is in my normal range.
- I have no muscle soreness or fatigue-like feelings.
- My appetite is normal.
- I feel happy, not moody.
- I am healthy.
- My lifestyle stress is low.
- I was not traveling yesterday.
- I am motivated to train today.
- I trained easily yesterday or took a day off.

KEY TAKEAWAYS

- You can probably recover sufficiently in the three to five days of an R&R week, depending on how stressful the prior training was and your lifestyle.
- You shouldn't need R&R periods in the Preparation and Base 1 periods as the training is quite easy, except for weightlifting.
- The most common way to include R&R in your training is by pre-planning it.
- The downside of pre-planning an R&R week is that you may experience fatigue well before the scheduled break.
- Pre-planned R&R breaks from training are usually scheduled after two or three weeks of serious training.
- A simple solution as to when to take an R&R break can be predicted by your age and level of experience.
- To determine pre-planned training breaks, decide how quickly you typically fatigue due to training load and how long it takes to refresh.
- Recovery on demand is theoretically a better way to take an R&R break from training.
- The downside of recovery on demand is that you must decide if it's time for an R&R break from training.
- Use heart rate variability to help you make R&R decisions—but realize that it is only a strong suggestion.
- Determine when it is time to return to a normal training routine after R&R by gauging your recovery status using self-perception guidelines.

DAY-TO-DAY RECOVERY

What about day-to-day recovery in weeks that aren't designated for R&R? This is when you are most likely to become overly fatigued. How do we prevent that? The simple answer is that your easy days should be easy so that your hard days can truly be hard. I realize that this is not very helpful when making daily decisions, though, so let's dig a little deeper.

HARD AND EASY DAYS

You may remember a table of training intensities from Chapter 3 (see Table 3.1), and in that table there were seven training zones: 1, 2, 3, 4, 5a, 5b, and 5c. Each of these zones had a corresponding description. Zones 1 and 2 were different degrees of "easy" and zones 3, 4, 5a, and 5b were variations on "hard." Zone 5c was "max effort" for very short periods of time. It's important that you understand this so that when the plan calls for an "easy" day, the workout is in zones 1 or 2. When it's a hard ride, it's zones 3, 4, or 5. That's what I mean by "easy days are easy" and "hard days are hard." Table 6.3 is a week in the Build period which illustrates this easy-hard planning method.

I explained the 5+2 weekly routine in Chapter 4 and I strongly suggest you follow it in the Build and Peak periods. You may recall that this means five easy days (including a day off the bike) and two hard ride days, just as you see in Table 6.3. My purpose in laying out the week like this is to make sure you come into a hard day rested and ready to go. That means the workout will be hard (zones 3, 4, or 5) and you'll become more fit because of it. To the contrary, a 4+3 routine in the Base periods with four easy and three hard days means that for two out of the three hard rides you are likely to be a bit tired from a hard ride just 48 hours prior. You're much better off doing two hard rides each week when recovered in 5+2 and ready to go than one workout that's fresh and two a bit tired in a 4+3 routine. Training while fatigued does not make you fitter or more mentally tough. It's simply wasted time—or worse.

I've also found that riders who follow the 5+2 pattern train more regularly than those who use a 4+3 plan, especially in the Build period when post-ride recovery is so important. I think the reason for this has to do with the excess accumulation of mental and physical fatigue over a few weeks, with each week having three hard rides. The accumulated fatigue negatively impacts performance. The 4+3 athletes also seem to frequently find reasons why they can't ride one day each week. That's because they are pushed to their limits too often. You may recall from Chapter 1 that consistent training is the key

Table 6.3. A typical weekly training plan for a Build period showing easy and hard ride days following a 5+2 routine

Monday	Tuesday	Wednesday	Thursday	Friday	Saturday	Sunday
Gym	Easy ride	Hard ride	Easy Ride	Easy ride	Easy ride	Hard ride

to successful racing. In the Build periods, 5+2 is the better routine. The reason for the 4+3 in Base is that your three most challenging days then are long rides and not high intensity, but rather more moderately high intensity.

I also want to emphasize the importance of a day off the bike (Monday in Table 6.3). While I suggest a strength maintenance (SM) gym session that day, it's very brief. And, of course, you could always move the gym session to another day, such as Thursday, post-ride, if you wanted a day completely off on Monday. Having a day off the bike gives you the option of having other things in your life besides sitting on a saddle and pedaling. This helps to offset the drudgery and boredom of training and is good for your mental health.

Speaking of boredom, your easy days should be somewhat boring. You simply ride, preferably on a flat course, steady and easy in zones 1 and 2. But interestingly, this is when most of your aerobic fitness is built, resulting in better race performances. I know it must seem contradictory to say that riding slowly will help you to race fast, but it does. Once you start training 5+2 you'll come to understand that.

The five somewhat boring days each week are offset by two hard rides for which you should be fresh and ready to go. That means they can indeed be hard. In fact, they may prove so hard that you go into them with a bit of dread. Your typical hard rides are in the categories of steady stamina rides, aerobic capacity intervals, sprint power repeats, fast group rides, and B and C races (see Appendix for workout details).

RECOVERY AND ADAPTATION

How can you decrease your recovery time following hard rides? The time between them is usually two or three days of easy riding in a Build period, 5+2 routine. That should be enough to allow for recovery, meaning you feel fresh and ready to go again on the third or fourth day. The greater question, perhaps, is *should* you try to accelerate your post-workout recovery after a hard ride? The argument against this is that recovery and adaptation are not the same thing. Recovery means you feel refreshed. Adaptation means the body is becoming more physically fit. Feeling ready to go hard again when the body is not yet fully adapted from a previous workout can cause you to make questionable decisions about training, such as inserting a third hard ride into your weekly plan in the Build period. That is how overtraining gets started, as Wes's story illustrates so well. Does this mean you shouldn't try to speed up your recovery? I see no downside to doing that so long as you don't decide to add another race-like ride to your week because you're feeling ready to go.

Adaptation is far more important than recovery, but recovery is not unimportant. It's a stage on the way to adaptation. When you feel recovered after a day of reduced training load, that's a good sign. But realize that your body may still be adapting and is not fully ready to go hard again. That's why I strongly suggest that you train with a polarized (5+2) routine in the Build period. That way, I know you'll go into the two weekly hard rides ready to go every week and avoid overtraining. And those rides will be truly hard, thus improving your race readiness.

Following a hard workout, adaptation needs three recovery modalities to occur quite quickly—sleeping, eating, and rehydrating. Anything else you do to speed recovery has only a relatively minor impact on your fitness, or none at all. The benefits of speeding recovery are mostly psychological rather than physiological. But that's not a bad thing. Being mentally refreshed and feeling ready to go, although you may not be physically so, is a good thing. Feeling tired, sore, and achy is simply not good for your training no matter what the next workout calls for. So, feel free to use whatever recovery tools you have available and like to use to relieve your feelings of fatigue. Sometimes this is all that's necessary to improve your sense of mental well-being. The most common recovery tools that have been shown by research to generally be safe are as follows. Some of these may be more effective for you than others:

- Cold-water immersion has long been accepted as beneficial for reducing inflammation short term, as in recovery between racing stages on the same day. But recent research has found that in the longer term, over several days, ice-cold water inhibits muscular adaptation. Alternating hot and cold-water immersion may prove more beneficial.
- Compression boots have not been found to have any direct physiological benefits, but many athletes feel more recovered when using them. There's no apparent downside to doing this.

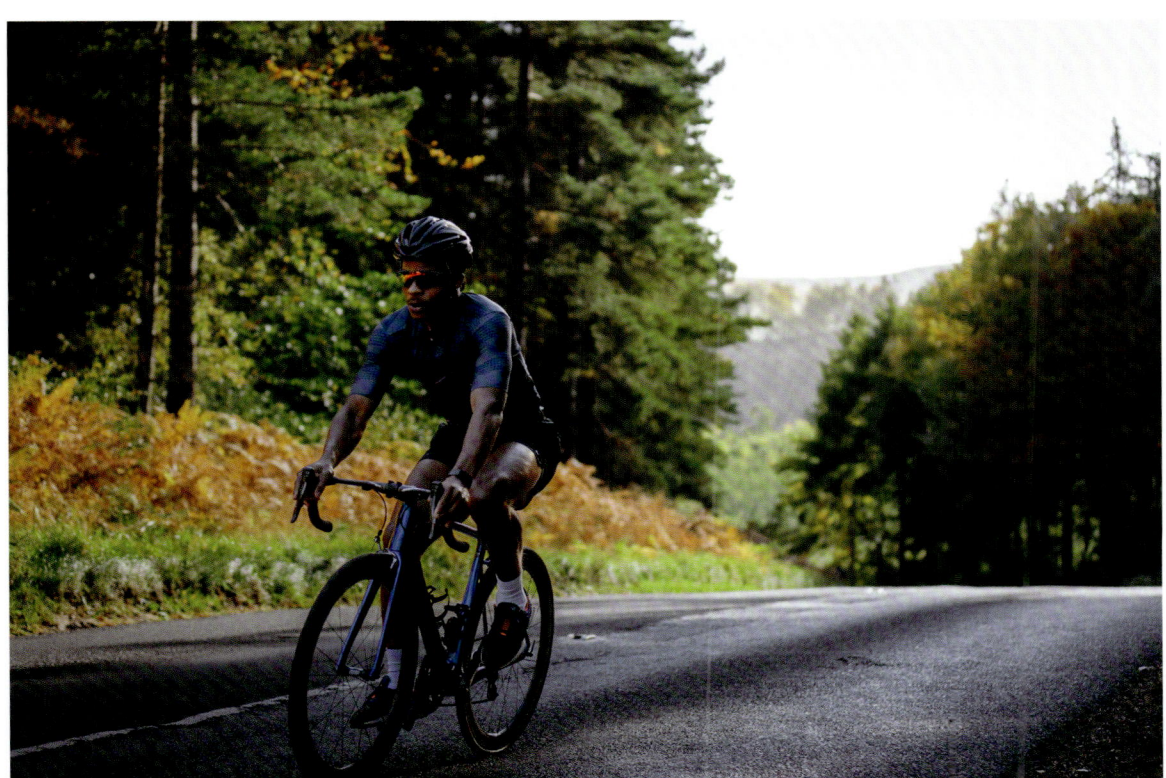

- Active recovery, such as going for a walk or swim, after a hard ride may relieve your sensations of fatigue. Running is less likely to be beneficial and may even be harmful. But be very conservative in how much additional exercise, even though it may be quite easy, that you put on your body after a hard ride.
- Gentle stretching, especially of the legs and lower back muscles, may reduce the feelings of stiffness or soreness.
- Massage is perhaps the most used recovery method in the pro ranks of cycling. The benefits appear to be mostly psychological, but that's okay.
- Foam rollers are commonly used by endurance athletes to relieve the sensations of leg and torso muscle tightness.
- Percussion devices (handheld devices that massage using rapid, repetitive pressure pulses) don't present any known downsides unless the user is overly aggressive.

The bottom line is that you can use almost any recovery tool you like so long as it doesn't interfere with sleep, nutrition, or fluid intake. If any one of these, for some reason, gets in the way of the three biggest contributors to adaptation, then it is detrimental to your performance.

Sleep is hands down the best recovery and adaptation modality available to you, as I explained in Chapter 2 and earlier in this chapter. I will cover nutrition and hydration in greater detail in Chapter 8, but the bottom line for enhancing recovery and adaptation is that what and how much you eat and drink has a lot to do with your daily training load. Your intake of food, and the types of food you eat, should reflect your training for that day. High-intensity and high-duration days require significant caloric intake to meet the demands of the workout. And, conversely, on days off, or when riding short and easy, you don't need as many calories.

As for hydration, drink to satisfy thirst. Your first choice should always be plain water. But there are times when calorically rich fluids and gels may be taken in, the most common being during long, intense rides and races. Short, easy rides require nothing more than water. Sports drinks may also be beneficial following a hard workout, but only in the immediate post-ride recovery time. Otherwise, sports drinks are best avoided. We'll take a closer look at the details of sports drinks and related products in Chapter 8.

When you eat is just as important as what you eat when it comes to recovery and adaptation. On hard ride days taking in carbohydrates immediately afterward is preferable to delaying intake. We're all used to the concept of day-to-day variations in workout types—a hard ride one day and an easy one the next. Following a highly intense ride, as you commonly do in the Build period, carbohydrate intake post-ride *may* be necessary for both recovery and

Recovery means you feel refreshed. Adaptation means the body is becoming more physically fit.

adaptation. But after a long, easy ride in the Base period, for example, the need for carbs after the ride is greatly reduced, assuming you rode as suggested in zones 1 or 2.

You may even take the opportunity to enhance your fat-burning by not eating any carbohydrates the morning of a long, easy ride, thus increasing your fat metabolism during the workout and after. Some riders even extend their carb avoidance after such a ride for a couple of additional hours, thus further enhancing their fat burning. That can be a good thing, but you need to be cautious with this nutritional restriction. If done too frequently you may overly stress your body, leading to excessive overreaching and perhaps eventually to overtraining, but in this situation, it would be due to under-recovering. This carb-restriction protocol done once-weekly in the Base period is probably sufficient to achieve the goal of improving your fat burning without risking a breakdown. But realize that the greatest volume of using fat for fuel is riding in zones 1 and 2. Restricting carb intake before and after a long, easy ride is just the icing on the cake.

PERFORMANCE MANAGEMENT CHART

If you use the TrainingPeaks app to record and analyze your workouts, you have a tool available to you that monitors your stress and rest relationships daily. It's called the Performance Management Chart and suggests the changes in your fitness, fatigue, and form throughout the season. This chart is based strictly on the data you upload every day from your power meter. To ensure the chart's accuracy your functional threshold power must be correct and up to date (see Appendix under Field Tests). That means testing every few weeks, as suggested in Table 5.6.

What I want to focus on in this chart is "form," which the app calls training stress balance (TSB). Form is simply another word for "freshness." Basically, this has to do with race readiness, and that's a reflection of how well rested you are. On your TrainingPeaks chart, as the yellow TSB line falls it means you are losing form, and becoming less fresh. As it rises you are becoming more fresh, and therefore more race-ready.

On the right side of the chart is the yellow TSB legend. Notice that there's a "0" (zero) in that legend about in the middle of the right side. That's the balance point for TSB. Above that is positive TSB/form ("fresh") and below it is negative TSB/form ("not fresh"). The more positive (the higher above 0), the fresher you are. The more negative (dropping below 0), the more tired you are. What we are concerned about on this chart is your TSB when it begins to fall below "0," meaning you are becoming tired. That's usually okay and, in fact, expected to happen when you are training seriously. The problem you need to be aware of is when your

TSB falls below -30 (minus 30). I call -30 and below "high risk" because if you spend much time here you will create great fatigue and are flirting with extreme overreaching that would likely become overtraining if continued for too long. This is the time to be cautious and to reduce the training load so that you exit this red zone quickly. How quickly you need to react depends on your unique capacity for training stress. It's usually best to stay there no more than two to three days at a time. You may only get into this zone two to four times in a season with, hopefully, an R&R break from training coming soon after.

The PMC is a great tool for monitoring your stress and rest status. But again, realize that your FTP must be accurate for the chart to have relevance to your status.

KEY TAKEAWAYS

- It takes a long time and a lot of focused training to become fast on a bike.
- Excessive fatigue starts with the attitude of "I can do anything I set my mind to."
- Many riders set a training load that is unsustainable and don't relent until they breakdown, which is too late.
- You must avoid excessive fatigue. At the first sign back off from high volume and intensity.
- The polarized (5+2) routine works well, in part, because you always come into a hard day of training recovered and ready to train hard.
- More important than adhering to "scientific training methods" is to learn to listen to your body and to act appropriately.
- A weekly day off from riding is good for mental and physical recovery.
- It's more important that your body adapts than it recovers quickly.
- Recovery, meaning a feeling of freshness, is an early stage on the road to physiological adaptation.
- The most important modalities for adaptation and recovery are, in their order of importance, sleep, nutrition, and fluids.
- It's during sleep that you become more fit.
- All other common recovery methods are trivial relative to sleep, nutrition, and fluids.
- Common recovery methods are likely more psychological than physiological, which is okay as mental recovery is also beneficial.
- How much and what you eat depends on what your workout is like on any given day.
- Occasionally doing long, easy morning rides without taking in carbohydrates before helps to boost fat metabolism.
- The TrainingPeaks Performance Management Chart is a good tool for managing your stress and rest status, but you must keep your FTP up to date.

THE REST OF WES'S STORY

The start of the next season after that Olympic year marked Wes's 10th anniversary since turning pro. There was little reason to celebrate, however, as the last three years had been quite a disappointment. He never fully recovered from the seven weeks of extreme overtraining a few years earlier. He was never the same athlete after that. And to make things even worse, the International Triathlon Union had made a significant change for the professional sport with draft-legal racing at about the same time, which they had no intention of changing. The combination was a double whammy for Wes's highly successful triathlon career.

After 10 years, Wes was in his 30s and recently married. Life was no longer about traveling the world and winning races. It was time to settle down and start a family. He left the sport he loved so passionately the year after the Olympics. He is now the father of two daughters and the owner of a real estate company in Boulder, Colorado, but still does occasional swims, rides, and runs for fun and fitness.

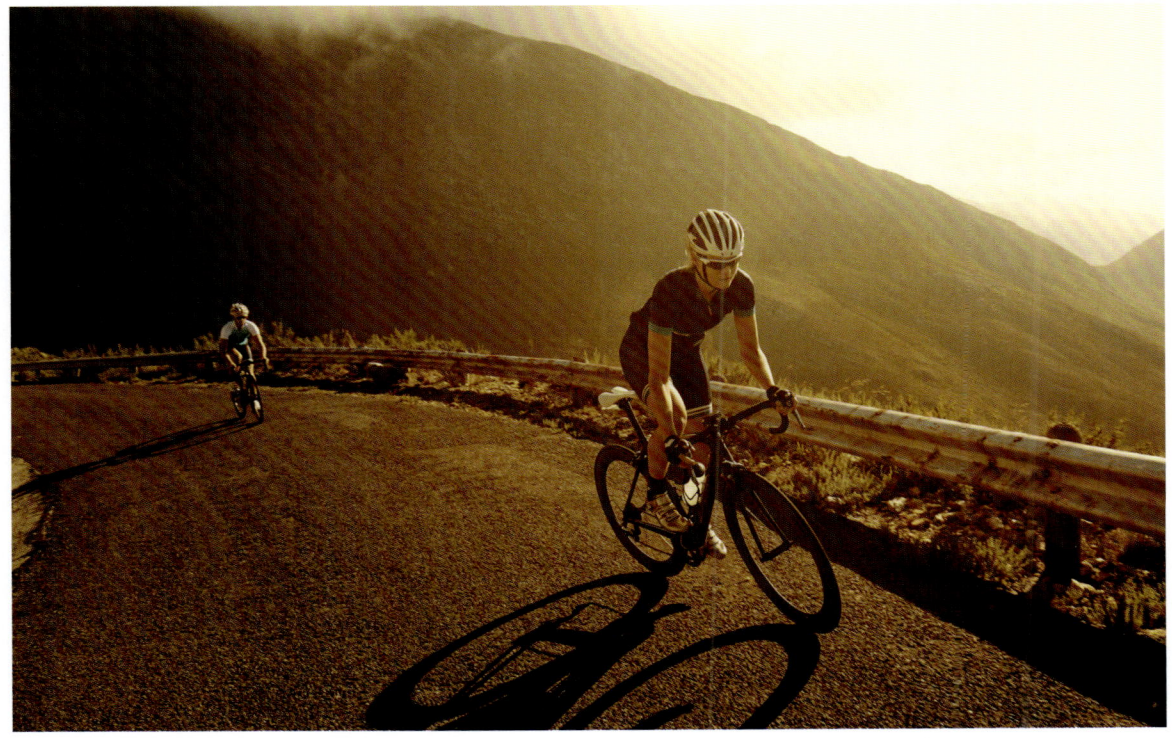

7. MINDSET

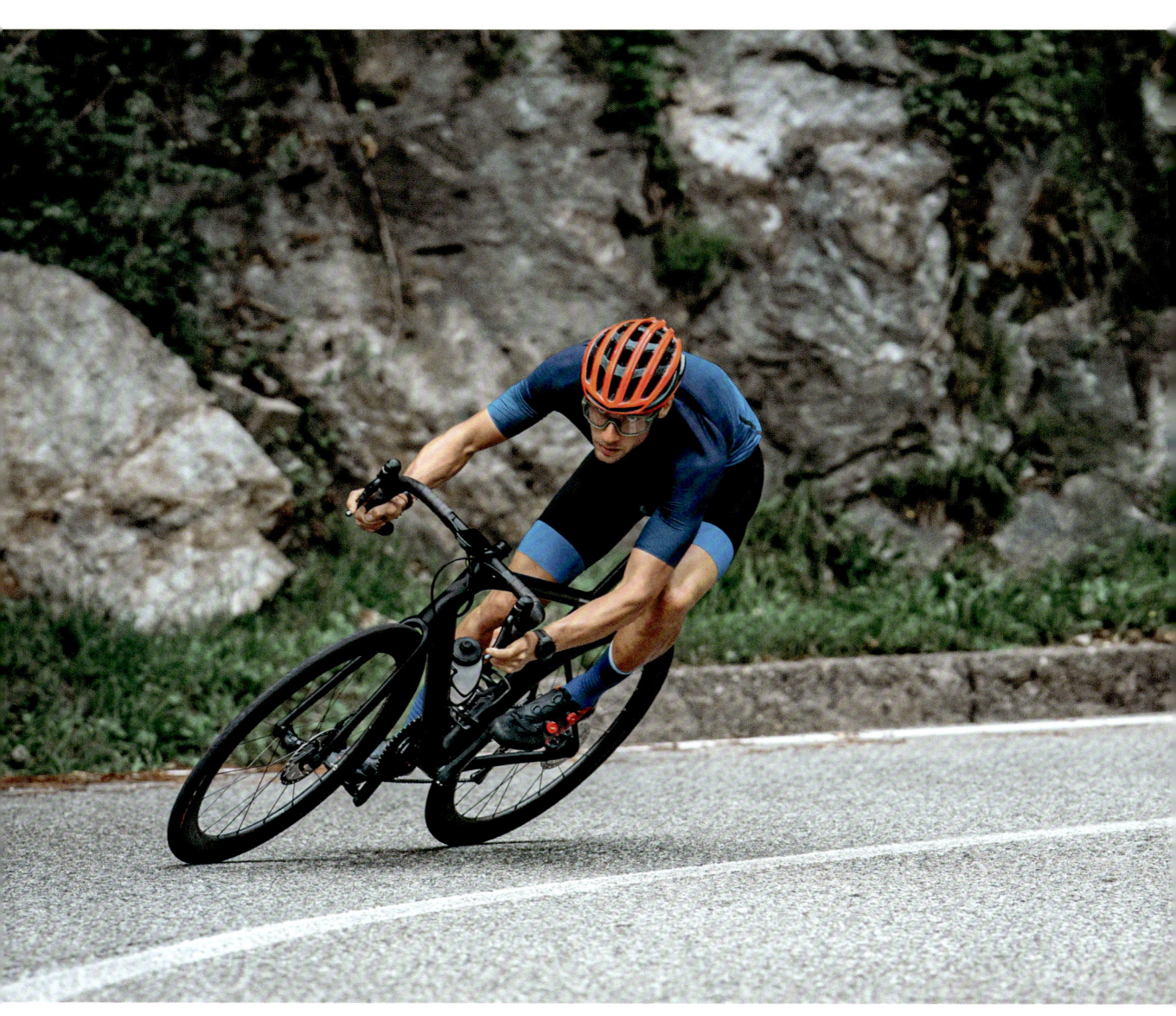

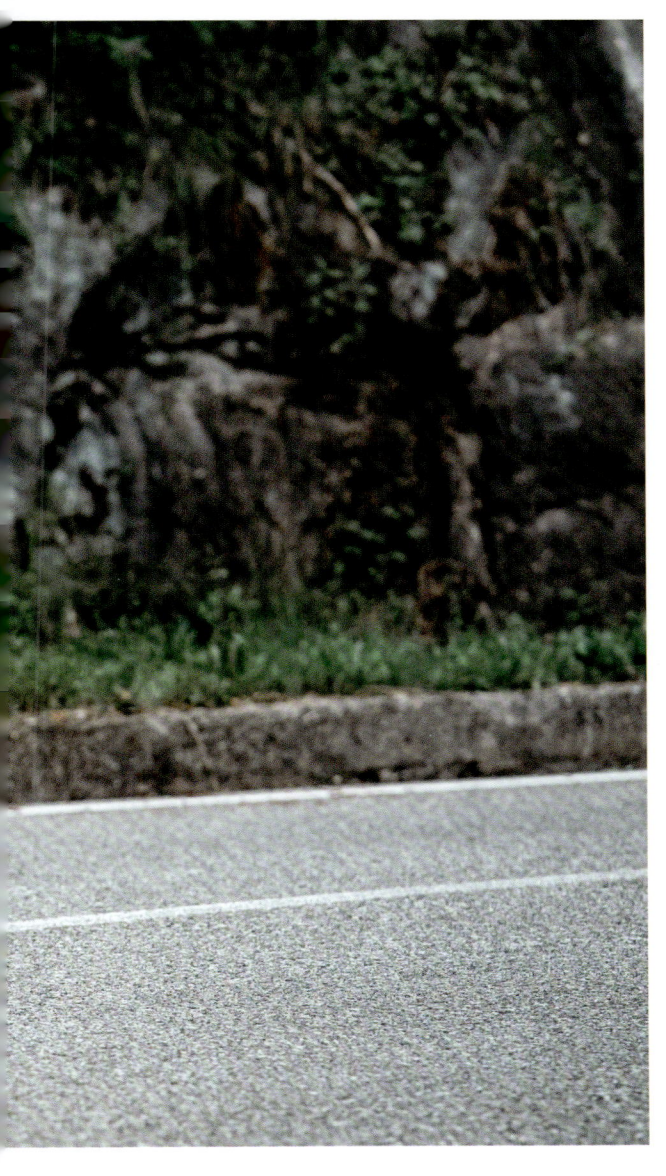

As you will see with Elizabeth's season, racing is not just grinding cranks and sweating. It also has a lot to do with what's going on in your head. Mindset, how you view and interact with the world around you, is critical to the success of the high-performance cyclist. With that in mind, let's get a big-picture view of where you are in terms of psychological readiness to train and race. Is there anything holding you back mentally? In previous chapters we looked at your physical readiness to perform. Now let's get an idea of where you are in terms of mental readiness to perform. We'll start with a simple self-assessment I use with my client-athletes.

ELIZABETH'S STORY

She called me in the early winter and introduced herself. As if I didn't know who she was. I followed women's cycling quite closely so the name was immediately recognizable. I also knew that she had done well in races.

Often a contender. Her real strength was the time trial. All of that came to me as soon as she said her name. What she wanted to talk about was coaching and asked if I would take her on for the coming season. Not only did I know who she was and how she performed, I also knew her coach quite well. He was respected in the cycling world, and I had a high regard for his coaching. He and I had a lot in common, including our training methodologies. What was popping into my head now was, "How could I be of help if her previous coach wasn't?" I'm sure I came across as a bit skeptical that I was the right coach for her. Nevertheless, I continued listening to what she had to say. My next question was, "Why me?" That started a long answer that took us back to how she got into the sport in the first place and evolved into the past season—with which she wasn't pleased.

Elizabeth came to road cycling quite late in life for a professional cyclist—her mid-20s. Before turning pro she lived and worked in New York City. She had always been active in a wide variety of sports, including soccer as a teenager, and had been on a bike a lot. As few New Yorkers did then, she rode a few miles to work every day. Her mother had read about the New York Cycle Club, a touring group, and suggested Elizabeth ride with them to meet people. Her first ride with the NYCC was an A ride—fast and aggressive. She was dropped and had no idea where she was. Not a great start. Her heavy commuter bike would have to go if she was to ride with them again. It did and she did. The club helped her grow as a rider and by the end of her first year she was one of the strongest riders in the group. In the coming winter she started riding with some mountain bikers. They also helped her to become a stronger rider.

She soon found herself inappropriately competing with the club's tour riders. So, with her rapidly improving skills and fitness, she decided to try racing with the local Century Road Club Association (CRCA), a competitive group. In the coming winter she also started riding with some male mountain bikers. All of this helped her grow even stronger as a rider. For the first year she raced in Central Park and in other local races with a CRCA team. She had gone from commuter to accomplished racer in a couple of years—not the traditional progression in cycling. This would eventually lead to her being picked up by a pro team. There are not many who move up in cycling that quickly.

As I do with all my athletes, I talked with Elizabeth by phone once every week, and something concerning began to stand out for me. She always pointed out that in her workouts she had not ridden to her expectations. And she was skeptical of her chances of racing well in the fast-approaching season. My impression was that her comments seemed fixated on faults. I soon got the impression that our challenge wasn't only race fitness. The best professional athletes I had coached were usually quite positive about their race expectations. I felt she needed a more positive approach to training and racing.

Once I came to this conclusion, I realized I needed help. I'm not a sport psychologist. I asked a friend for his professional thoughts. Gary was a client of mine at the time who had a broad background in psychology with a focus on counseling. He shared several ideas with me for how I could go about elevating Elizabeth's self-perceptions. Later in this chapter I will share with you some of his suggestions.

Much of our phone time that spring and summer had to do with Gary's ideas for boosting confidence in her training and potential for racing. That became a focus of our regular conversations. By our second year together I began to see some significant breakthroughs. We were now nearing the end of the season with the US National Time Trial Championship coming up. We began focusing solely on her race strength—the time trial. She had done well the previous year and I felt she had improved physically. I was more concerned with her self-perception.

As I always do, I spoke with Elizabeth the day before her National Championship race. We talked about the course, her bike setup, the weather, warm-up—all the usual stuff. I could tell she was nervous but there were no signs of lagging confidence. She seemed ready both physically and emotionally. That gave me good feelings about her podium chances. And again, as always, I asked her to call me after the race.

She did. And didn't even say hello. She started with, "I won!" I was thrilled. We had pulled it off! I started to congratulate her, until the next word out of her mouth made me stop. "But," she said with a short pause, "Mari took a wrong turn and finished second just 25 seconds behind me." Mari was considered the best time trialist in the country, having won Nationals a couple of times in her career. I could feel my heart sink. So close and yet so far.

I tried to reason with her that Mari could not have lost that much time as course marshals and spectators would have shouted about her mistake as soon as it happened. "Yes, she would have lost a few seconds but not 25," I said. And besides that, knowing the course is a part of racing. "She was second. You won," I told her. All to no avail. I had never heard a race winner be so upset.

The next A-priority race on the schedule was the UCI World Time Trial Championship in Spain that fall. We'd get another chance to prove her mettle. But when the US Cycling Federation announced the World's team, they left Elizabeth off the list. I was angry and called my contact at USCF. How could they not take the national time trial champ to Worlds? Apparently, others also thought it was a mistake and USCF soon announced that the team would instead be selected at a stage race, including a time trial, in Germany the week before Worlds. We now had an excellent chance.

As always, I talked with Elizabeth the day before that race with the usual topics. She told me she had reconned the course. It wasn't to her liking, she said. It wasn't just straight out and back. There were several corners, a few hills, a *steep descent on pavé with a tight lefthand turn at the bottom, and, to make matters worse, it was supposed to rain. It wasn't the course we would have liked. I could tell from her voice that she was upset. I tried to brighten her day by reminding her of all we had done in preparation to hone her race readiness. "Call me after the race," I said.*

She did. She started the conversation by telling me she crashed in the rain on the steep downhill at the lefthand turn. "That was it," she thought, "I wasn't going to Worlds." Then she told me how the mechanic in the team support car was there to get her back on the bike before she even stopped sliding. "I got back on, he gave me a push, and shouted something that got me charged up." I wanted to know the magic words the mechanic used to recharge her motivation. She couldn't remember. Long story made short: despite the crash she raced well enough to make the USA World Championship team.

Elizabeth went on to finish fifth in the time trial at UCI Worlds, the highest placing of any US woman that year in any cycling event. When she returned to NYC, we celebrated her successful season on the phone as best we could. And then I brought up the key question: "What about next year?" She said she was thinking about going after the hour record on the track. I commented that I had looked at the time for the US record only a few days ago and I was confident she could break it. "I'm not talking about the US record," she said, "I mean the world record." Wow! What a change. She had become one of the USA's top women riders.

CHALLENGE AND THREAT: ROB GRIFFITHS

"Every professional bike rider trains his legs, but very few train their minds, the only muscle they use to make decisions in races." (Mark Cavendish, *At Speed: My Life in The Fast Lane*, 2014)

Elizabeth's unexpected ascent into professional racing may have been a contributor to her mindset challenges, having not been afforded the typical developmental time of many years to prepare and build a well-rounded set of physical and mental skills.

That said, even multi-Olympic gold medallist, hour-record holder, and former Tour de France winner, Sir Bradley Wiggins, has recently been sharing his own psychological challenges with what's known as the "Imposter syndrome." In a UK-BBC documentary series (*Imposter Syndrome*, 2023), Wiggins described feeling a constant fear of being exposed as "not good enough," a fear of failure, and sometimes experiencing guilt about his success as he felt he was not worthy of it.

Developing a robust high-performance mindset is not only about being able to deliver consistently in the biggest of races, but also managing all the other inevitable life stresses and anxieties that come our way. From research we know that when taking on any task that we are motivated to do well in, like a race or a tough training session, we unconsciously appraise its potential demands. We consider things like distance, intensity, possible competition, and more. Then, again unconsciously, we match that against our perceived resources, such as current fitness levels, skills, experience, and more. We are in essence unconsciously asking ourselves, "Can I handle this situation?"

If we believe we have the resources to meet and exceed the demands being asked of us, we trigger several helpful physiological responses for our performance, such as increased cardiac output (heart rate), reduced total vascular resistance (blood pressure), and the release of hormones and neurotransmitters such as adrenaline, noradrenaline, and neuropeptide Y.

These responses prepare us for the competition. We might still feel nervous being washed with all that adrenaline, but we are approaching the event with a "challenge" mindset that supports performance. We are more likely to interpret our emotions positively as excitement for the upcoming event.

If, however, our appraisal of the event leads us to believe our current resources will not be enough, we can trigger a "threat" response. This raises different hormones, such as cortisol, induces smaller increases in cardiac output, and either provides no change or an increase in total peripheral vascular resistance. Such a physiological response makes it more likely that our emotions will feel debilitating, and we might feel unusually weak, distracted, and demotivated to the point of wanting to avoid the competition.

Psychologist Professor Marc Jones and his colleagues, researchers on the theory of "challenge and threat" states, have suggested that as part of our unconscious resource appraisal, we review our self-efficacy, what we might describe as self-confidence and self-belief. Their research along with that of others suggests that having self-confidence and self-belief are pre-cursors to a "challenge" state emerging, as it provides us with a greater sense of control and much more positive emotional responses.

One of the most recognized researchers in self-confidence is Albert Bandura. In his breakthrough work he described self-efficacy as, "how well one can execute courses of action required to deal with prospective situations." To put it in simpler terms, self-efficacy is a person's belief in their ability to succeed in any situation.

Bandura's work proposed four elements that can influence self-efficacy. Starting with the most influential, they are:

- Mastery experiences or performance accomplishments: this refers to the experiences you gain when taking on a new challenge and being successful at it.
- Vicarious learning: seeing others complete a similar task increases your self-confidence.
- Social persuasion: receiving positive verbal feedback while undertaking a complex task persuades you that you have the skills and capabilities to succeed.
- Emotional, physical, and psychological well-being: how you feel can influence how you feel about your personal abilities in a particular situation. For example, if you are feeling low or struggling with injury or illness, this is most likely going to negatively impact confidence in your personal ability.

Since Bandura's original work there has been a lot more research building on his findings. Psychologist Robin Vealey and her team of researchers in the USA developed a framework looking at the sources of self-confidence specifically in sports situations. They added four further sources of confidence: "successful preparation" for events and competition both mentally and physical; feeling good about one's "physical self-perception," such as body weight and image; "environmental comfort," including things like familiarity with the venue, equipment, and the ability to follow their routines and rituals; and finally, "Leadership," athletes having trust and feeling comfort in their coach's or team manager's ability to lead effectively and make good decisions.

Rob Griffiths has over 30 years' experience working with athletes at all levels in endurance sports. He has an MSc in performance psychology, and a special interest in mental skills and developing athletes' performance mindsets.

Figure 7.1 Mindset Skills Self-Assessment

Read each statement below and choose an appropriate response from these options:

1=Never 2=Rarely 3=Sometimes 4=Frequently 5=Usually 6=Always

___ 1. I believe I have the potential to race at a higher level.
___ 2. I train consistently and eagerly.
___ 3. I stay positive when things don't go well in a race.
___ 4. I know that becoming the rider I want to be will take a long time.
___ 5. Before races I remain positive and upbeat.
___ 6. I think of myself mostly as a success person.
___ 7. Before races I erase self-doubt.
___ 8. The morning of an important race I awake nervous but eager.
___ 9. I remain upbeat after a poor race performance.
___ 10. In a race I wait to make the critical move when the time is right.
___ 11. I'm able to race at or near my ability level.
___ 12. When suffering in a race I try to hold on as I know things will change.
___ 13. Staying focused during long races is easy for me.
___ 14. I stay in tune with my exertion levels in races.
___ 15. I control my emotions when things don't go well in a race.
___ 16. I'm good at concentrating as the race progresses.
___ 17. I'm willing to make sacrifices to achieve my goals.
___ 18. I know that my training will pay off if I follow the plan.
___ 19. I look forward to doing hard workouts.
___ 20. When having a bad workout, I remain calm and focused.
___ 21. I think of myself as a tough competitor.
___ 22. I tune out distractions in races.
___ 23. I set high but achievable goals for myself.
___ 24. When things aren't going well in a race, I quickly review my race plan options.
___ 25. When the race gets harder, I concentrate even better.
___ 26. In races I am mentally tough.
___ 27. When having a bad race or workout I remind myself of why I ride.
___ 28. I stay positive despite late race starts, bad weather, and changes.
___ 29. My confidence remains high the week after an unsuccessful race.
___ 30. I strive to be the best athlete I can be.

Scoring: Add up the numerical responses you gave for the statements above and total them for each mindset category listed below. Then determine your rating for each category by using the rating scale below.

Mindset Skills	Statements	Total	Rating
Motivation	2, 8, 17, 19, 23, 30	_____	_____
Confidence	1, 6, 11, 21, 26, 29	_____	_____
Focus	7, 13, 14, 16, 22, 25	_____	_____
Self-talk	3, 5, 9, 24, 27, 28	_____	_____
Patience	4, 10, 12, 15, 18, 20	_____	_____

How to determine your rating:

Total	My Rating
32-36	5 Excellent
27-31	4
21-26	3
16-20	2
6-15	1 Poor

The five mindset skills of Figure 7.1 should give you an idea of what your possible mindset strengths and weaknesses are. I consider scores of 4 and 5 for any of these as a good indication that the athlete's mindset for a given skill is sound and likely not limiting their training or race performance. A score of 3 raises some concerns while a 1 or 2 for any skill reveals a weakness that needs addressing.

With your mental strengths and weaknesses in mind, let's look at the mental tools that sport psychologists and coaches suggest help you broaden your strengths and improve your weaknesses.

MOTIVATION

I suspect your motivation to train and race is good or you wouldn't be reading this book. You probably deeply enjoy a ride that fits your demeanor for the day. I'm also sure there are days when you really don't want to ride. The weather is crappy, or you just aren't in the mood. It's the same for everyone, including me. Sometimes you must talk yourself into getting out the door and throwing your leg over a bike. But then there are also days when you really shouldn't ride because you didn't sleep well, your heart rate variability is quite low, you feel a head cold coming on, or you have a family or career commitment. These, and many more, are all valid reasons for not riding regardless of motivation. For those other days when you are not sure you want to ride there may be things that boost your enthusiasm.

SURE-FIRE MOTIVATORS

There are two things I have found that are great motivators for athletes. The most powerful is having a coach you report to daily. That "report" might be recording your daily workouts in your online training diary that you know your coach will read. Or it could be a conversation with your coach at regular intervals when you talk about how training is going. That is certain to incentivize you to follow the plan. Of course, hiring a coach can be expensive. The other sure-fire motivator—this one is free—is having a training partner or training group you ride with frequently. Knowing that someone is waiting to ride with you is certain to get you out the door on one of those "I'd rather not ride" days when everything is okay except your motivation.

CELEBRATE YOUR SUCCESSES

Celebrating boosts motivation. The bigger the success, the bigger the celebration. Consider including family, friends, teammates, and other supporters for the biggest successes. Celebrating reinforces your mental commitment to striving for success. As you've probably seen with other pro teams, Elizabeth's team celebrated successes the same day. If someone had a good race or the workout went exceptionally well, the team celebrated. Never pass up an opportunity to celebrate your successes in some way, no matter how big or small they may be. The same goes for others in your life. When they succeed at something—anything—celebrate with them. It could be as small as a pat on the back along with "Way to go," or it may be a party. Always celebrate.

A SECOND PASSION

Have something else in your life that you are also passionate about, such as a hobby, golf, art, music, your career, a non-profit, stamp collecting, or whatever turns you on. Having another passion balances your life. If one isn't going well, you can always fall back on the other for a short period of time to balance your mind. If cycling is your only passion, life is likely to become rather narrow and mundane. That's not good for motivation. A good example of a second passion is one of my best pro riders. She liked to read, especially fiction. When she wasn't on the bike, at a team meeting, eating a meal, or sleeping she was reading. Her passion for books helped to make her a well-rounded person and was a great fallback after a bad day on the bike. Having a second passion in your life is motivating.

KEY TAKEAWAYS

- Hire a coach if you need guidance; this is also good for motivation.
- The second-best motivator is a training partner.
- Your successes, no matter how small, should be celebrated in some way.
- Every rider should have a second passion in their life beside cycling to give them a balanced life.

CONFIDENCE

This the mindset slip I most often see in the athletes I coach—and at all levels of performance. The closer athletes get to a high-priority race, the more likely they are to doubt their ability to achieve their goal. I've seen this in Olympians and world-class performers in many sports, as well as back-of-the-pack, everyday athletes. I've had very few athletes, despite their level of performance, who were always confident. Most of the others are just hiding their doubts. I'm going to take a deeper dive into this topic as it's likely to be one of your mental skill weaknesses.

"Confidence" is from the Latin *"fidere"* meaning "to trust." And that's exactly what self-confidence is about—trusting yourself. It's believing deeply that you can achieve performing at your best on race day, and that you have all the abilities necessary for success. Or, if you currently don't have those abilities, knowing you have the capability and drive to develop them.

Your best mental tool for high performance is self-confidence. Confidence is a product of your motivation to succeed and your drive to achieve things that may be difficult to accomplish. Without confidence you are easily discouraged and likely to lose motivation. With confidence your chances of success are greatly increased and you can visualize accomplishment. If you sometimes sense even a slight lack of belief in yourself then there is room for your improvement as a high-performance cyclist. Signs that are *sometimes* indicators of lacking confidence are comparing yourself with others, joking negatively about yourself, self-doubt, sensitivity to criticism, feeling

Your best mental tool for high performance is self-confidence. The good news is that are there many tools to help you slowly build confidence and be more successful in cycling.

inferior, and being unable to comfortably accept praise. We all experience some of these from time to time. It's when they become a dominant theme in your interactions with others that they become a concern. The good news is that there are many tools to help you slowly build confidence and be more successful in cycling, and perhaps in life. Of course, our focus here is on cycling. The following are some mental-toughness tools that may help enhance your confidence as a rider.

YOUR SUPPORTERS

As I suggested in Chapter 1, to be highly successful as a cyclist you must surround yourself with other confident, successful, positive, and supportive people. This hopefully includes your family and friends as the starting point. These are the people closest to you who will have the greatest impact on your performance as a cyclist. In Chapter 1 I also suggested a rather large team of experts and supporters such as your teammates and others in your corner, who may include a sport medicine specialist, bike fitter, mechanic, sport psychologist, and nutritionist. These are people you have identified as those you will approach if their assistance is needed. It's all the better if you personally know them and have an established relationship. Elizabeth's pro team provided several of these experts, which took some of the pressure from her. And, of course, she was surrounded by teammates and team staff, some of whom were positive and, unfortunately, some who weren't. Knowing she had people who could help when needed made her breakthrough as a very high-performance rider possible. There's another side to this. Don't associate with people, no matter how smart they may be in their area of expertise or how well they may ride, if they don't believe in and support you. They will drag you down.

SUCCESS SAVINGS ACCOUNT

This was one of the most important confidence-building tools I suggested Elizabeth utilize. At bedtime each night I asked her to recall one thing she did on the bike that day that was good—no matter how small or insignificant it may have seemed. Some days you are likely to have a poor ride when it seemed nothing was significant. Perhaps on such a day just getting out the door to start the ride was a success. Discard the negative thoughts. Never dwell on them. There will be other days when something exceptional happens. You have a tremendous interval workout, or your climbing was the best it's felt in a long time, or you held the wheel of a strong rider, or some other significant achievement. Relive that day's success in your mind over and over, along with how you felt in the 10 minutes or so before falling asleep. This is the only time in your entire day when there are no interruptions or distractions. Do this *every* night. Make it a habit. Over the course of days, weeks, and months you will build a huge Success Savings Account of success memories.

There will be times when you need to take a withdrawal from your savings account. These are the days when a negative thought pops up ("I can't climb with these riders!"). That's when you reach into your account and pull out a big success and relive it over and over as you soldier on. This is a powerful tool, but you must remember to add to your account every night for it to work. Make it a bedtime habit.

"ACT AS IF"

Elizabeth had great respect for Jeannie Longo, with whom she raced, as well she should. Longo was without question the best rider of her era. I once asked Elizabeth how Longo looked before and during a race. She answered, "Jeannie looks like she thinks she's going to win." "I want you to look the same way," I said. "Before the race walk around *acting as if* you are going to win and ride *as if* you are going to win." We talked about exactly what that meant, and I continually pulled her back to recalling how Longo looked, how she walked, how she spoke to others, how she sat on her bike at the start, and more. Longo was the perfect role model. Physically pretend that you are confident and sure of yourself every day: head up, stand tall, look people in the eye. On the inside you will undoubtedly feel awkward, but if you keep doing it long enough it will eventually sink in. You probably know someone you can use as a role model. Take on that person's demeanor—their body language, their way of speaking, their posture, their interactions with others. *Acting as if* is a great place to start becoming more self-confident.

ACHIEVABLE GOAL SETTING

Set realistic goals that are challenging and within your grasp. Review your goal every day—after waking up, as you get on your bike, throughout the day. You may even write the goal on a piece of tape and stick it on to your stem. Or jot it down on a sticky note pasted on your bathroom mirror. Keep it fresh in your mind. A realistic goal that stretches you to a new level of performance is a strong confidence-builder. What doesn't build confidence is having goals that are too high or too low. Both will stymie your belief in self. I talk about my athlete's goals quite often in our weekly conversations. My question is always, "How are you feeling about this goal now?" I want to hear how the athlete is doing in regards to their confidence as the season progresses. But, at the same time, I realize there will be occasional setbacks that we need to talk about. This may be a good time to talk with a buddy over a cup of coffee.

REFLECT ON YOUR TRAINING BEFORE A RACE

Before an A race, talk with a teammate or close friend about the work and preparation you've done to get ready. This has been shown to lead to a more positive attitude about the race. You will confirm that you're ready for the challenge and that it is not seen as a threat. Elizabeth and I before each of her important races talked to help temper her thoughts and make sure all was going well in her mental preparation.

SUPERSTITIONS ARE OKAY

Do you have a pre-race superstition such as always eating the same food before a race, or putting your left shoe on first, or listening to certain music as you prepare? If so, then you're not alone. Most athletes don't admit to having superstitions as it makes them feel like kooks. But interestingly, research shows that there's a positive side to this. Your superstition may contribute to enhanced confidence that things are right. You're probably aware of the placebo effect in some studies when, for example, a sugar pill changed a person's health for the better because they were told it would. That's sort of what's going on with superstitions. You get a feeling of control and possible success when you engage your superstition. But if it becomes overly complex and a drudgery to perform then you may be affected negatively. Small superstitions build confidence.

KEY TAKEAWAYS

- To be confident you must commit to your plan, execute it as best you can, and be willing to accept the outcome.
- Surround yourself with positive and successful people, and avoid those who bring you down.
- Every night as you settle into bed, relive your greatest success of the day over and over until you fall asleep.
- Try taking on the composure of a successful, high-performance person even if it feels strange.
- Unrealistic goals do not take you to a higher level of performance; your goals must be realistic.
- Before your A race talk with a trusted friend about how your training has gone to help focus your readiness to race.
- If you are superstitious about something that is otherwise trivial, that's okay, so long as it doesn't complicate your readiness to race.

FOCUS

Bike racing, regardless of the type, requires a lot of concentration. For some races your focus must last for long periods of time, as in hours. It isn't just a sprint to the finish that's over in a few seconds. It's often the minutes or hours that got you to the sprint that are critical to your success. Focus also means reading your body throughout the race. You should always be aware of how you are feeling. Are your legs starting to feel tired? How's your hydration? Should you be taking in some food? How is the competition doing? Are they showing signs of fatigue? During the race you can't allow gaps in your focus to grow. Your race day success is significantly tied to how well you can focus for long periods of time. The starting place for improving your ability to focus is in long workouts. Especially those that are done in near A-race conditions, such as group rides, high-intensity workouts, and low-priority races. What can you do to improve your ability to focus if that is a weakness?

TRAINING OBJECTIVES

Staying focused on your seasonal goal can be difficult when you have several months until race day. It's easy to forget about exactly what you are trying to accomplish in working out and just ride your bike day after day. The key to avoiding this loss of focus is having several periodic objectives you strive to achieve in your training as the season progresses. With your training plan from Chapter 5 you should feel ready for the season ahead. There, you may recall, we included subgoals and objectives that lead to your season's goal. Your objectives are usually challenged with field testing at the end of an R&R week. These are all intended to maintain your seasonal focus. Periodically striving to achieve training-related objectives as the season progresses positions your reason for riding front and center.

RACE PLANNING

Having a well-defined race plan with a Plan B and even a Plan C as backups, just in case, keeps you focused on how the race is going. How these plans will play out should be something you give considerable thought to long before race day. For example, how will you know if you need to abandon the primary plan and incorporate Plan B? There could be a lot of reasons. Rehearsing the plans in hard group rides and low-priority races helps to ensure you know what's needed for your success. We'll work on your race-day plan in Chapter 9.

FOCUSED TRAINING

In the weeks and months before your most important races there should be considerable time spent building the fitness necessary to achieve your race goal. This involves being aware of the progress of your fitness and what your possible limitations may be on race day. It's never encouraging to recognize that you are lacking fitness in any area, but it is necessary to know what your limitations may be so that you are prepared.

KEY TAKEAWAYS

- Endurance events demand a mental focus; rehearse this in training.
- Training objectives, such as meeting certain standards in periodic testing, are indicators of how well your progress toward your seasonal goal is going.
- Learn how to develop a race-day plan by having plans for key workouts, such as your group rides.
- Pay close attention throughout the season to how your race readiness is progressing, and be prepared to make training and race-plan adjustments.

SELF-TALK

How you talk to yourself, especially in a high-performance situation, has been shown to have a significant impact on performance. It reveals how you think, particularly your self-perceptions, during a hard workout or race. Several studies using athletes have shown that self-talk influences performance in endurance athletes. A rider who is good at self-talk can pull a good race out of a mediocre one. Here are some suggestions that may help improve your self-talk.

POSITIVE SELF-TALK

In your thoughts always talk to yourself in a positive manner. Never self-flagellate when something goes wrong. Be willing to accept your failures while staying positive. Negative thoughts when things aren't going well deepen the mental hole and lead to low self-esteem and poor race performance. You must unconditionally believe in yourself and your decisions. Execute as planned. If you do well—or don't—accept it gracefully. Determine when your confidence usually starts to break down in a race, workout, or even just in your thoughts at home or at work. Be prepared to interrupt your negative thoughts with positive self-talk. This could also be the day before a race, the morning of, at the start line, or when something common happens in the race, such as a gap opening. (This is also a good time to make a withdrawal from your Success Savings Account and relive it.)

Research shows that positive self-talk reduces your perception of physical exertion when at a high-power output. In the same vein as positive self-talk are facial expressions, especially when they are made to the crowd at a race, such as a big smile when things are tough or sticking your tongue out to show you are working hard. Remarkably, this has been shown to reduce your feeling of effort. Learn to use some of the more common self-talk key words such as, "relax," "focus," "rhythm," and "calm."

USE AFFIRMATIONS

An example of self-talk in a race is saying to yourself, "Relax." An affirmation is a bit more personal and digs deeper into the details of the situation. An example could be, "Pedal smooth and steady." To make affirmations even more powerful say them to yourself as if you are an outside observer: "Tom, keep your pedaling smooth and steady." One Elizabeth commonly used was, "Throw your knees over the bars, Elizabeth." That was her code for smooth pedaling. Another one of my athletes used, "Relax your toes, Bill." Construct second-person affirmations that work well for you on training rides, especially when in a fast-riding group with different situations, such as, "Kate, you've done this before, you can do it again, stay focused and relaxed" or "Close the gap just like you've done before, Steve." Instead of, "My legs hurt," say, "Mary, your legs are doing the work they need to do so hang in there." Or you might say to yourself, "Jane, this is exactly how it's supposed to feel this far into a fast race." Another could be, "Alex, this is tough, but you've done it before, and you can do it again." Store your most effective affirmations into a separate Savings Account to be used when the time is right in a race or hard workout. Talking to yourself as an observer in such a positive manner has been shown to improve performance. Try it on your next hard ride.

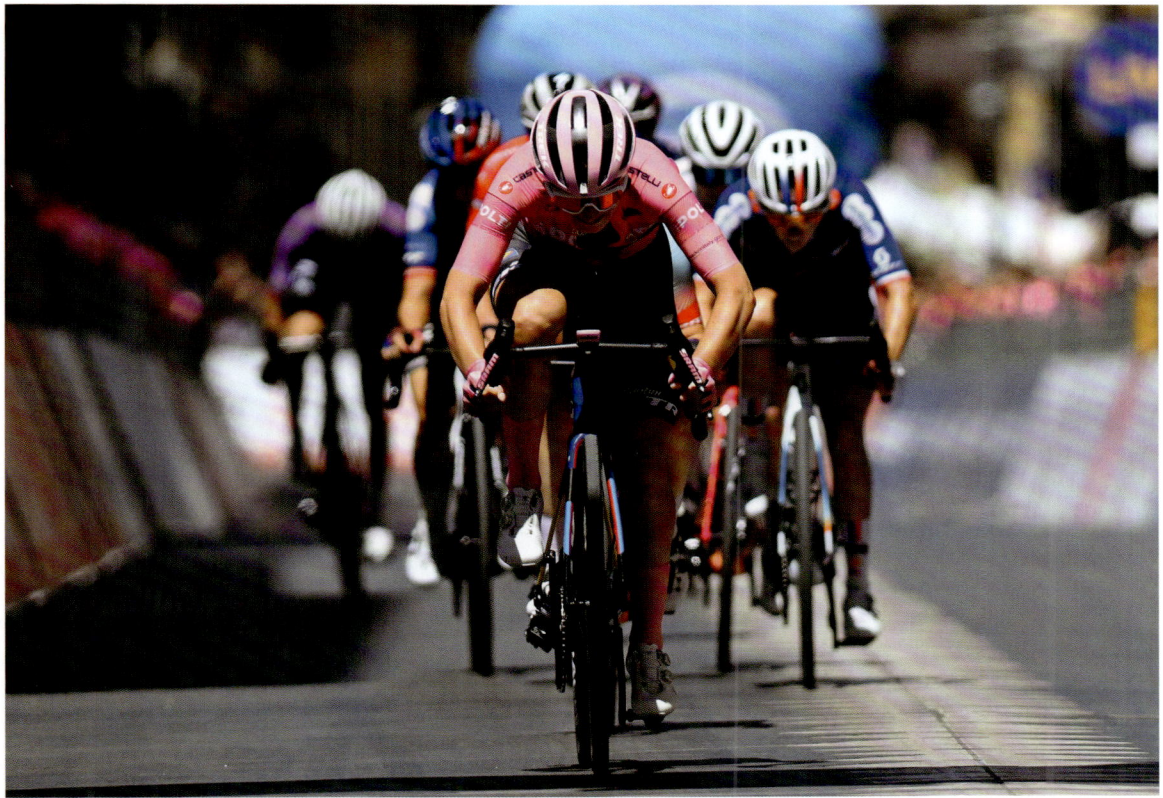

ASK YOURSELF CRITICAL QUESTIONS

You will come to a time in a race or hard workout when you know you're at your limit. This is where only the best riders excel. When such a moment occurs ask yourself the critical question: "Can I do this?" The answer will be either, "Yes, I can," or "No, I can't." If the answer is "Yes" then the next question should be, "How?" Answering that question is the key to your performance that day. Of course, all this thinking and self-talk happens in a split second because you've prepared for such situations during hard rides and low-priority races. Some workouts are more than just fitness builders, they are also race rehearsals. If the answer to the question of "Can I do this?" is "No," then you have found a weakness that needs to be addressed in training.

KEY TAKEAWAYS

- Self-talk is a powerful tool you should master.
- Plan, execute, and accept the results.
- Facial expressions are a form of self-talk.
- Include positive affirmations in your self-talk.
- Challenge yourself with critical questions when the going gets tough.

PATIENCE

Hard rides are challenging. Racing is even harder. Being a high-performance cyclist requires, first, knowing this and, second, being patient. After all, this is a very difficult endurance sport you're preparing for. If it was easy, anyone could just show up and win a bike race. But we know it doesn't happen that way. High-performance race results don't happen overnight. Preparation requires more than weeks or months of focused training. It takes years. The best athletes have a lot going for them, both physically and mentally. Observe how they perform in a race. They obviously understand patience. If this is a weakness for you, how can you develop the ability to persevere? Here are some suggestions.

REFLECT INWARD ONLY

As humans we tend to compare ourselves to others. Race competition makes that even more likely. In competitive cycling there is always someone you look up to as a standard for how you are doing. But that's a double-edged sword. Comparing yourself to others has some good sides, as when "acting as if." But comparisons, as when thinking about how you are progressing relative to another high-performance cyclist, can be emotionally damaging. There's always going to be someone better. It can turn out to be just another form of self-criticism. It's much better for determining who you are today by comparing yourself to a previous you—not to others. How have you progressed in the last two months? Or how are you riding now compared with last year at the same time?

Each of us is unique in many ways. What works for another person may not work for you, and vice versa. You've got to find that personal best way. When thinking about progress, compare yourself only with an earlier version of you. A good example of this is looking back in your training diary to see how you were riding and racing a year ago. Compare that with how you are doing now. What are the differences?

CONTROL EMOTIONS AND CONTEMPLATE SOLUTIONS

When things aren't going your way in a hard workout or race, don't lose your temper. When such a situation occurs, as they do for everyone, look inward. Ask, "Did I do something wrong?", followed by "If so, what do I need to work on?" You're not perfect. No one, including the best rider in the world, is. Was it just a dumb mistake or is the problem related to climbing, descending, sprinting, stamina, or planning? Whenever the weakness pops up, quell your emotions, and give it some thought. Accept that you have a weakness and decide how you will strengthen it. This is not a time to castigate yourself. Look for solutions—not excuses—and take a long-term approach to the fix.

MINDSET

MENTAL SKILLS SUMMARY

All your most effective mental tools must be repeatedly rehearsed throughout your daily activities—at home with your family, at work, at school, with friends, when you are riding, and especially when on a group ride or hard workout. B and C races are also a great time to learn. If you wait until your A race to use one of the above tools, it's probably too late. Discover which ones work best for you. Practicing these frequently will enhance their effectiveness, boosting your mental performance and ultimately your racing.

KEY TAKEAWAYS

- When the going gets tough, patience is a key to success.
- Compare yourself with how you've performed in the past—not with others.
- When things go wrong, control your emotions and learn from the situation so that it doesn't happen again.
- Identify which of these mental skills work best for you and practice them at every opportunity.

THE REST OF ELIZABETH'S STORY

Recall that I said early in this chapter that Elizabeth wanted to break the world record for the hour on the track? Unfortunately, she never got a chance, because that winter after her breakthrough season she was picked up by the top USA women's professional cycling team. That was quite a feather in her cap. They over raced her that first season—such a shame—but Elizabeth went on to win the Pan American Games Time Trial Championship twice, was on the USA Long Team for the next Olympics, and was also a three-time finisher of the Women's Tour de France. She was an exceptional athlete with whom I learned a lot about the mental side of endurance training and racing.

Now well past her professional cycling years, Elizabeth continues to be active as a supporter of women's sports. She produces a podcast—HearHerSports.com—which focuses on women in a wide range of sports.

8. COMMON QUESTIONS

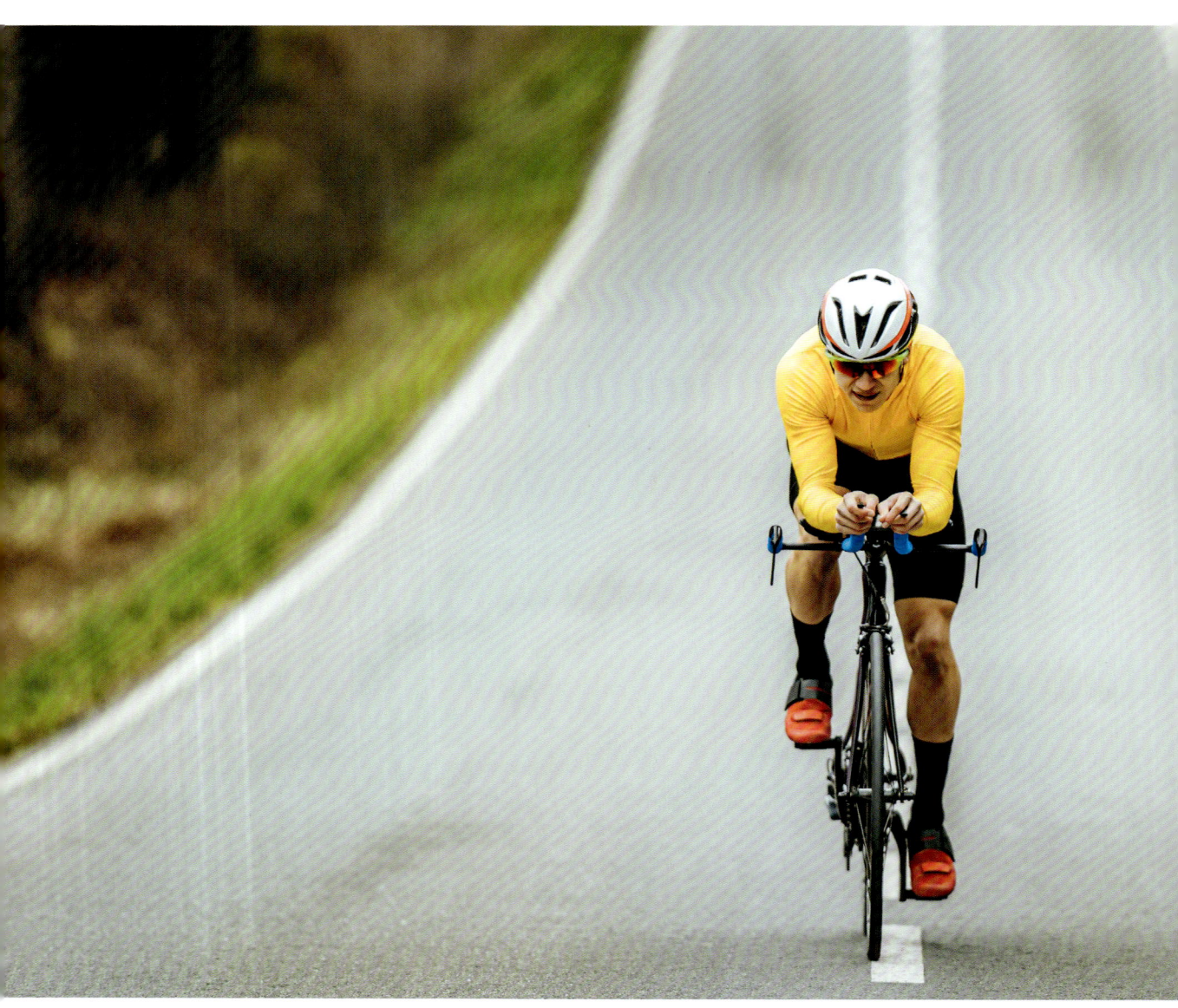

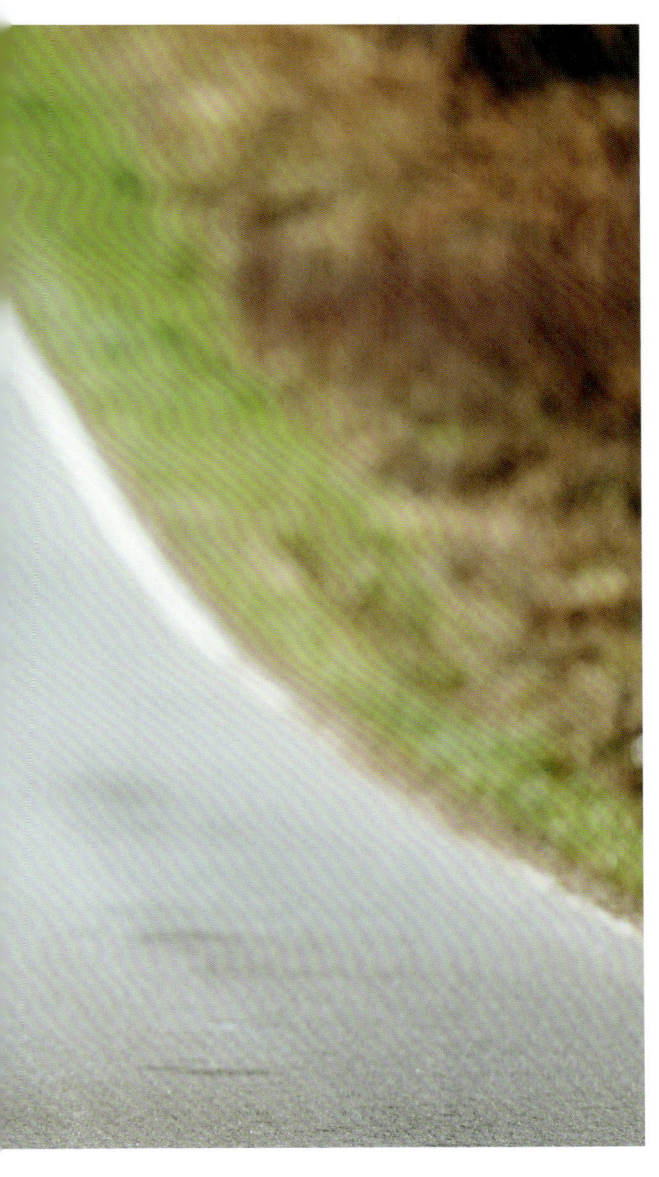

In this chapter I answer several questions that I'm frequently asked. The first is by far the most widely debated. It has to do with how to eat and drink to fuel your engine when on and off the bike. There are many options here supported by strong opinions. I'll tell you what I think. Second is another greatly concerning question for many riders: How do I lose weight? It's a simple enough question but loaded with lots of emotion. A somewhat less passionate question, but one that is of concern to many busy riders, has to do with how you train when you don't have much time due to other commitments in your daily life. A related topic addresses what you should do when you miss workouts. It's a complex matter and one that affects all of us. And finally, I'll answer a couple of questions that have to do with age—both old and young.

RALPH'S STORY

He called me on the day my wife and I were moving into a new home. I considered not answering and just letting it roll over to voicemail as I stood in the driveway giving directions to the movers. But I decided to take it. I'm sure my end of the call came across as a bit unfocused since my mind was in overdrive. It turned out the caller was an athlete interested in my coaching. I had done this same conversation so many times that I knew I could do it and still direct the movers. So, I started asking questions, the same ones I had done scores of times before with inquiring athletes. We started down my mental list: sport type, how long in the sport, experience, goals for the coming season, and more.

Everything was going very smoothly. I could tell he and I would get along great. But then I asked a question that threw a monkey wrench into the conversation: "Tell me about your diet." He said he was a serious vegetarian. And from what he went on to tell me, he seemed to eat a lot of bagels. Back then, the first was a red flag for me as I had never coached a vegetarian. My concerns were complications such as vitamin B-12 deficiency, insufficient vitamins D and K, inadequate protein, iron deficiency anemia, low calcium and zinc, and more. I assured him that eating a meat-free diet was healthy in many ways, such as lowering the risk of cardiovascular disease, diabetes, and some cancers, but I simply didn't know enough about what the diet of a vegetarian athlete should be. He sounded quite disappointed. I apologized and suggested a coach who I knew was a vegetarian who would give him great service. That was the end of our conversation, I thought.

Ralph called me again a few days later. We were now moved into the new house and were arranging things. He apologized for interrupting my day again. I assured him that it was quite alright and that I needed a break from moving furniture anyway. He went on to say he had been thinking about our previous conversation and that he was willing to make a dietary change. What if he included fish and occasional meat in his daily diet? "Would that help?" he asked. "Yes," I said. But I felt like a real heel for making him change his diet (and probably that of his family) because of my lack of experience with coaching vegetarians. We made an appointment to talk a couple of days later after I had the move-in finished. Then we would get down to the business of starting our coach-athlete relationship.

In our next conversation I found out more about Ralph's sport background and lifestyle. He did both triathlons and bike races, and had had some small success at both. But he was prone to back issues, which we later determined was related to poor core strength. And he overtrained when self-coached. That was nothing new as most self-coached athletes do too much, especially when it comes to intensity. I had been through this many times, so I knew his training had a lot of room for improvement. Primarily, he mostly needed more easy training days to be better prepared for the hard days.

I soon came to realize that he was more enthusiastic about cycling than multisport. He liked the always-changing strategies of road racing. I was somewhat relieved. It's quite a challenge to prepare an athlete for competition in two significantly different sports simultaneously. The cycling side of triathlon is more like time trialing than road racing. But even then, there are differences. A time trialist never has to dismount and run at high effort. And road racing is based largely on stochastic efforts— the pace and intensity is always changing. In triathlon the exertion is quite steady. All of this makes combining the two sports with high goals in each quite a challenge.

I shared all of this with Ralph and explained that it would be difficult to excel at both simultaneously. We had a long talk about what he hoped to get out of both sports. Again, I noted that he seemed to enjoy bike racing more. But he also had triathlon goals he wanted to achieve. One of those was qualifying for the World Championship in the coming season—a very high target. We started working toward that goal while keeping his road racing as sharp as we could.

SUPPLEMENTS—THE GOOD, THE BAD, AND THE UGLY: LOUISE BURKE

Supplements represent a multibillion-dollar industry, with athletes being enthusiastic contributors to the market. Until recently, most organizations in sports science and sports medicine took a conservative view on supplements, recommending that athletes don't need them and should avoid them. Fortunately, this has been replaced with a more pragmatic approach which recognizes differences in supplement types and uses.

The Good
Some products can make a valuable contribution to a cyclist's sport nutrition plan. These include the following types.

Sports Foods
Such products as sports drinks, gels, bars, chews, protein powders, electrolyte products, and liquid meals are all examples of tailor-made nutritional support for sport. Endurance athletes, such as cyclists, often need to consume large amounts of carbohydrate, fluid, protein, or electrolytes in scenarios where everyday foods aren't practical. Commercial sports foods continue to evolve for special populations or niche uses. These include plant-based protein supplements, and drinks and gels that can deliver even greater amounts of carbohydrate for high-fuel scenarios—such as stage racing in elite cycling. When used in the correct situations, the practicality of sports foods justifies their expense or their label as ultraprocessed foods.

Micronutrient Supplements
Iron, vitamin D, and calcium are some of the micronutrients that may be under-consumed by some athletes in their daily diets. Supplementation, under the guidance of a sports dietitian or physician, may be part of a plan to treat or prevent diagnosed nutritional deficiencies. Again, the focus should be correct scenarios of use. Athletes who self-medicate with these over-the-counter supplements often miss the opportunity to better address their nutrition needs.

Evidence-based Performance Supplements
Although many products claim to achieve outcomes that make athletes "higher, faster, and stronger," most are not backed by credible evidence. However, there are a handful of products with sound scientific support of their ability to target characteristics that would otherwise constrain training or competition performance. When used with correct protocols to address these scenarios, they can directly improve performance or contribute to factors that lead to it over time (for example, better quality training and improved recovery). Examples of the well-recognized products include caffeine, creatine monohydrate, sodium bicarbonate, nitrate/beetroot juice, beta-alanine and glycerol for hyperhydration. Other supplements that are receiving attention include ketone ester supplements, polyphenols from fruit (cherries, berries, pomegranates), and tastants (for example, menthol).

The Bad
A look at any supplement website or a visit to a supplement store will identify that there are literally millions of products on the market that don't fit the categories identified above. Some involve ingredients that are enthusiastically marketed, but have failed to gather scientific evidence. Others involve multi-ingredient products with some of the characteristics or ingredients

identified above, but in doses that are unlikely to achieve the potential benefits or in the presence of unnecessary ingredients.

Why is this bad? At best, it presents a drain on an athlete's resources. We all have a limit on our budgets, our time, and our beliefs. Focusing attention on products that have poor potential to enhance a sport nutrition plan or contribute to performance outcomes means we've lost the opportunity to work with something that does. Sometimes, people justify the use of non-evidence-based strategies with the theory that even if it doesn't really work, the placebo effect (our belief that it does) will still provide a benefit. However, this approach misplaces the opportunity to add confidence in a sport nutrition plan to the real benefits it could provide! And any use of supplements contributes to a risk of an "ugly" outcome.

The Ugly

Despite the professional appearance of commercial supplements, in most countries, the supplement industry is not regulated or enforced to the same level as its food or pharmaceutical counterparts. One of the resulting dangers is the presence of ingredients that are harmful to the health or sporting goals of the athlete. This includes ingredients that are harmful—for example, impurities, chemicals that are in trials for medical purposes but have not been declared safe, or excessive amounts of stimulants. Some of these ingredients are not declared on the label so the athlete may be unaware of what they are consuming. Others may be simply contaminants resulting from impurities in the raw ingredients or from cross-contamination in the manufacturing process. The use of such supplements can lead to health issues, including severe outcomes on occasions. Even if these ingredients are in minute quantities, they may be banned for use by anti-doping regulations such as the World Anti-Doping Agency (WADA) code, and detectable in anti-doping testing protocols.

Strict liability rules in anti-doping codes—meaning that the athlete is responsible for any banned substances detected in their blood or urine samples, regardless of how they were ingested—have caused some athletes to receive anti-doping rule violations as the result of inadvertent intake from supplement use. High-performance athletes should avoid higher risk supplements (for example, multi-ingredient muscle gainers, fat burners, and pre-workout products) and only use products that have been batch-tested by third-party schemes. Many agencies, such as the Australian Institute of Sport (ais.gov.au/nutrition/supplements) and USADA (usada.org/athletes/substances/supplement-connect/), provide great resources regarding supplement effectiveness and safety.

Professor Louise Burke is a sports dietitian with more than 40 years' experience in counseling, education, and research with high-performance athletes. She is now a full-time researcher at the Mary Mackillop Institute for Health Research at Australian Catholic University in Melbourne.

FUELING THE ENGINE

What should you eat and drink for high-performance cycling? That sounds like a simple enough question, but this is a thorny topic with many "it depends." Let's start with an *it-depends* example. Should an athlete of Australian Indigenous descent eat the same diet as a native-born Norwegian athlete? That's kind of a far-out question. Let's close in on what's a more likely situation. How about an athlete who has been diagnosed as pre-diabetic? Can they eat the same diet as non-diabetic athletes? And even more common: what if the athlete has high blood pressure? Should their diet differ from the diet that is commonly recommended for endurance athletes? And more: what about a rider who has dietary allergies, such as to nuts? How should an athlete who is lactose or gluten intolerant eat? Or my dilemma at the start of this chapter—how should a vegetarian athlete eat? How about a vegan athlete? The questions are simple, but the answers are complex because "it depends" on so many individual variables. To some extent, each of us is unique when it comes to nutrition. There is no one-diet-fits-all answer to how you should eat. But it's not possible to talk about this topic without making some suggestions and then leaving it to you to adapt it to your unique situation.

So how about you? What should *you* eat? As your coach, I would need to know a lot about you before recommending a dietary plan. Even then it may be quite complicated and well beyond my coaching knowledge and experience. That's why I initially declined to coach Ralph. What *you* should eat is a question best answered by a registered dietitian or, better yet, a sport nutritionist who has a solid background in both nutrition and endurance training.

The athlete's diet is not only a broad topic, but also deep as there is a tremendous amount of research on it. All of this is to make the point that I will only touch the surface of this topic. To dig deeper I'd suggest reading one of the many books available for athletes written by authors with a great depth of sport nutrition knowledge and experience.

> **RECOMMENDED SPORT NUTRITION BOOKS**
>
> *Advanced Sports Nutrition*, Dan Benardot (Human Kinetics).
> *The Endurance Diet*, Matt Fitzgerald (Da Capo Lifelong Books).
> *Nancy Clark's Sports Nutrition Guidebook*, Nancy Clark (Human Kinetics).
> *Nutrition Periodization for Athletes*, Bob Seebohar (Bull Publishing Company).
> *The Plant-Based Athlete*, Matt Frazier and Robert Cheeke (HarperOne).
> *Sport Nutrition,* Asker Jeukendrup and Michael Gleeson (Human Kinetics).

In this chapter I'm not going to examine the broad range of topics that so many sport nutrition books address, such as the micronutrients, how your body stores and accesses each nutrient type during a ride and when at rest, energy systems, nor the details of human digestion and metabolism. It's not that these are unimportant subjects. They certainly are, but such subjects are better addressed in a book devoted to the many detailed essentials of nutrition. Instead, I want to take a big-picture view of a healthy, sport-specific diet with reference to daily food choices, workout nutrition, and the important details of a race-day diet. This section is aimed at most riders who have no particular dietary needs, such as those mentioned at the start of this topic. This will hopefully get you pointed in the right direction as you seek to balance your diet with high-performance training. To fine-tune it to your unique needs and lifestyle, educate yourself by reading or speak with a nutritionist.

DAILY FUEL

It's important to have a foundational philosophy when thinking about all things related to performance. I would suggest that such a philosophy must begin with the principle that health comes before fitness. I realize that sounds quite elementary. The reason I even bring it up is that I come across many athletes who assume that since they train seriously and with lots of saddle time, they can eat anything they want. It really doesn't work that way. In the long term, you can't out-train a poor diet. It will eventually catch up with you. While frequent and regular exercise has a lot to do with your overall health and longevity, it is not a surefire cure-all for any other lifestyle issues.

And as you become older, the risks from eating an unhealthy diet increase. Riding a bike does indeed make you healthier. There's no doubt about that. But it doesn't make you immune to diseases and conditions that also threaten the health of your sedentary neighbors. I've known many older athletes who have experienced serious health setbacks despite years of serious training. Exercise, while quite beneficial to your well-being, does not make you invulnerable to the downsides of an unhealthy diet. It just delays them. If you want to be healthy and still riding strong in your 60s, 70s, and 80s, you had better have a healthy lifestyle, including diet, in your 30s, 40s, and 50s.

What is a healthy diet? I believe it's one that is quite basic, consisting of *natural* foods, such as vegetables, fruits, whole grains, and animal products. I believe frozen meals, soft drinks, chips, candies, cookies, margarine, crackers, sweetened cereals, processed meat products, breakfast cereals, candy, and desserts, mostly in boxes and plastic packages, don't belong in a healthy diet, which should avoid ultraprocessed foods with high-fructose corn syrup, added flavorings, hydrogenated fats, colorings, and multi-syllable chemicals—and a lack of fiber. Does this mean you should never eat a cookie or a few crackers? Not at all. What's important to your daily refueling is to eat a diet that is made up, primarily, of natural foods. An occasional bit of junk food will not threaten your health.

How much of your daily caloric intake should be natural versus highly processed? I can't put an exact figure on this. But I can tell you that it should be heavily weighted to the natural-food side, as in around 90 percent. Researchers in the USA and UK have found that about 50 percent of foods consumed in those countries are highly processed. That's a sad situation. Should you try to "grade" your diet based on such numbers? No. It is much too complicated and varies from day to day. I suggest, however, that you are always aware of what you are eating and strive to make it as natural as you can. That's the diet you will excel with and the one that will lead to a long and healthy life as a cyclist.

I'm sure you are aware of carbohydrates, fats, and proteins as the nutritional basis of diet. What are the best *natural* sources of these nutrients? For your carbohydrates I recommend vegetables, fruits, berries, whole grains, beans, and brown rice. Among the best sources of natural fat are olive oil, avocado, fish, nut butters, and Greek yogurt. Natural protein foods include animal products such as lean meats, fish, milk, and eggs. Other natural sources of protein are legumes, nuts, and lentils. These types of food will fuel your training and racing while not threatening your long-term health.

WORKOUT FUEL

Notice that I didn't mention above any of the sports supplement products we are all used to as endurance athletes. Should you eat these? Well, first, they are not natural. In fact, far from it. They are foods (if we can use that word for these products) that are highly processed, meaning they have been stripped of their natural ingredients, mixed in unnatural ways, loaded with sugar, contain food additives such as artificial colors and flavors, and are often replete with unpronounceable chemicals. Does that mean to never eat them? Probably not. They can prove useful in a very long ride or race when carbs are needed to fuel the effort. And it doesn't matter which of these supplements you use. Research has shown similar results from fluids, gels, chews, bars, or any mix of these. It just comes down to which you prefer and which don't upset your stomach.

Are there other real-food sources you could use on a long ride instead that are natural? Most certainly. It wasn't too long ago that riders carried bananas and even small sandwiches in their jersey pockets. Some still do. These foods were a bit of a hassle to prepare and carry, but they did the job in a healthy way. Sports supplements are certainly more convenient, but not as healthy. The more frequently you do very long rides, the greater the benefits of using packaged nutrition products.

I would strongly suggest that the only times you use such foods, if you use them at all, are when you are on the bike and riding more than two hours. They are best avoided after the ride or at any other time in your day.

Many riders eat too much carbohydrate at the expense of fat and protein. You need only replace the carbohydrates you burned that day in training. So, of course, the higher intensity riding you do, the more carbs you should eat. But bear in mind what you read about in Chapter 6. There I told you about overtraining and that one of the most common causes of this is too much high-intensity training. Another contributing factor, which I didn't mention, is a diet chockfull of ultraprocessed, high-sugar foods. If you are going to eat more carbohydrates than are necessary, the preferred selections should be from the natural food choices mentioned above.

Perhaps the most neglected food type in the rider's diet is protein. These types of foods play a key role in the rebuilding phase of recovery, especially when it comes to muscle and bone development and immune system function. Endurance athletes need considerably more protein than what government agencies recommend. Most of the research on this sport-specific topic now recommends about four calories per pound (2.2 kilograms) of body weight per day.

Now let's look at this topic of workout fueling from a different perspective. A fit and well-nourished athlete's body stores approximately 2,000 calories of carbohydrate. But even the skinniest rider's body stores about 53,000 calories of fat. Tapping into that fat storage for fuel is one reason I recommend so much zone 1 and 2 training time. It not only conserves carbohydrate for those times when you need it for an intense effort, but it's also metabolically healthy.

Figure 8.1 demonstrates how these two primary fuel sources are utilized during all your rides from zone 1 to zone 5. The slopes of the fat and carbohydrate in this figure vary with the individual but are highly trainable. Note Crossovers A and B. These are the intensity at which the athlete goes from primarily using fat to drive the pedals to carbohydrate-dominant fueling. Crossover A in Figure 8.1 is the rider early in the season whose fat metabolism is overly dependent on using carbohydrate for fuel. Note that Crossover B is well to the right. This is late in the Base period when the rider is well trained to burn fat for fuel due to considerable training in zones 1 and 2. Moving the crossover to the right is a result of spending lots of saddle time doing Aerobic Endurance workouts. It's possible to improve your metabolic fitness to enhance fat-burning while sparing your carbohydrate by pushing the crossover point to the right. The most metabolically fit athletes have a crossover which is very far to the right.

Some athletes are wholly dependent on carbohydrate during exercise—and life in general. A gradual rise in their heart rates as they ride at a steady power output is due to this dependence on carbohydrate. This enlists very little fat for fueling the ride. They are wasting the fuel source they have the least of to ride easily. That will come back to haunt the rider late in the race when carbs are needed to fuel high-intensity efforts. Those who train a lot for fat metabolism move the crossover far to the right, thus sparing carbohydrate as a fuel source for later when they can use it to take a commanding position in the race. Along the same line, a rider who eats a very high carbohydrate diet will also tend to be carb-burner with a crossover on the low-intensity side of Figure 8.1. That's why I recommend that riders eat a diet with fewer calories from carbs, and more from fat and protein than is common in Western society. That would be very roughly 50 percent carbohydrate, 25 percent fat, and 25 percent protein as an average for the season. I've known of many endurance athletes who have reduced their carb intake even more, down to 40 percent, and still race at a high level due to their nutrition periodization strategy.

Figure 8.1 Fat and carbohydrate utilization relative to training zones

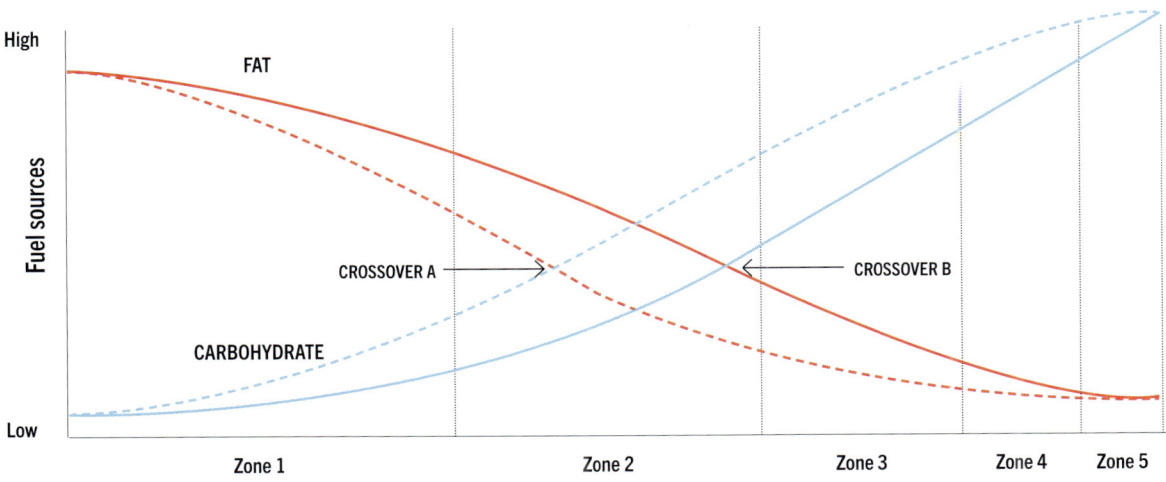

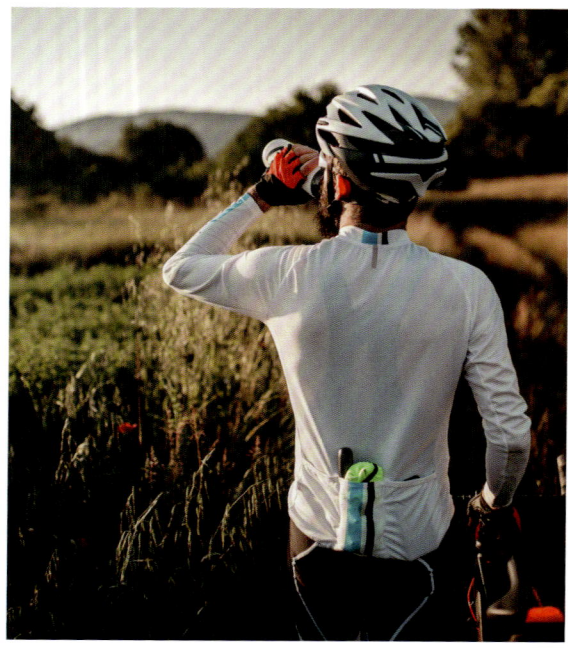

NUTRITION PERIODIZATION

Chapters 4 and 5 described how to periodize your workouts by building a base of fitness starting with training frequency, progressing to duration, and then topping off your race readiness with race-like intensity training followed by a taper. You should look at diet from the same perspective as your workouts. Workouts and diet should fit together like the gears and chain on your bike. In other words, diet should change throughout the season to meet your nutritional needs as determined by your workouts. This is a relatively new concept in endurance training. To understand it let's first explore the topic from a big-picture, seasonal training perspective.

In previous chapters I've explained the significance of sleep for recovery and adaptation. It's just as important to emphasize the importance of nutrition for both recovery and adaptation. Because of this, periodization of nutrition has become an important piece in the quest to achieve a high level of performance. The basic idea is to eat a diet that reflects the demands of your training. Just as greater sleep is common following a hard training day, eating must also reflect your biological needs. In other words, your diet should not necessarily be the same day after day and month after month. It should vary just as your workouts vary. How does nutrition do this? It plays a key role in restocking carbohydrate stores, muscle repair, restoring body fluids, controlling excess inflammation, and boosting general health.

Figure 8.2 offers a look at how calories, carbohydrates, fats, and proteins may vary from period to period throughout the season. There are periods when your intake of calories is low, moderate, or high. In the same way, the sources of those calories—carbs, fats, and proteins—also vary throughout the season. All of this depends on the volume of training and the intensity of the workouts. As volume increases, calories should also increase. As the intensity of training increases, your intake of carbs increases. Note in the figure that the only fuel source that remains relatively constant throughout the season is protein.

Figure 8.2 is not intended to be a precise gauge of how to regulate your diet, but rather as an overview of how nutrition generally blends in with your riding. This figure doesn't address all issues, such as how much and what to eat during R&R weeks. Nor does it get into the daily changes that are necessary due to the combination of hard and easy training days. But the obvious solution of how to eat when following an undulating workout calendar is to eat relatively more fat and less carbohydrate when rides are low intensity and more carbs and less fat when high intensity is the focus.

Figure 8.2 Periodization of nutrition throughout the season

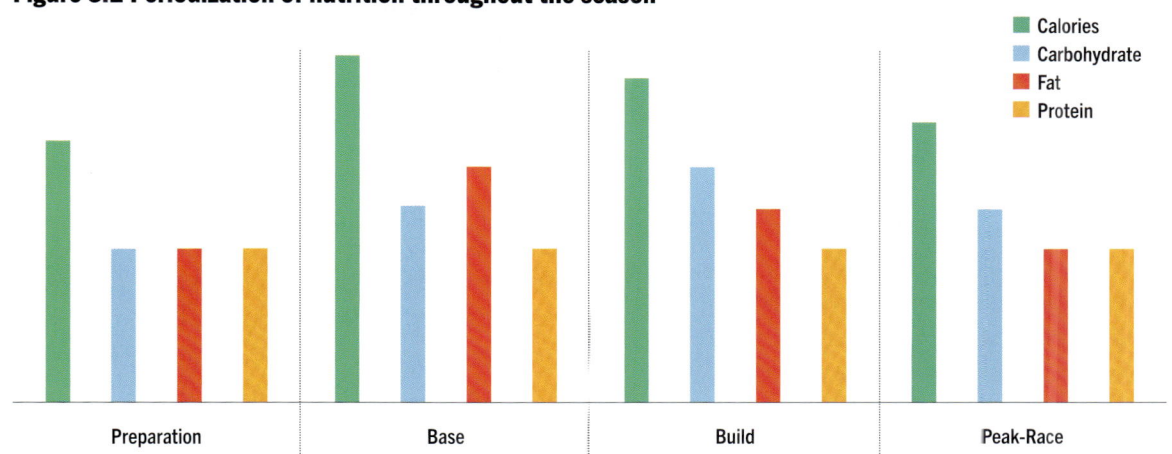

HYDRATION

As for what to drink during a ride, I'd suggest water only for rides shorter than 90 minutes to two hours. The type of workout you are doing will determine when to make the switch to a sports drink, gel, or other carbohydrate source. If it's to be a long and easy ride, I'd suggest drinking water only for the first two hours. Be aware that dehydration over a two-hour ride reduces cardiac output, and thereby aerobic capacity, by up to 8 percent. But if it's an intense ride, taking in carbohydrates starting at about 90 minutes is the way to go. You should have enough carbohydrate stores in your body to manage the early, water-only, portion of the workout. This carb restriction period at the start of a ride will also help boost your fat-burning metabolism.

Besides the need for hydration while riding, also be aware of your fluid intake throughout the remainder of your day. Avoid feeling thirsty in the hours after a ride by drinking plenty. Also, there's no need to buy expensive recovery drinks for use immediately after hard or long rides. Chocolate milk, fruit juices, and vegetable juices make good post-ride recovery drinks—and they are much less expensive.

In the last few years there has been a trend in professional racing to increase the amount of sugar-based sports drink riders take in. For decades sport scientists have advocated taking in no more than 60 grams (240 calories) of carbohydrate per hour, since that had been shown to be the upper limit for a rider's gut to process during a race. That's about one large bottle. But recently that's been pushed upward with some pros consuming 90 grams (360 calories) or even up to 120 grams (480 calories) by training their guts to handle ever-greater amounts. You may be capable of making such a switch, but I wouldn't recommend it. Nausea in the middle of a race is not fun.

Also, with sports drinks be attentive to the effect of high-carb intake for hours at a time on the saddle relative to general health. Be especially aware of your dental health. Frequently rinsing your mouth with water and brushing your teeth post-ride may well save you some trips to your dentist.

BODYWEIGHT

KEY TAKEAWAYS

- Your health is more important than your race performances—choose your diet accordingly.
- Most of your food should come from vegetables, fruits, whole grains, and animal products.
- These natural foods should make up 90 percent or more of your diet.
- Use sports supplement products only when working out, and then only after 90 minutes to two hours in the saddle.
- As a serious athlete you need more protein daily than those who don't exercise.
- You, and all athletes, have a tremendous amount of fat stored—this should be your primary source of fuel when riding.
- By riding in zones 1 and 2 you are using fat to fuel your ride and training your body to become better at fat burning.
- Aim for a diet that is roughly 50 percent carbohydrate, 25 percent fat, and 25 percent protein.
- Your diet should change throughout the season to match the fueling demands of your workouts.
- Eat more fat and less carbohydrate on days when you rode slow and easy and more carbs and less fat when the ride was at a high intensity.
- For the first 90 minutes to two hours of a ride drink only water.
- Drink enough fluids to avoid undue thirst during a ride.
- For long races drink a large bottle of a sports drink with 240 calories every hour after the first 90 minutes.

How can I lose weight? This is among the most asked questions I receive from cyclists. A better question, perhaps, would be, *should* I lose weight? Before getting into the pros and cons, let's examine the theoretical details of bodyweight and performance.

How does bodyweight affect performance? It all comes down to this: dropping a few kilograms may boost your aerobic capacity since VO_2 max is a measure of the maximal amount of oxygen you can deliver to your working muscles per minute *divided by your body weight* (in kilograms). For example, if a rider weighs 70 kilograms (154 pounds) and loses two kilograms (4.4 pounds), and assuming the oxygen delivery to the muscles of 4.2 liters per minute stays the same, then their aerobic capacity would increase from 60 to 61.8. That's about a 3 percent improvement in a basic fitness metric for having lost about 3 percent of bodyweight. Bottom line: the cyclist would ride faster—maybe.

THE WEIGHT-LOSS DILEMMA

Common thinking goes like this: "If I could improve my aerobic capacity by 3 percent by losing just 3 percent of my bodyweight, what if I lost 5 percent of my bodyweight? That would mean an improved aerobic capacity of about 5 percent. That's a big change."

This certainly sounds promising to most riders and seems a lot easier than putting in hours and hours of training to get faster. The greatest benefit, of course, would be when climbing as that's when bodyweight is truly an impediment to performance. However, there would be no performance benefit for riding on a flat road or even when time trialing all-out on a pancake-flat course. In fact, it may be a disadvantage due to a potential loss of muscle.

The possibility of muscle loss when losing weight is the problem here. If you are already very lean (less than about 14 percent body fat for a woman and 6 percent for a man), you should expect this to happen. You may, however, be able to hold the muscle loss at bay if you really understand diet or work with a sport nutritionist. When trying to lose even a small amount of weight in a short period of time, the loss of muscle is a common problem. When your body isn't getting adequate energy to meet all its need due to calorie restriction, it first takes the needed calories from stored fat and then turns to muscle protein. To avoid this, you would need to increase your protein intake; continue to ride easily; and lift weights, especially for the legs. To avoid a breakdown, I would suggest losing no more than a half kilogram or one pound every two weeks. That's quite a slow change, but this may help prevent the loss of muscle while making the process easily manageable. If you make a mistake in weight loss, make it on the conservative side. Rapid weight loss can be disastrous.

HOW TO LOSE WEIGHT

It's apparent that both weight gain and loss come down to calories in versus calories out. Calories out has to do with your workouts—cross-training, riding, lifting weights, along with your normal daily activities. Calories out, by itself, is usually inadequate for losing weight. Most riders must also restrict calories in. This is the big challenge. It requires continuous self-monitoring of what and how much you eat.

Let's start by looking at what causes bodyweight to creep up, so you know what the enemy is. The greatest contributor to weight gain is usually eating ultraprocessed foods—the kinds that are found in the central aisles of your grocery store, as explained above. These are the foods typically stored in plastic or cardboard containers. Their taste and texture are hard to resist. That's the manufacturer's goal. If you can't resist it, you will buy and eat more. Once again, the place to start losing weight is to eat only natural foods, as described above. They are much less likely to cause a weight increase.

Another common contributor to weight gain is mental distress. Such stress could be related to your job, family relations, an overly demanding work schedule, or other psychological challenges that keep you on edge. There simply may be too much going on in your life. Such stress causes your body to release a hormone known as cortisol. This in turn triggers the release of another hormone known as ghrelin, which arouses hunger. Unfortunately, in our society today, extreme hunger often leads to eating more ultraprocessed, fake foods. Trying to lose weight when daily stress is overwhelming is next to impossible. The bottom line is that there is too much in your life that causes pressure. Not only your training, but your health is at risk. If this describes your lifestyle, what must be done to simplify your daily routine? The starting place is to say "no" more frequently. This will not only improve your health and ability to lose or manage weight, but it will also take your training to a higher level.

What riders often do to shift the calorie-in, calorie-out balance is to include more high-intensity workouts in place of easy rides. This is not a good idea as it upsets the 5+2 ratio of easy and hard training days and is unlikely to make a dent in your body weight. Another common "solution" is to greatly restrict calories. Again, not a good idea as this will negatively affect workouts and recovery. I wouldn't recommend frequent fasting either as this is also likely to negatively impact your training.

Instead, take the long-term approach to losing weight by slightly reducing daily calories-in for a few weeks. The time to do this is early in the season in the Transition, Preparation, and Base 1 training periods. That will give you eight to 12 weeks to take off a small amount of excess fat. If you are considering reducing your weight by more than 5 percent, you need to devote most of your season to the project. This usually can't be done in only a handful of weeks as it requires a gradual and conservative approach to prevent overtraining or perhaps even illness. You can still train and race while focused on restricting calories but don't expect good results. A much better way to shed a large amount of weight is to spread it over two seasons. At the start of your Base 2 period, assume you have lost all you can this season. Maintain and then come back at the end of the season and start another weight-loss project for a few weeks. This requires patience and persistence but is much healthier.

> **Understanding *how* to lose weight doesn't mean you *should* lose weight. If you are already quite lean, the potential downsides outweigh the benefits.**

You must also come to accept that your weight will vary daily, perhaps by a kilogram or a couple of pounds. This mostly has to do with water retention and is not a problem. Eating a carbohydrate-rich meal plays a role here as for every gram of glycogen (the storage form of carbohydrate) stored you also store about three grams of water. Such a weight change should normally rise and fall from day to day. If it doesn't and only increases over several days, then an adjustment to your diet or lifestyle is necessary.

Of course, understanding *how* to lose weight doesn't mean you *should* lose weight. If you are already quite lean, the potential downsides outweigh the benefits. But if you are carrying excess body fat, small adjustments to your diet carried out over several weeks at the start of a new season should make a difference.

HOW ABOUT SNACKS?

Eating between meals can be good or bad. It depends. Too little food intake after a ride is likely to reduce your resting metabolic rate. Some snacking is okay if it's healthy food and the timing is right. But be aware that training is not a ticket to eat junk food. Snacks you should entirely avoid are those high in sugar. The best snacks for managing bodyweight and meeting your training needs are protein-based snacks. Good sources are unsalted nuts, hard-boiled eggs, unsweetened Greek yogurt, Cheddar cheese, and cottage cheese.

These types of food are high in both protein and fat. Getting additional protein in daily is typically a good thing for a serious athlete. And foods containing some fats are satiating, meaning they satisfy your hunger quickly.

THE BOTTOM LINE ON WEIGHT LOSS

If you need to reduce your bodyweight there are four things I'd suggest. The first, if you don't mind counting calories, is to reduce your daily food intake by a relatively small amount, such as 200 to 300 calories. That's the equivalent of one potato, three bananas, two large apples, two slices of Cheddar cheese, one fried chicken leg, or three slices of bacon. That should be easily accomplished daily. If you average a reduction of 250 calories daily, you will theoretically lose a pound or a half kilogram every two weeks. That's not enough to impact your training, but enough to have a measurable effect on your bodyweight over the course of your early season. The second suggestion is to increase your aerobic endurance training volume by 10 percent in the Preparation and Base 1 periods. That's not a lot but it will add up over the eight or so weeks early in your season. Third, eat more protein, not only in your meals but also in snacks. If there are times in your day when eating a small amount between meals is common for you, be prepared with a cup of nuts or other protein-rich foods as listed above. And, finally, adjust your mindset about eating. Rather than thinking of this as a time for enjoyment, shift your thoughts to food as fuel for your tank.

KEY TAKEAWAYS

- Losing weight *might* improve your climbing but has no benefit for riding on flat terrain.
- If you are already very lean, losing weight is likely to cause a loss of muscle and therefore power.
- To lose bodyweight, some dietary restriction is necessary.
- The most common cause of weight gain is eating ultraprocessed foods.
- Psychological stress is a common contributor to weight gain and must be reduced to manage your weight while improving training in general.
- A small, daily decrease in calories consumed in the early season can result in a significant change in your bodyweight.
- Daily bodyweight variations are to be expected largely due to water storage.
- Snacks between meals are best if they are mostly protein with some healthy fat, such as unsalted nuts.
- Take a slow change, long-term approach to weight loss to maintain training.

TRAINING TIME

There are two questions I see a lot of when it comes to training loads. The most common is, how do I train if my lifestyle is very busy with only a few hours available to ride weekly? The other is, what do I do if I miss a few workouts? Both questions imply deeper problems that are often very personal and unique to the individual rider. Let's examine both.

THE TIME-LIMITED RIDER

What if you have a very busy lifestyle and find it difficult to train as you would like to? I understand. It can be difficult to meet the daily challenges of life. The most common obstacles are the ones that are most important to you—family and career. Riding comes in about third for serious, but time-limited riders. Perhaps you only have about eight hours weekly to spare for saddle time. That's about as low a weekly training volume can go and still allow you to race competitively. At such a level, every workout must have a well-defined purpose and be followed precisely. This also impacts the types of racing you do. With such a low weekly training load, I'd suggest focusing on short races such as criteriums, cyclocross, and time trials.

How can you build race-day fitness for such events with so little time to train? The following is what I suggest. Ride 60 to 90 minutes on any days you can, striving for a total of about eight hours weekly—and more when possible. Start every day with a ride in zones 1 and 2, but on two days each week of the Build period finish with about 30 minutes of higher-intensity efforts. These could be stamina, aerobic capacity, or sprint power sessions (see Appendix). One of the weekend rides in the Build period may be fully devoted to group rides or races. The other rides are steady efforts in zones 1 and 2 to build and maintain aerobic endurance. This would allow you to get in about six hours of aerobic endurance training, which should still give you a sound fitness base. With these suggestions, your training weeks in the Base and Build periods may look something like the training weeks in Table 8.1. If you have more or fewer hours available, adjust the daily durations while always striving to get at least one hour on the bike. For the Peak and Race periods you may still use the proposed weekly plans in Tables 5.5 and 5.6, along with Table 4.2.

For most busy cyclists the best time to fit in a ride is usually in the morning before that day's scheduled activities start and potentially go longer than expected. That will usually mean some rides, if not most, will be indoors. You will need a good bike ergometer.

MISSED WORKOUTS

The question that is usually asked right after the time-limited question is what If I miss a few workouts? It would be nice if this never happened, that you trained consistently, and all workouts were completed. But in the real world, that's not going to happen. The question should be, what can I do about missed workouts?

First, you need to accept that everyone misses a workout or two on occasion, including pro

Table 8.1. Suggested training weeks in the Base and Build periods for a time-crunched rider

	Base period	Build period
Monday	Gym 45 minutes (Base 1 only) or off	Off
Tuesday	Ride 1 hour Aerobic Endurance (zones 1–2)	Ride 1 hour Aerobic Endurance (zones 1–2)
Wednesday	Ride 60 minutes of Aerobic Endurance (zones 1–2). Then ride 30 minutes including Muscular Force and cool-down	Ride 90 minutes with 60 minutes of Aerobic Endurance and 30 minutes of Stamina, Aerobic Capacity or Sprint Power
Thursday	Gym 45 minutes	Gym 30 minutes
Friday	Ride 1 hour Aerobic Endurance (zones 1–2)	Ride 1 hour Aerobic Endurance (zones 1–2)
Saturday	Ride 60 minutes of aerobic endurance (zones 1-2). Then ride 30 minutes including Muscular Force and cool-down	Ride 90 minutes with 1 hour aerobic endurance and 30 minutes Aerobic Capacity, Stamina, Sprint Power, or a group ride or race
Sunday	Ride 2 hours aerobic endurance (zones 1–2)	Ride 2 hours aerobic endurance (zones 1–2)
Volume	8.5 hours	7.5 hours

riders. While I'd like to see everyone I coach never miss a ride, it just isn't realistic. We have things in our lives beside cycling and they often find a way to intervene. As mentioned above, cycling is third behind family and career, so it's bound to happen. The only issues are how many workouts are missed and how often. At some point consistency becomes an issue. And as mentioned in Chapter 2, consistency is the best predictor of performance. But being realistic, what you really need is guidance on what to do after one or more missed workouts. The following may help.

Three or Fewer Workouts Missed

This is probably the most likely scenario. It's a simple one to fix. Return to training as if nothing happened. Don't try to make up the missed rides. Cramming more workouts into a few days creates the potential for a breakdown and another loss of time. It's simply not a big deal to miss a couple workouts if it happens rarely.

Four to Seven Workouts Missed

This is the one I dread the most. It is, undoubtedly, the hardest scenario to deal with.

If the lost time was due to illness, as is quite often the case, you probably won't be ready to return to normal training right away even if the symptoms are gone. Your body's chemistry and physiology have changed, which will affect your capacity for exercise. This will show up when you start back as a high heart rate or a high perceived exertion at a relatively low power output. If this is the case, you will need to treat it as more than seven days missed, even though you are starting back into training right away. If the lost workouts were due to illness, once back on the bike, your rides for the following week, and possibly longer, should be in zones 1 and 2 only. No higher intensities at all Give your body a chance to get back to normal. Watch your efficiency factor (EF) for these rides very closely. EF will probably be much lower than it was before the illness. When—and only when—EF is normal (what it was for AE1 and AE2 rides before the illness) you are ready to start training "normally" again. You'll need to evaluate how you feel as you start back into two hard rides weekly. And being conservative, gradually work them back into your weekly training. This will certainly affect your race preparation, depending on when in the season it happened, and how sick you were.

If the missed training was *not* due to illness and you are ready to start right away, you will need to make some adjustments to the plan. The first change is to consider the lost training time a rest week. This is necessary, but will throw off the scheduling of training for your A race. Your training blocks will no longer be synchronized to bring you to a peak of form on the day of the race. There are a couple of ways to resolve this dilemma. The first option, if you are in the Base or Build periods, is to reduce the length of the current three- or four-week period by one week. If you still aren't synchronized, do the same for the following period. The second option is to reduce the Peak period from two weeks to one. Neither of these is perfect. Both are going to result in less fitness being developed. But that's the reality of missing a week of training. You can't have it both ways: miss several workouts *and* have the same fitness as if nothing happened.

Once you are ready to train again you will need to step back and make up probably two or three key workouts. Decide which were the most important ones missed, given your limiters, and reschedule them. This may well mean pushing other workouts farther ahead into the plan. Eventually something will have to give. You'll either miss one of the culminating workouts or decide you are progressing well enough to skip or modify one of the sessions remaining in the plan. There are simply too many variables here for me to be able to tell you exactly how to handle your situation. Give it a lot of thought.

Up to Two Weeks of Workouts Missed

If this was due to illness and you were in Base 3 or either of the Build periods, start back into training with a Base 3 training period. If you were in the Base 2 period, go back to Base 1 or even Preparation period training. Stay with that until you feel normal when working out. You will know because heart rate and perceived exertion will match power as they did before you got sick. This will be reflected in your EF being normal compared with when you were last in this training period. If in doubt, include another few days of only easy riding.

When your training vigor returns, repeat the last week of hard training you did before the interruption. If that week goes well then begin moving forward with your "normal" training from that point. If it doesn't go well, repeat that week again. At some point you will need to leave out one to three weeks, or even more, of planned training. That could mean omitting a couple of weeks in Build 2 or the first week of the Peak period. It's more important at this point to make sure your Base period fitness is back to normal than to press ahead into the Build period when not ready.

More Than Two Weeks Missed

If you were in the Build period when this training pause happened, then return to the last Base period you previously completed and start over again from there. If you were in the Base period, then go back by one three- to four-week period from where you left off. As with the previous scenarios you will have to leave out some significant portion of your remaining plan. The priority for omissions is the first one or two weeks of Peak, portions of Build 2, and Build 1, in that order.

Late Season

If any of your training time is lost in the last week of Build 2 or the Peak period continue with your training as if nothing happened. But as with all these scenarios, if the lost time was due to illness be conservative with intensity as you start back, opting to train primarily in zones 1 and 2 until your EF is back to normal. If your EF does not return to normal quickly and you still feel rather run down and weak, then consider not doing your A race. Should you decide to do it anyway, then race conservatively, considering it a hard workout while realizing that fitness was lost and you may still be experiencing rather weak feelings from having been sick. Be cautious not to push yourself to your limits, thus increasing the risk to a return to being ill.

KEY TAKEAWAYS

- If you can only train fewer than 10 hours weekly, focus on short races.
- If time is limited, twice each week in the Build period, after an hour in zones 1 and 2, do some high-intensity training for a portion of the last 30 minutes.
- In the Build period a group ride or low-priority race should be done on the weekends if you are pressed for time.
- Missing workouts occasionally is unfortunate but highly likely for every rider.
- If you miss one to three days of training, don't sweat it; press ahead as if nothing happened.
- Four to seven workouts missed due to illness is of great concern; start back with AE1 and AE2 rides focused on getting EF back to where it was pre-illness.
- If you miss up to two weeks of training, repeat your last fully completed week, paying close attention to your EF for easy rides.
- Missing two or more weeks requires stepping back to the last Base period you fully completed and repeating it in its entirety.
- If you must back up and repeat your last fully completed Base period, make up for the lost two or more weeks by omitting the Peak, Build 2, or Build 1 period, in that order.
- Efficiency factor (EF) in easy rides is the key to assessing your readiness to train "normally" again when training days had to be omitted.

AGE

How does age affect training and racing? The number of master and senior riders is increasing faster than the number of new, young riders coming into the sport. How should older athletes adjust their training as they age? By the time you are in your 50s you are usually aware of the need to make changes, but you may not be sure of what those changes should be. On the other side of the coin, parents, especially those who are cyclists, often encourage their children to take up the sport. How is this best done so that the kids become cyclists and aren't turned away from the sport by overly enthusiastic parents?

OLDER RIDERS

Aging questions I often hear: I just turned 50 (or 60 or 70). Should I cut back on my training? Another common question: how should I change my training as I get older? At some point young riders become old riders and training must be adjusted accordingly. This often takes care of itself as the physical effects of aging place limitations on what we can do. Let's start this topic by examining what those changes commonly are, first from a physiological perspective, and then from a mental point of view.

At some point in one's early 30s, aerobic capacity, one of the best indicators of performance, begins to wane. From a peak in their mid-20s, by the time they are in their mid-30s a consistently trained, high-performance rider can expect a roughly 6 or 7 percent loss of VO_2 max in a decade. The annual change of less than 1 percent is so small at this age that the loss is often not even noticed. In fact, many 30-something riders do not experience any drop in performance at all, despite this physiological change. Wisdom based on years of experience is a great compensation for the physiological downturns at this age.

By the time these same wise riders, now in their 40s, start to become fully aware of an additional 7 percent or so of VO_2 max having been lost, it becomes too great to ignore and make up for with wisdom alone. Now the loss of aerobic capacity has become roughly 14 percent lower than it was in their mid-20s. This aerobic capacity drop is also reflected in functional threshold power (FTP), which is in an obvious decline, along with other performance markers such as sprint power and stamina. Wisdom by this

Osteoporosis is certainly a concern in cycling. The best solution for a dedicated cyclist is weightlifting.

point is found in how decisions are made about training rather than on-the-fly race decisions with younger riders.

When most riders become 50-something it's apparent that racing with those in their 20s and 30s is no longer a challenge they are up to. Too much of their fitness has gone south. Racing is largely confined to their peers by this time. Oh, there are some riders who can still challenge the best youngsters, but they are few and far between. However, every club seems to have one. These are the "super agers."

By the time we're in our 50s there are a lot of changes taking place in the body. The most concerning are the early stages of osteoporosis and sarcopenia. The first has to do with a decrease in bone density and the other with the loss of muscle mass.

Osteoporosis is certainly a concern in cycling. Even riders in their late 20s who have been riding since their early teens are sometimes found to have the bones of a 70-year-old person. That's because riding a bike does not place enough stress on the bones to fortify them the way running does. A 50-year-old rider crashing often results in an extremely serious condition that may negatively affect the rest of their life. What can be done to reduce the seriousness of such a situation? The best solution for a dedicated cyclist is weightlifting. You may recall from an earlier chapter that I recommend all riders include strength work in their training primarily for the legs. That will keep lower body osteoporosis at bay. By the time riders are in their 50s that needs to also include some upper body bone-building. Think of upper body strength exercises as being push or pull. Include one of each in your weekly gym workouts. Examples of such exercises are bench press (push), bicep curls (pull), lat pull downs (pull), weighted rows (pull), and tricep extensions (push). Just as with the leg exercises I described in Chapter 4, vary the weight loads seasonally.

Sarcopenia is not likely to be leg-related for the serious rider. This is one time when riding a bike is greatly beneficial. Cyclists of all ages tend to have very muscular legs. But the aging rider's upper body musculature may well be in decline. The exercises recommended to offset osteoporosis will also help turn around the drop in above-the-waist muscle mass. Something else that has been shown as beneficial for rebuilding muscle is a dietary shift toward more protein. There are several studies that have found older riders benefit from eating a protein-rich diet. Of course, you can't just increase calories for obvious reasons. If you take in more protein then something needs to be trimmed back. I'd recommend eating less carbohydrate, especially starches and sugars, to take in more protein.

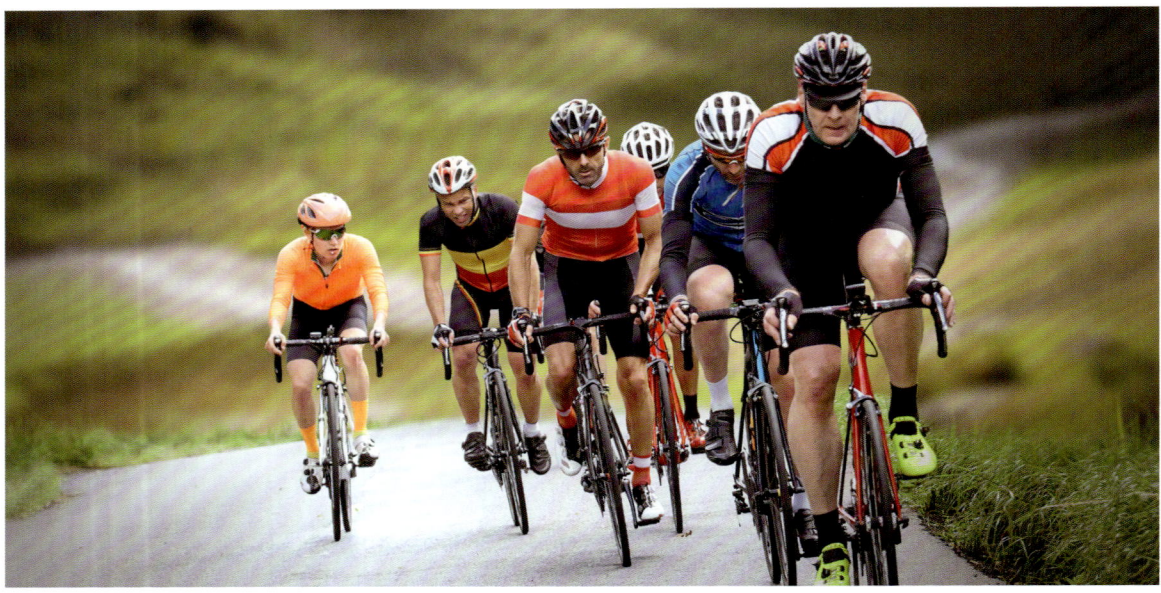

YOUNG RIDERS

I once had a father call me to ask if I would coach his son as, "He's the next Lance Armstrong!" Needless to say, I didn't agree to coach the teenager, and I never heard of him again. There are lots of father-child stories like this. My son, Dirk, once told me of a very good junior cycling buddy whose father was his coach and drove him to train at the highest level possible, much as a pro. The workouts were exceptionally demanding for a young rider with extremely long and hard sessions. Dirk said that his buddy often didn't follow his dad's training plan. He knew, even as a teenage rider, that the workouts were over the top. The story goes that he would start out on a long, demanding ride, stop under a tree to take a nap, and then ride home several hours later. I've run into lots of stories like these. Such tales exemplify the worst thing about coaching juniors is often their parents. The kids are usually a lot of fun to work with.

How do I get my kid into cycling? That's a great question and I certainly encourage parents to help their children take up a sport such as cycling—if the child wants to. This is something you can't force. The best way to do this, I believe, is to be a good role model by being a cyclist, runner, triathlete, swimmer, Nordic skier, or regular participant in some other sport that you obviously enjoy. If you truly love your sport, it will likely rub off on your kids. This is something you can't make happen.

If you'd like examples of how other junior cyclists became top competitors on the world stage, I'd suggest reading the biographies of some of the sport's best, such as Eddy Merckx, Laurent Fignon, Greg LeMond, Bernard Hinault, and others. I'd also suggest treating your child's involvement in sport as a lifetime activity, not as a short-term attempt to be the next Tadej Pogačar. And most of all, have fun riding with your child. In later life you'll come to see these times together as the highpoints of your life.

KEY TAKEAWAYS

- Aerobic capacity typically begins to decline when an experienced rider is in their early 30s.
- For a very active athlete the rate of decline of VO2 max is less than 1 percent per year.
- Training and racing experience often offset the loss of physical fitness for the 30-something rider.
- By the time we are in our 50s the physical performance changes are usually too great to overcome with experience.
- Two of the greatest physical changes for the aging athlete are osteoporosis and sarcopenia, which can both be offset by doing strength work.
- A shift toward more protein in the diet helps to offset sarcopenia when combined with weightlifting.
- Parents of promising junior riders are often overly involved in their child's progression as an athlete.
- The best way to get your child started in cycling, or whatever sport they most enjoy, is to be a good example as a lifetime commitment to your sport.
- Research supports the idea that participating in a variety of sports as a junior is preferable to specializing for later success in a sport.
- To learn how the young cyclists became world class, read their biographies—you'll learn a lot about growing up as a cyclist.
- To encourage your child, continue to participate in the sport and train together often.

THE REST OF RALPH'S STORY

I coached Ralph for more than seven years—the longest I coached any athlete. During that time, he won his age group in a local triathlon, an accomplishment he had never achieved before. And later that season he finished second at a national-caliber race, qualifying him for the Triathlon World Championship. Goal achieved! That fall he finished 12th in his age group at Worlds. He was ecstatic. Despite his multisport success, he eventually moved away from triathlon and began to race his bike more often. That was his first love.

Ralph became a very good cyclist in his region and was often on the podium, including a silver medal at the Wisconsin State Road Championship. He and I are still great friends and in frequent contact. He's a full-time cyclist now and has a coach who is doing a good job for him. While I've never brought up the topic of nutrition since we worked together, he has told me that he still eats a varied diet, including vegetables, fruits, and animal products—with an occasional bagel.

9.
RACE DAY

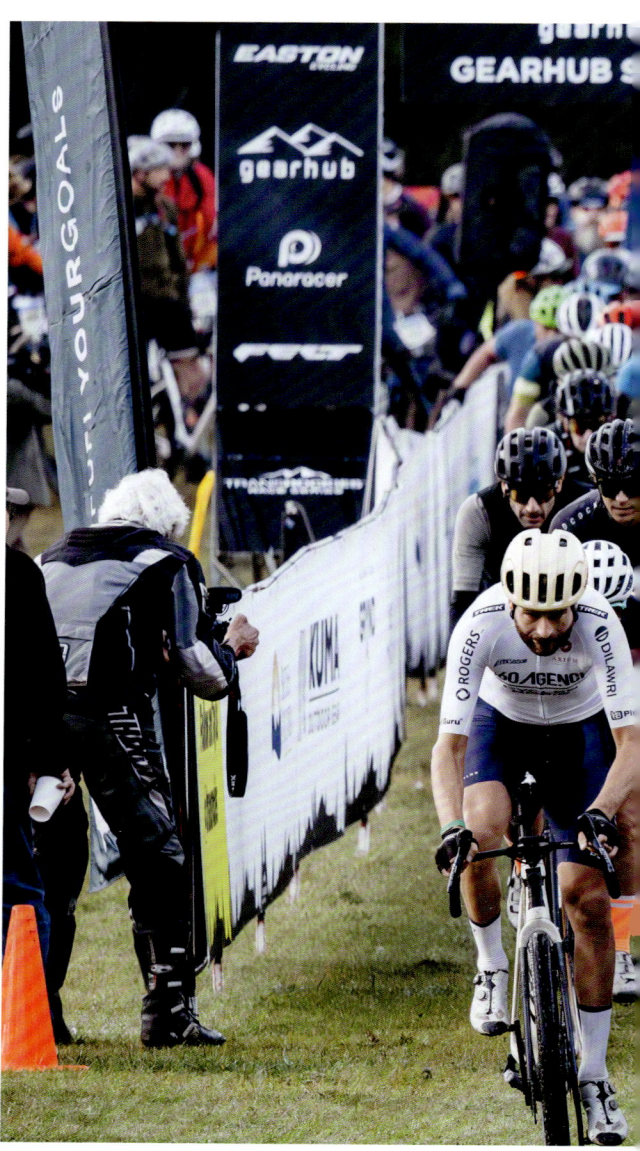

In this chapter we'll investigate two race-day conditions over which you have no control, although they can seriously impact your performance. Here I'll give you some ideas on how to prepare for two of the worst scenarios that you are likely to experience at a race—heat and high altitude. Then we will dig into the details of your Race period, including at how to be ready on race day, and finish with post-race considerations that wrap up your season.

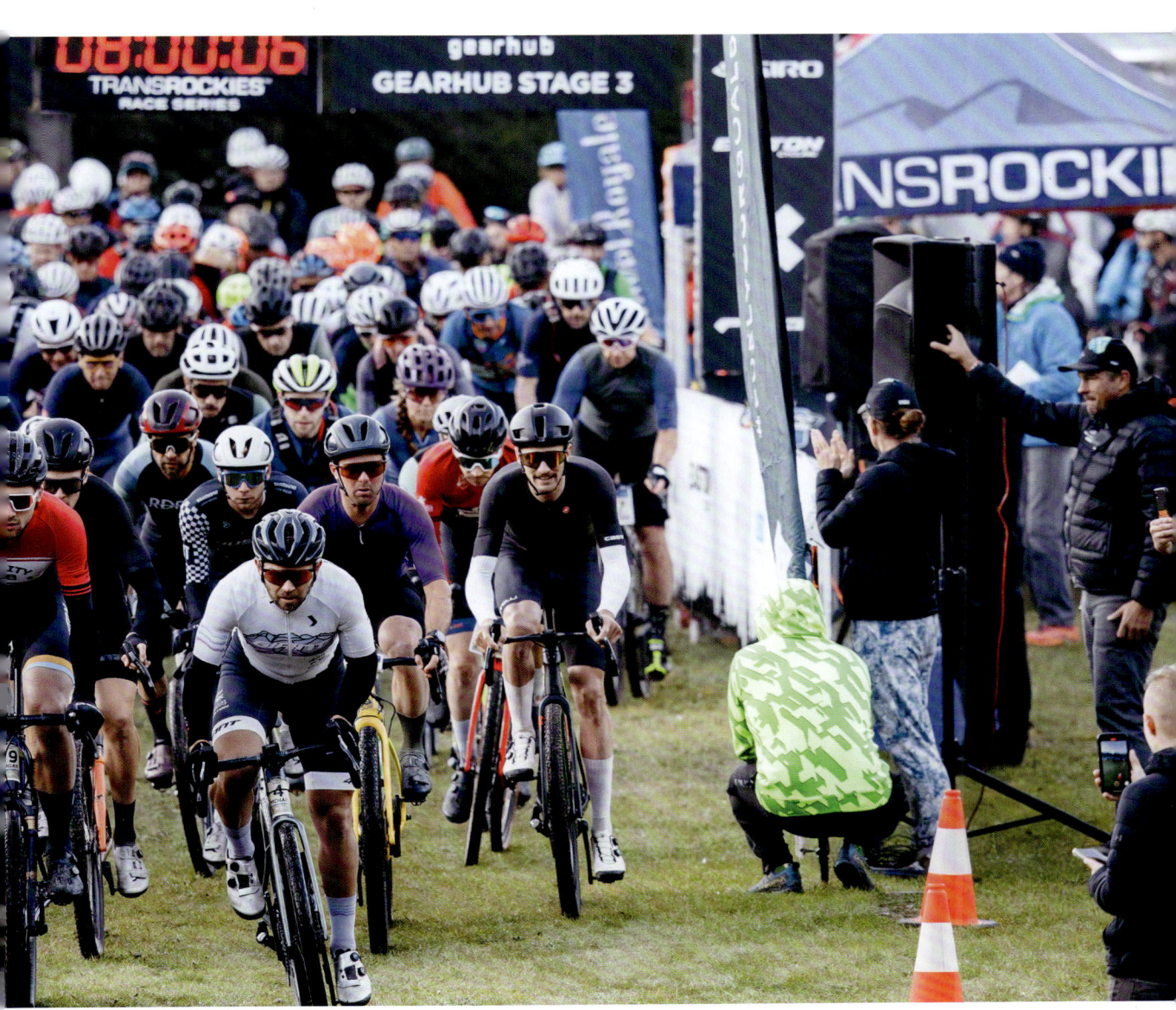

JOHNNY'S STORY

Seen from a very broad perspective, and from a coach's point of view, there are three types of athlete. First, there is the high-motivation, limited-ability athlete. This category makes up most amateur, age group athletes. They are a great pleasure to coach as they try hard to excel. But nature just wasn't on their side at conception. As hard as they may train, they just can't seem to achieve at a high level. It's very frustrating for them. The second type of athlete has great ability but is lacking in motivation. This athlete frustrates the coach. When training consistently they can race at a very high level. They may never realize an excellent performance, however, due to sketchy training. Third is the high-motivation, high-ability athlete. This is the rider who performs consistently at a high level.

Such an athlete is the coach's dream client. But there are very few of them. There's a fourth type of person, but they seldom take up sport, unless it's strictly about "health and fitness." But even then, it is rare. This is the low-motivation, low-ability person. They make up a huge chunk of the population. Their most-common connection with sport is watching it on television. As a coach, I've never had such a client. They are common in the general population, but rare in coaching.

Johnny was a type two rider. He was very talented—perhaps the most talented rider I have ever coached. Before I started working with him, he had won the National Junior Cycling Championship. But by the time he came to me for coaching, he was a few years older and his drive to succeed was beginning to fade considerably, as I later discovered. When we first talked about a coach-athlete relationship for the coming season, I could tell he was mostly going through the motions of training at a high level. When we talked about racing, he was all ears. But he didn't seem to have the same enthusiasm for riding day after day. As a coach, what I saw when we first met to talk about working together that day was that he had tremendous talent. It was hard to turn down such an athlete. They are rare.

He was quiet and a bit introverted. I realized this at the time, but I had coached many such athletes before. That's not a problem. In fact, I'm much the same way, only without the national championship on my palmarès. But as I coached him, certain things became apparent. I learned that he had very strong support from his parents, and that this seemed to be his primary reason for staying in the sport. It was expected of him. That wasn't obvious at first. I agreed to coach him and was excited to have such a talented athlete to work with. Then we got down to business.

We began working together just as the Base period was starting a few months prior to his first A race. At the time it was winter in Northern California, where he lived. I noticed little things in his training that raised red flags. Interestingly, the most concerning had to do with the weather. When the weather prediction was for snow, he'd decide ahead of time to skip the next day's workout. If it even looked like it might rain, he took the day off. He almost never rode indoors on a trainer. Too boring. Workouts were often abandoned due to a flat, equipment failures, late arrival for a group ride, or "just didn't feel like it today."

He missed most of the gym workouts. It was becoming quite frustrating for me, and we were only in the Base period.

Then as we came to early spring and the start of the Build period with better weather and occasional races, Johnny began to come around. Whenever there was a B or C race coming up, which was quite frequent in the spring, he trained much more reliably. He had two A races that summer. In the last few weeks before each his training improved considerably. And he was always considered a podium contender whenever he raced. He seemed to come to life as the season progressed. In fact, I had never had a client who was so focused in the late Build, Peak, and Race periods. For about six weeks he was on top of the game. He seemed to be intent on making up for time lost earlier in the season. His tapers were always excellent. And he really came to life the morning of a race. But I knew there was a price to pay on race day for the substandard Base period. And it happened over and over.

THE SCIENCE OF THE WARM-UP:
TREVOR CONNOR

Warming up is as ubiquitous to cycling as having a bike or cycling shoes. Coaches and athletes have perfected the warm-up routine over decades of trial and error. It has become dogma, but a growing body of science is showing the traditional warm-up doesn't work nearly as well as we think and, in some cases, may actually hurt performance. And what the research shows does work, isn't catching on.

To understand this disconnect it's important to first know why we do warm-ups. One of the most cited reasons is to heat or literally warm up our muscles. Having warmer muscles is also believed to prevent injury. A third reason is VO_2 priming, which is a fancy way of saying a warm-up gets our aerobic engine fully revved up before the race. Finally, there's post-activation potentiation or PAP. Our muscles won't contract fully when they're rested. We need to do a few explosive efforts to get our muscles to activate or "potentiate" fully. For a track cyclist who needs to put out maximal wattage off the line, having fully potentiated muscles is critical.

What the research shows is that while the traditional warm-up generally accomplishes all four of these things, it still frequently doesn't help performance. So why is that?

One explanation is that these benefits aren't as important as we traditionally thought. VO_2 priming has been shown to only last 10 minutes and has no impact on performance. PAP has similarly been questioned. Some think the benefits of a warm-up are actually more anaerobic in nature and only help in the first few minutes of an event that starts hard. If an event is long or starts easy, it really doesn't matter if you warm up at all.

Another explanation is the impact of fatigue. While the traditional warm-up produces many benefits, it can also raise lactate levels, lower pH, and increase other markers of fatigue. The result is that the side effects can outweigh the benefits.

In other words, the traditional 45-minute warm-up with several ramp-ups and six to eight sprints is too long and too hard.

What is best? First, remember that a warm-up only helps in the first few minutes of a race. So, a true structured warm-up is only needed for events that are explosive or hard from the start—criteriums, time trials, and track events. To avoid too much fatigue, keep it to 15 to 20 minutes of moderate riding to warm your muscles. PAP and VO_2 priming are important, but it doesn't take much. Three or four six- to 10-second sprints will get you there. That's it.

If you're doing a three-hour road race, rolling around the parking lot is all you need. Use the time to assess the other riders. The experienced riders understand they don't need anything if the race starts easy, so if you see them on their trainers with a look of concentration on their faces, they're probably planning to blow up the race off the gun.

When doing a structured warm-up, you need time to recover after your last hard effort, but not so long you lose the benefits of the warm-up. Fatigue markers such as elevated lactate and lower pH take 30 minutes to fully recover, while the benefits of PAP and elevated muscle temperature only last 20 minutes. VO_2 priming is even shorter at about 10 minutes. Putting together the best balance seems to be finishing your last effort 10 to 12 minutes before your event start.

Wrapping your head around such a short and simple warm-up can be tough, but it consistently wins out in the research. The most important message is to avoid fatiguing yourself with too much intensity. Just remember that we are all individuals, so start with a shorter warm-up and then experiment.

In regard to where to warm up, there is nothing magical about the trainer. It just gives you more control and allows more focus—especially when you don't know the local roads. That said, if you're getting ready for a crit or time trial, nothing beats warming up on the course.

Finally, remember that hot and cold weather can have a big impact on performance and the fatigue or damage they cause can far outweigh a warm-up's benefits. Using heated clothing on your core and legs after a warm-up in cold weather has been shown to help. But, sometimes forgoing the warm-up altogether to stay in a warm car or an air-conditioned room is the best thing you can do.

Trevor Connor is a physiologist and coach who worked at the Canadian National Centre. He is now the owner of Fast Talk Labs, which produces top-quality information on endurance sports training science, and The Paleo Diet, a healthy eating science company.

CHALLENGING RACE CONDITIONS

It's always a good idea to choose A races that match your strengths and avoid your weaknesses. For example, riders who climb well are advised to enter races that have hilly terrain. But if you are not a climber, then such races are best avoided. For those who have excellent endurance and thrive on multi-hour events, long races are an obvious choice. But if you excel at short, fast races it's probably not wise to do long ones. Unfortunately, however, there are times when you have no choice. You've simply got to do a race that's not right for you. For example, you're not a climber but your local championship will be held on a rollercoaster course. Or the most important event of the series you're doing well in is a very long race, but you're more of a short-course specialist. So, what do you do? Just ride the best you can, and hope things go your way? That's not a practical race plan. It's just wishing and hoping. You need to prepare for whatever conditions are expected. That may mean working on your climbing or building more endurance. Such limiters must be realized early in the season, so you have time to prepare.

Let's take it up a notch by examining a couple of the worst race conditions, that are also quite likely, and putting together a plan for each. What if your national championship, a race that comes at the peak of your season and which you've been focused on, happens to be in a very hot location this year? Or perhaps it will be contested at high altitude. And you live and train in a relatively cool place at sea level. Heat and altitude are probably the harshest race conditions imaginable for your A race. These are the conditions most riders would like to avoid, but sometimes you have no choice. The only consolation is that the two almost never occur at the same event as high-altitude races usually have cool weather. How do you prepare for such challenging race conditions? Let's take a deep dive into each.

PREPARING FOR A HOT RACE

Here's the bad news. Your A race this year is at a very hot location and your start time is in the hottest part of the day. What will you do? The bottom line is that there's only one way to prepare for a hot race—you must train in the heat. That sounds simple enough, but what if where you live and train is comparatively cool? Perhaps you could travel a bit and train for one weekend where it's hot. Or perhaps you could spend a couple of back-to-back weekends training there. Unfortunately, it's not that easy. That strategy just won't work. Training for a hot race day is not simple. In fact, the more you learn about heat adaptation, the greater the challenge becomes. For example, research has shown that it takes 10 to 14 days of near-continuous exposure to heat to acclimatize. Why so much time? Heat is one of the most challenging conditions you can encounter for a race. That means going somewhere that's hot to train for a couple of weeks. While that may be the best way to prepare, it's probably not realistic for you. You're simply not going to take two weeks away from your family and career to train at a location where it's hot every day. So, what can you do? Let's take a look.

If you don't adapt to the expected race venue's heat your chance of having a high-performance ride is highly unlikely. A rapidly rising core temperature on race day is the basic problem. It only needs to rise about one degree above normal to cause a catastrophic problem. This causes early fatigue in even the most fit riders. And the less adapted to the heat you are, the greater your chance of an elevated core body temperature and early race exhaustion. Depending on the severity of the heat on race day and the degree of your lack of adaptation, extreme fatigue may occur within the first 20 to 30 minutes after the gun. Your race could be over quite early. No amount of positive thinking or sodium-laced sports drink will rectify this. Your long season of focused training on this race was for naught.

But what if there's a way you can adapt to heat without leaving home? That would sure help. All you must do is get your core temperature to rise on most rides during a 14-day period. The simple explanation is that you need to sweat massively in training. And you would need to maintain that high-sweat rate for 60 to 90 minutes on most days for up to two weeks. The best time to do this may be in your two Peak period weeks. How might you go about training in the heat at home? Let's look at some options.

One adaptation strategy that may work for some riders who live in a moderately warm environment is to train in the hottest time of the day. The temperature needs to be in the range of 95 to 100 Fahrenheit (35 to 37 Celsius) for an hour or more over a two-week period. This could make the heat-adaptation challenge somewhat easy to manage. You could follow your training plan by doing easy rides in the hottest part of the day. This *must* be an AE1 workout that's truly easy. But since heart rate rises in the heat, it is probably better to think of this intensity as "very slow." Do not ride even moderately fast or use the higher power zones, including zone 2. It must be quite leisurely. Heat adaptation is not very responsive to intensity and is more a product of duration. Just get in saddle time on these days. Two days each week of the Peak period are hard days (see Table 5.5). These hard rides should be done in a cooler part of the day. This means that over a 14-day period you will get in eight heat adaptation rides. But your goal is to get a minimum of 10 such workouts. This means you need to get in two more hot rides at the end of the Build period or the start of the Race period. Or one in each of them right before and right after your Peak period.

Another heat-adaptation option if your locale is not hot enough is to wear layers of clothing to increase body temperature and promote heavy sweating. A cycling raincoat is a good option as they typically don't "breathe" much. Or you could simply dress for a winter ride even though it's summer—long sleeves, a jacket, leg covers, booties, and full-finger gloves. You'll get weird looks, but cyclists are used to that. Be very cautious when doing this. You're setting yourself up for possible disaster. Keep the rides no longer than one hour initially and up to 90 minutes at most in the second week. Make the duration increase in small bites over the two-week period. Don't rush it. And, as described above, keep the intensity slow. Again, these rides should be AE1 workouts only. No exceptions. You can still do your two hard rides weekly without the extra clothing.

Here's a third option, which is not quite as beneficial as the previous two but may better fit your lifestyle. Sit in a sauna or steam room for an hour daily for 10 to 14 days. This is not as effective as riding in the heat, but has some heat-adaptation benefits. This can be done before or after your daily rides. To make this even more effective, avoid air conditioning in your car, workplace, and home throughout the day. You may get some pushback on this from your fellow workers and family. After all, they probably aren't preparing for a hot race.

It's quite possible that none of the three options above will work for your situation, so let's look at a fourth option. The plan here is to simulate a hot environment. In a small space such as a laundry room or walk-in closet, set up your indoor trainer along with a space heater. Turn it on well before you plan to start your ride so that the room reaches 95 to 100 Fahrenheit (35 to 37 Celsius) prior to the workout. Then start your AE1 ride for an hour or so. If you don't have such a small room, another option is to use a tent that is tall enough to sit inside of on a bike and trainer. This could be done in a basement, garage, or even outdoors on a patio in the summer. If the room or tent doesn't get hot enough, wear extra layers of clothing. If everything is going as it should, you will sweat heavily throughout the ride.

Besides sweating, how do you know if you are adapting to a hot environment? Your heart rate monitor will tell you. Even though you are doing an AE1 ride, within a few minutes of starting, your heart rate should rise to 20 or more beats above your zone 1. And your rating of perceived exertion (RPE) will also go through the roof. As you adapt over the two-week period both will come back down at the same power output. They will undoubtedly remain high, just not as high as when you started doing such hot rides. This change is a good sign that you are adapting. Do not ride for more than an hour with your heart rate elevated by 20 or more beats per minute. When it comes down to less that 20 bpm high you can start extending your time in the hot environment regardless of which of the above methods you are using. That should happen within 10 days. Again, the upper time limit for a hot ride once this occurs is 90 minutes. And, of course, the workout remains as a slow and low-power AE1 even when going longer.

Regardless of which method from the above you use, it's imperative that you drink cold liquids throughout your hot rides. This will not only help you avoid a physical breakdown on the ride, but also keep your hydration level high enough that your blood does not thicken due to a heavy sweat rate. Highly condensed blood lowers aerobic capacity and power, making the ride harder than necessary. This also increases your risk of heat exhaustion while riding. At the first sign of excessive fatigue for such a slow ride, stop the workout. If you feel you are at your limit, regardless of how little time you may have ridden, stop the workout. No exceptions. Heat adaptation is not worth a trip to the emergency room.

As mentioned, the *hard* rides each week should *not* be done in a hot environment such as a small room or tent. But these rides may be followed by a "cool down" in your hot environment, on the bike or in a sauna, to help expedite the adaptation. In this situation, reduce the hot duration to 30 minutes or less.

Should you ever feel lightheaded, dizzy, or gasping for breath, stop the hot ride and cool off immediately. The best way to do this is to peel off extra layers of clothing; go to a cool, well-ventilated, or airconditioned room; sit or lie down; and sip an ice-cold glass of water or sports drink. Put ice packs on your head and torso. You'll need someone to help you do all of this. "Heat exhaustion" feels just as it's named—exhaustion. Should this happen, it means that something was wrong with your hot training environment that day. The conditions may have been too hot, you started the ride with too much fatigue, you were dehydrated at the start, or you overdid the workout intensity or duration. If this happens it is a serious situation. Do not do another hot ride until you've determined the cause and corrected it. If you return to heat training after a few days away from it (highly recommended), be very conservative with temperatures and ride durations.

When it comes to refueling in the heat, you're facing a double-edged sword. On the one hand, the need for carbohydrate increases during a hot ride, but the body does not process consumed carbs well in the heat. What the body does in this situation is to rely heavily on its storage form of carbohydrate—glycogen. Most of this glycogen is stored in the muscles. If you start feeling lightheaded late in a ride or race on a hot day, it may be because your body is running low

Training in a hot environment not only prepares you for a hot race, but also boosts your aerobic capacity, stamina, and economy by increasing blood volume.

on glycogen. In other words, you're bonking. This is a common problem in a hot race or ride. As you gradually adapt to the heat your body will become better at processing fluid sources of carbohydrate, and you'll be able to avoid the dreaded bonk.

How long does your adaptation to heat last? This is important to know the week of the race, especially if you must travel to the event. It may also open the door for other options in heat training. Research suggests that heat adaptation lasts, at most, about 14 days after the culmination of heat-adaptive training. There will undoubtedly be a rapid loss of adaptation in the last few days of that two-week period. This means that you could heat-adapt for the first two weeks of a Peak period and then train as normal in your Race week. Another option is to start your 10- to 14-day, heat-adaptive training in the last Build period and then do easy, heat simulation rides three times weekly in the Peak and Race periods to maintain your heat adaptation.

Besides adapting to the heat and staying well hydrated in a hot A race, is there anything else you can do to keep your body heat under control on race day? Absolutely. Avoid the excess heat by staying out of the sun. Also, stay as cool as possible before the start. Wear an ice vest or frozen jersey, drink cold liquids to satisfy thirst, stay in the shade, and use a fan to keep your body temperature down during your warm-up.

To keep your core temperature down as much as possible during the race, pour cold water, if available, on your skin. That's been shown to be more effective than drinking cold water. But doing both is a good idea. Also, if available during the race, place small ice packs at the base of the back of your neck to dissipate heat. What you're trying to do is lower your core temperature by one degree or so. Some combination of these methods will help do that.

The good news from all this heat preparation, as mentioned in Chapter 5, is that training in a hot environment not only prepares you for a hot race, but also boosts your aerobic capacity, stamina, and economy by increasing blood volume. A hot race could be a blessing in disguise. Just be cautious with heat exposure both in training and on race day.

PREPARING FOR A HIGH-ALTITUDE RACE

How does the health risk of racing in the heat compare with the health risk of high-altitude racing? Hot races are dangerous due to the possibility of heat exhaustion and even heat stroke. Heat exhaustion results from the loss of fluids and sodium. Heat stroke is a serious medical emergency marked by the body being unable to control its internal temperature. This makes a race in a very hot environment extremely dangerous. It is not to be taken lightly. Racing at a high altitude can also result in an emergency that must be dealt with immediately. The common symptoms are shortness of breath, fatigue, headache, nausea, dizziness, and more. Being unprepared for a race at altitude can be just as dangerous as not being adapted to the heat of your race. With both conditions we are no longer talking about just race performance, but rather your health. Both are serious and can be life-threatening. Neither should be taken lightly.

Just as the best way to prepare for a hot race is to train in the heat, to prepare for a high-altitude race the best strategy is exposure to high altitude. The latter is a bit more challenging as you can't quite as easily simulate altitude in your home as you can a hot environment. For races at the most common high-altitude locales, such as the Rocky Mountains in the USA and the Alps in Europe, preparation usually requires several weeks spent at altitude to allow for adaptation. For the highest common race elevations of 6,500 to 8,200 feet (2,000 to 2,500 meters), that may require as much as three to four weeks of living and possibly training at the targeted altitude. I say "possibly" because preparing for high altitude is mostly dependent on total daily time spent there as opposed to doing workouts at the goal altitude. In fact, the most effective way to get ready for a race in the clouds, besides living there, is to train at a much lower altitude. That's because workouts at high altitudes will always be low intensity. You simply can't ride as fast in an endurance race at a high altitude as you can at a low altitude. Fitness may be lost by training at a high altitude. For example, in northern Arizona where I live it is common for elite runners to have multi-week camps in the city of Flagstaff at 7,500 feet (2,280 meters) and drive 45 minutes to do intervals at 4,300 feet (1,300 meters) in nearby Sedona. That way they can easily get 22 hours at altitude daily and yet still train fast at a lower altitude. Any workouts done at the higher altitude are very slow and easy. "Live high, train low" is the standard for altitude preparation.

Why would a workout—or race—at high altitude have a low intensity? It's because air pressure at high altitudes is lower than in your lungs. That makes it difficult to ingest gases, including oxygen, and pump it to the muscles. You breathe deeper and faster. The higher the elevation, the thinner the atmosphere and the harder you must breathe to inhale oxygen. Since most of the atmosphere's gas molecules are close to the earth's surface, the higher you go, the less there are. But the good news is that your body will adapt over about a three- to four-week "live high" period to this condition. You still won't be as fast as you have been at, say, sea level, but you'll breathe somewhat easier and lower your risk of altitude sickness. The bottom line is that your aerobic capacity will be lower the higher you go to race. But, of course, it's the same for everyone, including the competition.

At high altitude your body's iron stores are likely to decline. This, in turn, decreases the body's hemoglobin, which transports oxygen to the muscles. If deficient, it is very difficult to get an adequate iron intake from food alone. Supplementation is usually necessary. If you go to high altitude to train, I highly recommend having your iron status checked by your doctor three months prior to travel. If your iron level is low, talk with your physician about using a supplement. It's best to arrive at the high-altitude camp with a normal iron level as altitude is likely to negatively affect your capacity for adapting to a higher altitude. Adaptation is based on increasing your red blood cell count to carry more oxygen to the working muscles. Iron is a necessity for that change to happen.

Another commonly used option, besides living at high altitude for several weeks, is to purchase and sleep in a high-altitude tent. These are legal according to the World Anti-Doping Agency (WADA), but they are banned by some countries, including Norway and Italy. However, to entirely reap the benefits of such a tent you would need to spend most of your hours every day in it for at least three weeks—eight to 10 hours of sleeping in the tent daily is not enough time to cause an adequately adaptive response by your body.

That leaves a camp at altitude as the most effective way to prepare for your high-altitude race. If you live at a moderate altitude in the range of 5,500 to 6,500 feet (1,600 to 2,000 meters) and will be racing at an altitude of less than 7,500 feet (2,300 meters) you may find that you have little difficulty on race day, which makes all this discussion about adapting unwarranted. But if you live and train at sea level, 7,500 feet can be disastrous to performance—and health. You must adapt.

If you are fortunate enough to be able to travel to a high altitude to train, what should you do? In the first few days at your camp keep workout intensity low, zones 1 and 2 only. Sleep during those first few days could be difficult. Afternoon naps may help. Excessive training at altitude, especially intensity, can block adaptation. Again, keep your rides easy at first. After three to five days, you should be able to increase both your workout durations and intensities. Workouts will be considerably slower during your entire stay at altitude. If doing intervals, your power and speed will be noticeably lower than at home. If you can't come down to a lower altitude for your interval rides, adjust by making the hard portions shorter and the recovery intervals longer.

If you are simply unable to travel to a higher training venue for at least three weeks, here are some other high living and training possibilities. If you live at sea level and your race will be at 1,600 to 6,500 feet (500 to 2,000 meters), arrive at the venue three to five days before the race. If your race will be at 6,500 to 9,800 feet (2,000 to 3,000 meters), arrive one to two weeks prior. And if your race is higher than 9,800 feet (3,000 meters), arrive at least two weeks prior. While these options are minimal to get at least a bit of adaptation, they may still be unrealistic for you. So, what is another option?

If you simply can't take the time to attend a high-altitude training camp, and the race isn't extremely high relative to where you live, you may be able to make the most of your situation by determining when you will arrive prior to your race. This mostly has to do with those times when high altitude just makes you feel run down and possibly sick. The time when most athletes feel terrible is in the range of one to three days after arrival. Arriving four or more days early could give you all the exposure you need to still produce a good race. You may still feel somewhat under the weather for a few days, but you should come around prior to race day. If it's not possible for you to arrive at the race venue four or more days prior to the race, plan to arrive no more than 24 hours before your race start time. The typical range for feeling poorly at altitude is 24 to 72 hours. So, if not adapted, get there either the night before the race or just prior to the start, leaving only enough time to settle in and warm up.

KEY TAKEAWAYS

- To prepare for a hot race you must be exposed to heat for 10 to 14 days.
- Racing well in extreme heat without first adapting is dangerous.
- Heat adaptation workouts should be, at most, 60 to 90 minutes long.
- If you can't train outside in high temperatures where you live, you can simulate and achieve the same benefits by training indoors.
- All workouts in hot conditions must be slow and low power, although it may feel hard.
- Your heart rate in hot workouts will give you feedback on how well you are adapting.
- Stay well hydrated during hot rides to avoid heat exhaustion.
- Hard rides should only be done in cool environments; do not do them in high temperatures.
- A common problem when riding at high ambient temperatures is bonking; start such rides after digesting a high-carbohydrate meal.
- Heat adaptation training lasts, at most, about two weeks.
- Prior to the race, stay as cool as you can by staying out of the sun, wearing cool clothing, and drinking to thirst.
- During a hot race stay cool by putting ice packs on your upper back, by pouring cold water on your head, and by staying well hydrated.
- Training in the heat has been shown to boost fitness by increasing blood volume.
- Racing at high altitude is as threatening as racing in the heat.
- To fully prepare for a high-altitude race you must train at high altitude.
- At high altitude, your first sign that things aren't right is deep breathing.
- A common problem that interferes with adaptation to high altitude is having low iron status; have this checked prior to arriving.
- High-altitude tents are legal (with a few exceptions) but not as effective as traveling to high altitude.
- Be very cautious with training load and sleep for the first three to five days at altitude; err on the easy side for workouts and take naps.
- If you can't take the time to adapt to a high-altitude race, arrive at the venue either four or more days early or less than 24 hours before your start time.

RACE WEEK

With a week to go until race day there is still a lot you must get right to be fully prepared. The first is honing your "form"—readiness to race. How do you ensure that you are both physically and mentally ready to perform at a high level? We'll investigate that in the following sections. The racecourse and expected race day conditions must also be scrutinized. These both play a key role in your race strategy and tactics, and must be determined well before the start. You also must be dedicated to your personal needs, such as sleep and diet.

RACE-WEEK FORM

The week of the race is when your form usually becomes palpable. You'll sense it happening. If you are following the taper suggested in previous chapters, you should feel fresh and itching to race hard. As explained in Chapter 5, form means the absence of fatigue combined with the physical and mental readiness to race. When the peaking process works you will sense feelings you rarely experience. In fact, when riding in Race week, you may find it hard to hold back when the plan calls for an easy workout. What you are experiencing happens, at most, only a couple of times in a season. It's a rare sensation that must be treated with care and caution so as not to ruin it with only a few days until your A race. It would be very easy for you to screw up months of race preparation by wasting your new-found form on long, high-intensity group rides that are uncalled for. You must be cautious with your enthusiasm and patient with your workouts. Save it for race day.

As you shed fatigue by doing short rides in the race period week, you must also include some high-intensity, race-like efforts to maintain fitness. See Table 5.6 for details. These few high-intensity rides are necessary to come into form. Just as bad as overdoing it with hard rides, doing only easy rides with no high intensity at this point can also ruin your race day. Your form will be lost. You now need a blend of short, hard, and easy rides to sharpen your race readiness. Just be cautious not to make your high-intensity rides also long rides—you will be tempted to. Your endurance is now well established and won't fade in the last few days before your race unless you stray from your purpose during the week. If you are patient, you will come to feel indestructible. Hold back.

RACE STRATEGY AND TACTICS

To define your race strategy and, eventually, your race-day tactics, you need to start with the desired outcome—it should match your goal—and then work backwards. What must you achieve along the way from the finish back to the start? If this is a team race, the starting place is talking with teammates about what to expect and your team's tactics from start to finish. This should have been mostly decided within the last few days. Now you only need to put a ribbon on it. Of course, the primary goal of the team is to assist this race's team leader. You must precisely understand your responsibilities and how they blend in with your teammates' race-day roles. Of course, your team role should also fit nicely alongside your personal goal for the race. They must not conflict. You should already know what your strengths and weaknesses are relative to this course and your competition. It's time for the team to discuss how the pieces should all come together.

What if something happens early in the race that hinders or even negates your plan? This could be the loss of a key teammate due to a crash or other unexpected situations, such as a big breakaway that your team missed. The possibilities are many. If this means you can no longer achieve your primary goal, then it's time for Plan B. What is your team's next best alternative outcome for the race? How do *you* fit into Plan B? These are the sort of things your team should have discussed well before race day. Coming up with a last-minute Plan B during the race is next to impossible. Be prepared.

Also, realize that it's not always the fittest and fastest rider who wins. The race outcome is often decided by who prepared the best. It comes down to who stayed the most focused for weeks on exactly what is necessary to achieve a specific goal and then carried out the tactical plan with precision. In cycling, success often comes to the smartest, not the fastest. The smartest rider is well positioned in the pack and expends energy at only the appropriate times. Energy is never wasted. The smart rider sees well in advance how the race is likely to turn out and prepares for the expected situations. Race-day preparation is both physical and mental. Physically, the rider strives to be situated in an

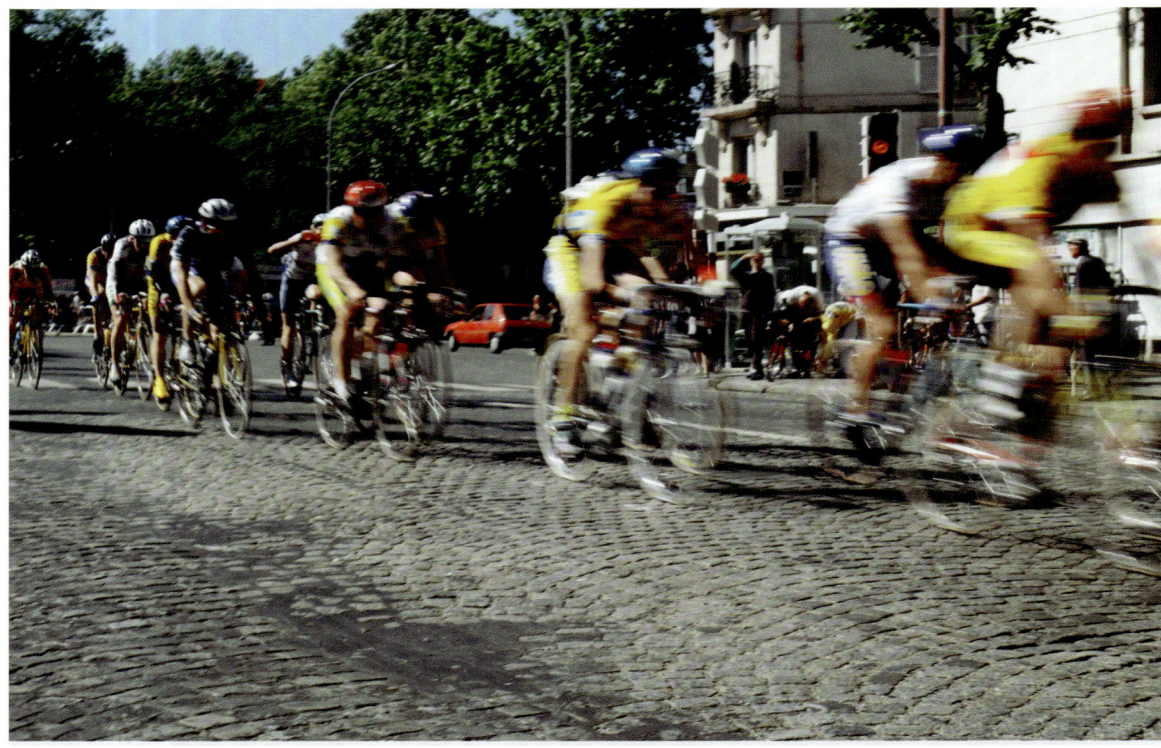

appropriate place in the pack. Mentally, the rider is always considering what is happening throughout the race. There is little time for a physical or mental break. Stay focused.

The reason for all your group rides and B and C races throughout the season was to put you in lots of situations in which you had to make quick decisions. What you've learned in these situations forms the basis upon which your decisions will be made on race day. You seldom have time to ponder all your options in the heat of battle. Decisions must be made very quickly. There is rarely enough time to analyze. Experience is the foundation for fast decisions. Trust your preparation on race day.

Prior to race day review how the race has played out in past years. Were there strong teams that dominated from the start, or did it come down to a sprint? Who won? How did prior years' riders win? How did weather in previous years affect the outcomes? Do your research on all such critical questions several weeks prior to Race week. Be prepared.

If your A race is a time trial, mountain bike, cyclocross, gravel, gran fondo, cyclosportive, or other more individualized event, what do you want your race outcome to be? This also reflects your goal for the season. Is your goal to win the race, podium, finish with the leaders, finish within a certain time range, or just finish? Or something else? The week of your event, review your tactics in support of your strategy. Start by considering the race terrain—climbs, descents, corners, wind, course conditions—and their impact on *your* race performance. Also, consider your competition. What are their known strengths and weaknesses? Be realistic. All of this should have been addressed well before race day so your training would be focused on the event outcome.

RACE WEEK SLEEP

Riders often have poor sleep as they get closer to race day. This may be compounded by flying to the race venue, especially if traveling east. A step toward improving your sleep is to arrive at the race venue at least two days before the event and become comfortable with your sleep quarters. Sleep is often the greatest problem when not at home. Traveling east by three or more time zones can be very hard on your normal sleep and other lifestyle patterns. You can, however, at least partially adapt to the new eastern time zone in advance of your travel. Begin by adjusting your daily schedule to your event's time zone by changing your daily routines—especially sleeping and eating patterns—by 30 minutes daily for three- or four-days prior. Going to bed earlier each night, awaking at an appropriate race-venue time, and eating a bit earlier in the last few days before traveling will help you adjust your internal clock. The more time zones you cross traveling east makes this quite challenging. But even a one-hour adjustment helps. In contrast, traveling west is usually much less difficult and the lifestyle and sleep adjustment can usually be made quite easily. Why is this so? Relative to your internal clock, traveling west essentially makes the days longer and traveling east makes them shorter. Shorter days are difficult to adapt to.

If there is no time-zone change, sleeping in a new environment can still be a challenge. Arriving at the race venue two days or more early and becoming accustomed to the new conditions, especially where you will sleep and what you eat, can be the difference between a poor and good performance on race day. Should you have to arrive on the day prior to your race, the cards are stacked against you.

One night of poor sleep has been shown to affect next-day race performance in several types of endurance sports, including a cycling time trial. And the negative effects of poor sleep prior to a race are not limited to just the physical side of riding. Loss of sleep has also been shown to negatively affect decision-making ability.

THE DAY BEFORE THE RACE

The most important activity for this day is to check out the course. Depending on your event, you can probably preview at least a part of it on your bike. The rest may be done by car. Take special note of the locations of challenging course conditions, such as the grades and lengths of hills, corners and especially a series of tight turns, off-camber turns, roundabouts or street "furniture," and road surface or terrain conditions. Check your weather app the day before to see what wind speeds, directions, and gusts are expected, along with predicted temperatures and the possibilities of precipitation. Also note how far you are staying from the race start. Plan how you will travel there on race day while taking into consideration how long it will take to ride or drive to the venue. Plan to arrive earlier than necessary—just in case.

What you do with your lazy day at your temporary quarters is also important. After getting in a ride and checking out the course, there may be other activities planned for this day by the race director and, possibly, by your team or coach. Your team meeting should include a review of the course, the anticipated weather, strong teams, the fastest and smartest riders, and the team's race-day plan. Make sure you fully understand your role in the plan.

All of this is likely to take at least a couple of hours, if not more. What you do with the remainder of the day depends on what you know works best for you the day before a race. You may hang out with friends, watch television, go to a movie, take a bus tour of the city, or go out for meals. Other than a short ride with a few, brief high-intensity efforts, stay off your legs for most of the day before the race.

What you eat today should be light and easily digested, and preferably the types of food you typically eat. Now is not the time to check out new and unusual cuisine. The evening before the race, lay out your race kit and check your bike by looking for loose connections, tire wear, chain lubrication, and smoothness of shifting. Get to bed at a time which is normal for you with considerations for the time zone and optimal sleep conditions you noted from the night before.

The day before also review your race day fueling and hydration plan. What food and fluids will you carry in your pockets and on the bike? Where are the course feed zones? You may also remind yourself of how important taking in adequate fluids is to race performance.

Throughout the day prior to the race your mind is likely to be active with a lot of random, race-related thoughts. These commonly fall into two broad categories: things you *can't* control and things you *can* control. Those that are out of your control include the competition, weather, what's happened in the past, and the race outcome. Do not waste your time on these thoughts. They offer no benefit to your race mental readiness. Dismiss them immediately. Instead, give your attention to those things you can control, such as commitment to your goal, strategy and tactics, course conditions, accepting the results regardless of the outcome, and positive self-talk. Your mind must be as ready to go as your body.

Before calling it a day and crawling into bed, I'd strongly suggest reviewing what you've done in the past few months to prepare for this A-priority race. You've focused for several months on doing the appropriate workouts at the right times, getting adequate recovery, including quality sleep, eating the right foods, and managing stress. You've left no stone unturned. You are ready for this race.

When you go to bed that night, review recent successes you've had in training and racing. Mentally relive one of your greatest accomplishments on the bike, whether in a race, group ride, or hard workout. Repeat this success over and over until you fall asleep.

KEY TAKEAWAYS

- By following the tapering plan you will begin to come into form—do not be inspired to train longer and harder.
- Your team's race strategy should be formed well in advance of the race and not conflict with your personal race goal.
- While you and your team should have a plan for the race, it's a good idea to have a Plan B (and maybe C) as well.
- The smart rider is constantly reading the race to be prepared for when something critical happens.
- The hard group rides, and B and C races, over the course of the season should have mentally prepared you for this A race.
- Before the start, review how the race progressed in previous years and be mentally ready for such situations.
- Come to the start line well prepared; know your strengths and limiters, and those of your competition.
- If traveling to your race, particularly if it's over several time zones, have an arrival lifestyle plan that addresses sleeping and eating.
- Even if you've done the race before, check out the course just in case something has changed.
- What you do off the bike in Race week is based largely on your past race experiences, but a key maxim is *do not waste energy*.
- The specifics of race day have to do with what you know works for you, especially when it comes to eating; try nothing new.
- Prior to the race, your mind should *only* be focused on those things you can control.

RACE DAY

Start your day, as much as you can, as any other day. That may include what you eat and drink and any other common morning routines such as stretching, checking your heart rate variability and pulse, reading the news, checking the weather, or whatever gets your day going comfortably. Plan to arrive at the start in plenty of time to become acquainted with the venue setup while leaving time for a warm-up. Realize that things on race morning often take longer than was expected the day before. Allow for some spare time. It's better to have a little too much time on your hands prior to the start than to rush around trying to get things in place at the last minute.

WARM-UP AND START

On the way to the start, review where and how you should warm up. The exact location should have been determined the day before. Continue to keep your thoughts positive while considering only that over which you have control. Mentally review a checklist of your race strategy and tactics several times. Tactics should include how you will react in expected situations. Once at the start venue take a few minutes to speak with friends and teammates about life in general. Be upbeat and positive in all conversations. When the time is appropriate, prepare your bike for the warm-up. This is when your mind begins to narrow the topics you think and talk about as you become more focused. Let other non-race matters fade into the background. Now is when you start getting your mind ready to race.

Warm up as you usually do before a hard workout or race. This is also a last chance to review your race strategy and tactics. While warming up remind yourself how you will know if you had a successful race. Also, review what it is you most want to achieve in the race and how you are going to do that.

Once the race starts, be patient. Charging away from the start line of a long road or gravel race is usually done by those who are new to the sport and have little race experience. Patience is the key. Review your tactics once again. Regardless of your race type, wait until the time is right before making a decisive move. Consider in advance how you will know the right time.

On the other hand, some event types, such as criteriums, cyclocross, and mountain bike races, usually require a hard effort of several minutes right from the start. Expect this and have a plan for how you will manage it. For some events and course types this can be a make-or-break moment.

RACE REFUELING

Eat and drink in the race just as you have done in hard workouts, and in B and C races. Try nothing new. Stick with your race-day nutrition and hydration plan. All of this should have been refined in your training, especially on days of high-intensity workouts, fast group rides, and low-priority races. Now is not the time to try something new. Stick with what you know works, even if it's not perfect. Save the experimenting in search of perfection for training rides and low-priority races. The longer your race, the more critical fueling is to your success. Long races, especially, are a refueling competition.

THE MENTAL RACE

In a mass start event, it always comes down to reading the race. This means paying attention to other riders, especially in the latter half of the race. Listen to their breathing—labored or light? Pay attention to their pedaling—circles or squares? How often and how much are they drinking and eating? Are they staying adequately fueled and hydrated? Who is wasting energy? Watch for signs of fatigue on climbs and coming out of corners. Decide who looks weak and who appears strong. Stay in the moment but sense what other smart riders may do, given what you've observed in the current situation.

If your event is a time trial, you must come to it with a well-rehearsed pacing plan. It's common to use intensity metrics, such as heart rate and power, to help assess your race effort. Just be aware that in the first few minutes you will feel unbelievably powerful. That feeling, however, will soon fade away. If you accepted your super-fitness at face value and went out too hard, you'll eventually fade and finish poorly. This can't be avoided. Have a plan for how you will pace your race and constantly remind yourself that you must stick to it. Also remind yourself throughout the warm-up exactly how you will get the early intensity right. Then be sure to stay with your plan regardless of how great you feel. If you truly are experiencing a great leap of new fitness, still hold back at the start. You can always call on your new-found fitness later in the race.

What if you are doing a cyclocross or a mountain bike race? How do you pace that? In such races there is no time for looking at numbers on your handlebars. It's all mental. Constantly gauge how you feel, realizing that your sensations early on will be misleading. Racing based on feel is very difficult to do, especially early in the race. This is a mental skill that comes only from experience. That's one reason you train. The more such races you do, the better you will become at gauging perceived exertion.

KEY TAKEAWAYS

- Arrive at the race start with plenty of time to spare.
- During the warm-up, review your race strategy and tactics.
- Be prepared physically and mentally for how you expect the race to start.
- Refuel in the race just as you have planned based on your experience of what works well for you.
- Pay close attention during the race to your competition.
- When racing a time trial, have a pacing plan that you have rehearsed and stick with that.
- For cyclocross and mountain bike races, intensity is gauged strictly by perceived exertion.

POST-RACE

There are three or four things that must happen in the 24 hours following your race. The purposes are to make your world of bike racing a friendly place, tighten your team's bonds, and analyze what happened in the race. That's three. The fourth is entirely up to you, as I'll explain.

IMMEDIATELY AFTER THE RACE

On finishing, the first thing you should always do after greeting and praising your team members is find your primary competition and congratulate them for a good race or offer consolation for a poor outcome. They are the reason you raced so well. Treat other riders with the same level of respect you expect from them. Do not, under any circumstances, be a poor loser. There is nothing to be gained and it will always come back to haunt you. That does not rule out speaking with race officials about something illegal or at least questionable that was done to you or your team. Condense your complaint and present it to the proper officials in a calm and concise manner. Otherwise, regardless of the outcome, be kind and friendly with the officials and with your competitors. You are all in this together.

The next thing to do right after the race is to share thoughts on how you and the team did. You can get into a deeper analysis later. For now, what initial thoughts come to mind about how the race went? What did you do well? Were there obvious mistakes that could be easily corrected? Ask others for their opinions. What could *you* have done better? Learn something, no matter how small, from every race. This also goes for hard group rides. Grow as a rider from your errors and those of others. Never stop learning.

COOL-DOWN?

While it is quite common, not everyone accepts that a cool-down post-race is beneficial. Some see it as a waste of energy that will result in greater fatigue. Others believe it is necessary for the body to gradually return to a calm state, both physically and mentally. The roots of the cool-down go back to the days long ago when athletes, coaches, and sport scientists believed that lactate was the cause of exhaustion and to prevent soreness and fatigue the following day it had to be removed by easy pedaling post-race. Nobody in sport science still believes this, yet the cool-down remains popular. I doubt if it will cause you any harm, so feel free to ride easily for a while after finishing if you want to. While it may do nothing for how you feel tomorrow, it might help you to relax now.

CELEBRATE!

The last thing to do on race day is to celebrate what you and the team accomplished today. This could be a meal together or a brief meeting. No matter how marginal the outcome, there are always things that were done well. Build your team around these positive examples. Bringing the team together to share stories and show appreciation for what was accomplished is a step toward even greater outcomes in the future. Save the deep analysis for later.

IN-DEPTH ANALYSIS

Immediately after the race is not a good time to analyze how you or the team did. Emotions are running high and there may still be some confusion about what occurred. Of course, exactly what happened may be painfully or happily obvious. Still, give it a day to sink in. Avoid making changes to anything right away. Deep analysis is best done the following day so that you and others have time to let the many details of the race simmer. Be reluctant to draw immediate conclusions. You may think you know exactly what happened and why, but after talking with others and thinking about everything yourself, you may find things look different the following day.

The reasons for a good or poor race performance generally fall into some combination of seven broad categories: knowledge of the racecourse and conditions, the race plan, physical readiness, mental readiness, strategy and tactics, nutrition and hydration, and equipment. These form the crux of what you and the team need to consider going forward. Why did we race well or what explains our lackluster performance? What could we have done better?

If the race was not a team event—it was a time trial, mountain bike, gravel, cyclocross, gran fondo, or another more individualized event—the process described above remains the same.

KEY TAKEAWAYS

- Immediately after the race share thoughts and opinions with your teammates and then talk briefly with your main competition.
- Following the race, a cool-down at a very easy intensity is common, but not necessary; it's your call.
- Always find a reason to celebrate following a race.
- The day after the race is the time to do a deep analysis, but never on race day.
- The key question to be answered: why did the race turn out as it did?

THE REST OF JOHNNY'S STORY

Johnny was among the most talented athletes I ever coached. And in many ways, the best. He could do things on a bike that most good riders wouldn't even attempt. Despite his lack of motivation in the Base period, he always came to life the last few weeks before a big race. He had race smarts and knew how to read the peloton. He was an all-rounder who was good to great at sprinting, climbing, and time trialing. He was always in the right place at the right time in most race situations. But he still didn't perform as he should, given his talent. He was lacking an aerobic base. It always came back to haunt him late in a long race. He would have been nearly unbeatable if his motivation to train earlier in the year was greater. That season coaching Johnny was one of the gloomiest of my coaching career. He was a tremendous athlete but so much talent was wasted. I decided not to repeat it.

EPILOGUE

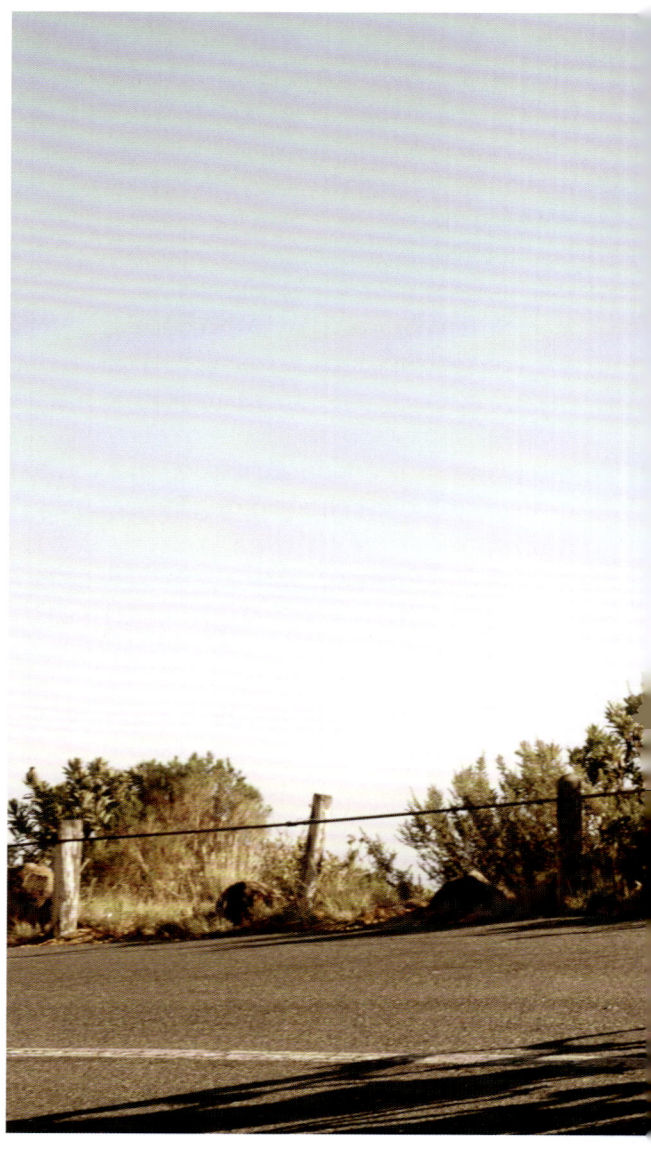

I've coached a lot of athletes. They've ranged from novice to elite. Regardless of ability, each had the same basic goal: to perform at a higher level. The nine athletes featured in the book's chapters are good examples of those I have coached. All ranged from good to great in their sports, and each, in their own way, was a high performer. You don't have to climb to the top step of the podium to get that label. However, you certainly need to put in the time and effort. But there's more to it than that. In those nine chapters I tried to narrow your focus to what must be done in training to race faster. I only touched the surface, I left a lot out. As I conclude this book, I want to comment on just a few topics that I also see as contributing to high performance. They probably aren't what you would expect.

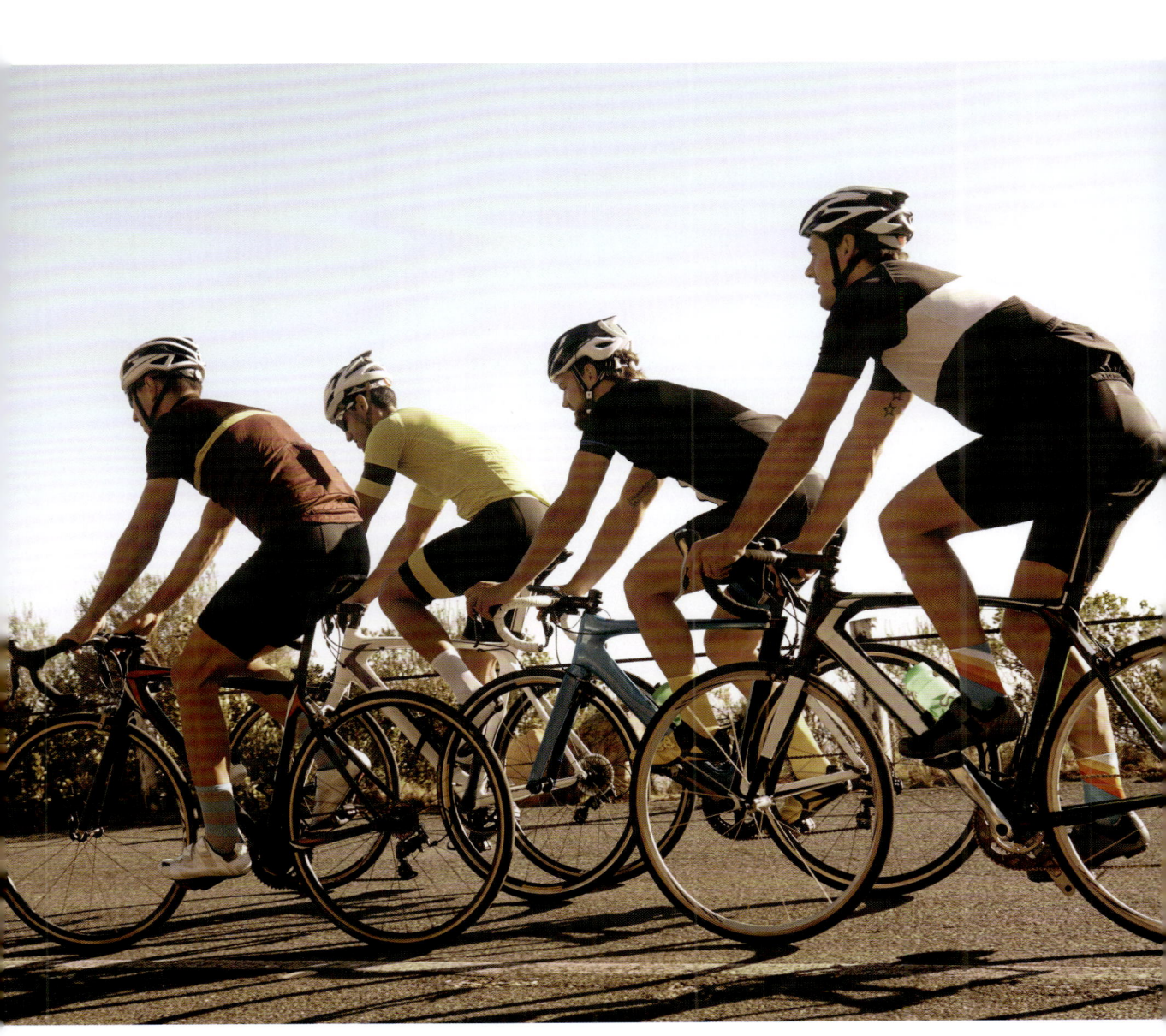

SIMPLICITY

This book is sure to make some riders think that training is complicated, especially planning the season. I apologize if that's the conclusion you've drawn having read it. My intent wasn't to make it difficult to understand. You may see it that way because I pointed out most all the details needed to help you get your training plan aimed directly at your goal. That adds a lot of complexity. Perhaps if I boil the planning part of the book down to one paragraph, you'll begin to see why I say that it doesn't have to be complicated to train for a high-performance race. Here is how I would condense the chapters on planning, which is a sizeable chunk of the book, into a single paragraph.

Focus on aerobic endurance and muscular strength in the Preparation and Base 1 periods. In Base 2 and 3 continue to grow your aerobic endurance while cutting back on weightlifting and including three *somewhat hard* rides weekly. Space them with easy, aerobic endurance rides mostly in zone 1 and some in zone 2. In the Build period maintain your aerobic endurance and do two race- and limiter-specific workouts weekly separated by easy rides. For the Peak period begin gradually cutting back on volume as you taper for the race while still doing two hard rides weekly. In the Race week period do short rides with a bit of high intensity to maintain sharpness. At the end of the season rest a lot and when you go for a ride, make it short and easy with no high intensity. Take one day off the bike each week throughout the season.

That's the heart of your training plan as described in this book in a single paragraph. Keep it simple.

CONSISTENCY

I've used the word "consistency" a great deal throughout this book. I've referred to this as being the core of success in endurance training. I've defined it as not missing workouts. It goes well beyond that, however. On the previous pages I've described how short-term fitness comes from high intensity and long-lasting fitness comes from consistency. My point was that if you train consistently and are patient, you are certain to improve. Now, at the end of the book, it's time to step back and look at this word from a different perspective.

Here's its dark side. There is a narrow divide between consistency and obsession. It doesn't take much to move from the first to the second. Obsessive behavior is marked by seldom taking a day off from training, refusing to ride easy when the training plan calls for it, frequently pushing your limits, denying you are tired when it's obvious to everyone that you are, and putting training above health and life in general. By doing such things you will, undoubtedly, train consistently, but high performance may not be the result. You are more likely to end up overtrained and, perhaps, unhealthy. Obsessive training often leads to burnout and the eventual abandonment of the sport. Unfortunately, this step from consistent to obsessed is a small one that happens so slowly you may not realize it.

As I write this, I have just learned that Dave Scott, arguably the greatest triathlete of all time, is facing open heart surgery. I've followed Dave's career since the 1980s when he won the Ironman© Triathlon World Championship in Hawaii six times. Now at age 70, and still very active and fit, he admits that he "exercised like a maniac" throughout his life and has learned that "more does not mean better." Sadly, his training went beyond consistent over a lifetime. He suggests that this is at the root of four serious heart conditions and the reason for his surgery. As you saw in Wes's story in Chapter 6, overtraining should not be taken lightly. Wes's experience led to an early end to his racing career. Dave's experience takes us well beyond overtraining.

The bottom line is that exercise is strong medicine. It's also quite good for your health—if you treat it with the respect you would any other powerful medicine. Unfortunately, some don't. Let's look at this from a different perspective. If your doctor recommended taking one pill daily for an ailment, I expect you would stick with the prescription dosage. Right? You surely wouldn't take two pills daily, believing that would end your health problem sooner, would you? Exercise should be seen in much the same way. There is a dosage which is right for you. That's not easy to nail down, but I tried to help you get it right in Chapters 4 and 5 (see Tables 4.1, 4.2, and 5.2). As you learned early in your reading here, there are three "pills" for athletic training—frequency, duration, and intensity. There is a dosage for each of these which is right for you. Taking more than is prescribed may be merely a problem in the short term. Doing that weekly, month after month, year after year, is sure to present health problems.

Keep your training consistent but avoid obsession. It's okay to ride very slowly, miss an occasional workout (everyone does), and take a day off. Riding should be one part of your life—not the reason for your life.

TRAINING BALANCE

The number one problem I run into with athletes who are determined to excel, which at its root is a good thing, is that they overtrain and under-rest. Workouts are too hard and rest is too infrequent. This is like obsessive training but is usually focused on one of the training "pills"—intensity. Such an approach to training usually leads to frequent fatigue and, possibly, a short cycling career. It's hard to keep high-intensity training going year after year. The Greek philosopher Socrates advised, "All things in moderation." That comes down to avoiding the extremes and choosing the mean in training as in life.

The bottom line is that you must go easy most of the time and hard only occasionally. The easy rides allow for R&R while building your aerobic fitness. And they result in your hard rides being truly hard and beneficial to your race readiness.

I certainly understand why riders train too hard. It seems logical that if you want to race fast, you need to train fast. I'm not opposed to that concept. It's how this solution is applied that is the problem. Your training should be mostly easy to develop an aerobic fitness base while the easy rides prepare you for the hard efforts. The easy part happens when you train in zones 1 and 2. So most of your training should be in those zones. A small amount of your training time should be planned to prepare you for the fast speeds of a race. It's easier to develop speed than aerobic endurance. Two or three fast rides each week will do it. I've proposed that in the Base period you include three weekly moderate-intensity rides, and in the Build and Peak periods you do only two weekly, high-intensity, hard rides (see Table 3.1). That will ensure that you come into the hard ride days fresh and ready to push your limits, and in the days after you have adequate time to adapt.

Also, riding in zones 3 and 4 when the workout calls for zones 1 and 2 will *not* make you faster. This will just make you tired, so that when you come to a truly hard-ride day you don't have the legs to test your limits. Of course, when you're tired the hard workout will feel hard. But the power numbers won't be what they could have been. I might also point out that the pros don't overtrain themselves by going moderately hard on what was meant to be easy days. Even they take it easy to fully develop their base aerobic fitness. They just ride faster than the rest of us when training easy. Their rating of perceived exertion (RPE) is quite low on easy days, as yours should also be. You must hold back. There is nothing to be gained by half-wheeling your training partners and trying to "beat" riders you encounter on the road. By riding more slowly on most days you will ultimately become faster. I've explained this phenomenon in multiple ways throughout this book. It's a critical lesson you *must* learn.

THE MOST IMPORTANT DATA

As you've probably figured out by now, I am a big believer in training-specific data analysis. With the athletes I've coached I've always tried to determine their limiters and then decide how I can measure progress in that area from their daily workout data. For example, a rider benefits from a bigger base of aerobic fitness by moving their carbohydrate-fat crossover point to the right (see Figure 8.1). That's a common need early in the season for everyone. I watch their efficiency factor (EF— a measure of how many watts per heart beat you produce when riding at a low intensity) methodically throughout the Preparation and Base periods to make sure we're making gains in that regard. When EF for similar rides is rising over several weeks you have a great indicator of improving aerobic fitness. But there's another EF which is even more important, and it needs to be monitored throughout the entire season, not just in the early season periods. Unfortunately, it's hard to measure precisely.

This EF is your "enjoyment factor." When you stop enjoying riding your bike and begin looking for reasons why you shouldn't train today, this EF is in decline. Something is wrong psychologically. I hope this doesn't happen to you. If it does, you've become a low-motivation athlete as described in Johnny's story in Chapter 9. What are the signs of a declining enjoyment factor? As with Johnny, the weather may become an excuse to skip a workout. Or you just don't feel like riding today. Or perhaps you have more important things you need to do. The list of excuses can be very long. But they all point in the same direction—the enthusiasm which you once had for the bike is in decline. There could be lots of reasons for this. A common one is that you've been pushing yourself too hard and not realizing the expected gains. Others may be lifestyle stresses, a crappy diet, lack of sleep, failure to achieve a goal, or unclear goals. This list goes on and on. You're burned out.

It could also result from the pressure of aiming for a very high goal. Perhaps it's a goal that you realize, deep down, is not realistic. A narrow focus on a goal you believe can't be attained often requires something akin to living the life of a Buddhist monk—only without the Buddha part. You're fried. To achieve high performance certainly does require deep commitment. But the goal must be realistic. To achieve such a goal will certainly mean setting aside other things in your life that you also enjoy. If the mental pressure continues even though the goal is within reach, the signs of a wavering enjoyment factor may simply be an indication that this is the wrong time for you and this goal. Perhaps you should let it go. Take a break.

Regardless of the underlying reason, something must be done about your low "EF." For some strange reason, you have lost the desire that you once had. A common solution is to take a break from training. I can't say how long that should be. The old saying, "absence makes the heart grow fonder," usually leads to a fix. But it may take a long time. Other solutions may be changing your daily routines, such as getting more sleep, eating healthier food, changing the people you hang out with, altering your daily workouts, or taking a spur-of-the-moment unplanned vacation. Or just pay attention to your feelings. What change do you think you need? If it means setting aside your training for a while, that's okay. Do it.

When you think it's time to start back, do so in a different way. Find a training partner you can ride with several times each week who will not half-wheel you. Change your training routine entirely. Eat a healthier diet and stay well hydrated. I'm somewhat biased on this one, but the best solution may be hiring a coach. Make sure the coach understands your dilemma. Search for someone who shows at least sympathy, if not empathy, for what you have been going through.

Also, be aware that the timing may not be right for you to train for a high-performance race. Put it on the backburner and just ride for fun. Your enthusiasm will return when it's time.

ROLE MODELS

Most people are not aware of this, but everyone is a role model. That includes you. If you are like most people, over the course of your life you have looked up to others who strike you as acting in a way you'd like to act. It could have been a teacher, a coach, a friend, a boss, a workmate, a family member, or someone you didn't know but observed from a distance. My role model was a high school coach. He personified how I wanted to talk, behave, and treat others. That was more than 60 years ago, but I still ask myself when in a high-pressure situation, how would coach Scotten handle this? We all need role models to help us shape our lives in positive ways.

You probably don't realize this, but there are others who are watching you—the things you say, how you treat others, what you eat, how you train and race, your attitude to life in general, how you express yourself, if you are friendly or not, your composure, your sense of humor, and a lot more. You are probably not aware of who these people are. They may be other riders, friends, acquaintances, work or schoolmates, children, neighbors, or people you just pass in the street. Such people are there, and they pay close attention to how you interact with the world. Make the world a better place—be a good role model, both on and off the bike.

HIGH PERFORMANCE

Every rider would like to be thought of as a high-performance racer. I've never coached anyone who aspired otherwise. I certainly hope you have success from what you have learned here in your reading. But that excellence goal, at its core, presents a never-ending task. When you have finally achieved a high-performance goal, you immediately have a new challenge. You move the bar higher. Like most serious riders, you are never truly satisfied. I suppose there is a lot that is good about that. But it can also become a burden. Season after season the high-performance rider is always striving for excellence. I think that the true essence of high performance is not about who you beat, how fast you raced, or how fit you were, but rather how much you enjoyed the journey. Striving for high performance and excellence as a person can be a long, long ride. Be sure to have fun along the way!

EPILOGUE

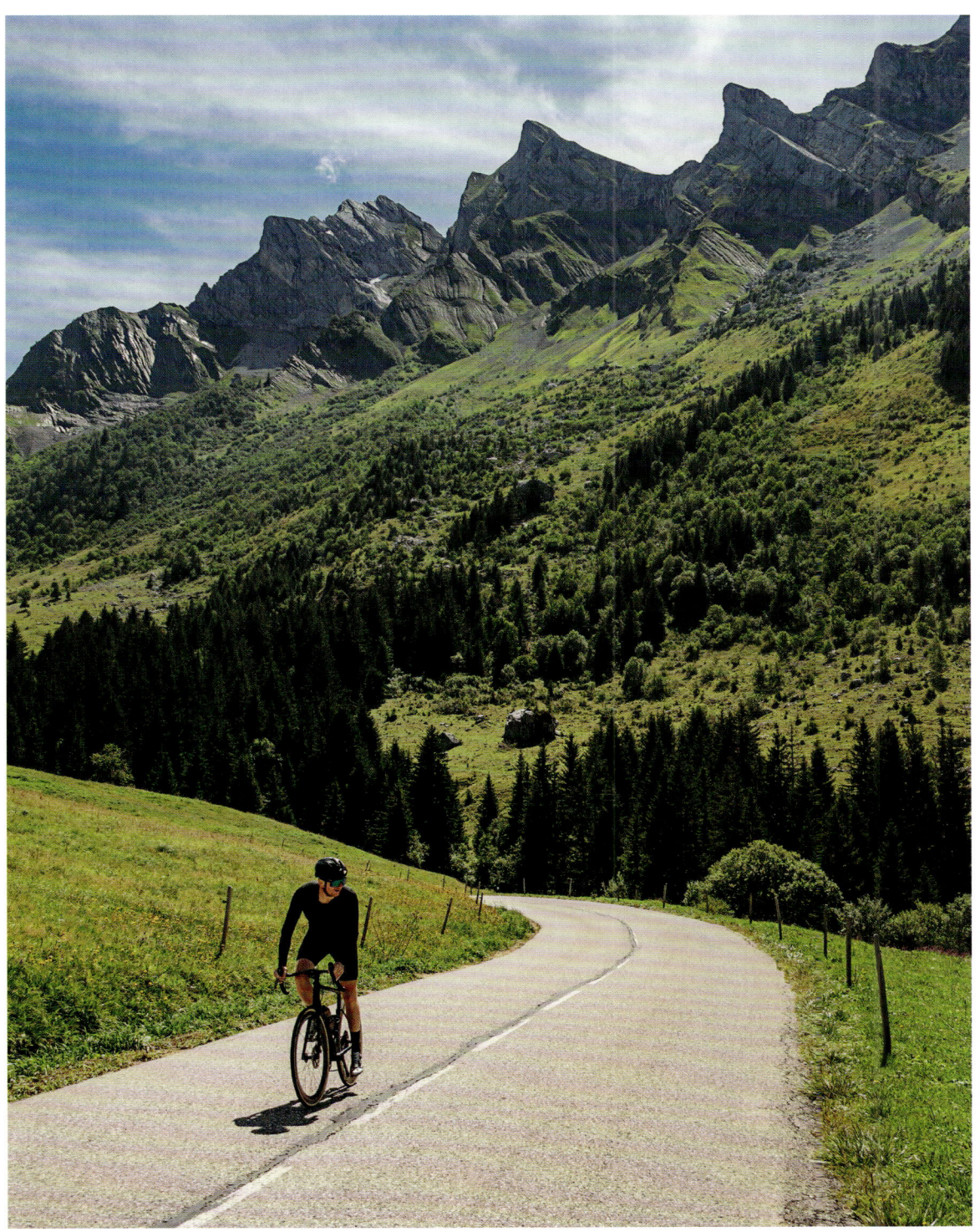

APPENDIX

The following are workouts sorted into the six abilities according to Figure 3.1: aerobic endurance, muscular force, speed skills, aerobic capacity, stamina, and sprint power. Also included below are field tests. This is not intended as a catalog of all the possible workouts, but rather a listing of common and basic workouts. Additional workouts may be designed by changing the structure of these sessions. Or you may combine two or more workouts from the list below to form a new session. In fact, this is recommended in the Build and Peak periods when preparing for the demands of a race which seldom have a singular focus. Mass start races are especially unpredictable as an initially disordered group places numerous demands on you, often in quick succession.

All the workouts below should start with a warm-up and finish with a cool-down. In between is the "main set." The warm-up is intended to prepare you physically for the demands of the main set while the cool-down gradually returns your body to a normal, recovered state. Typically, low-intensity rides need a relatively short warm-up. As for the cool-down, markers of appropriate efforts are a lowered heart rate and reduced breathing. The higher the intensity of the main set, the longer the warm-up and cool-down should be. For a high-intensity main set, especially for zones 4, 5a, 5b, and 5c, the warm-up should gradually build into the higher zones, but with durations as short as a few seconds to a minute done as repeats with long, easy recoveries between. Such warm-ups should be 20 to 30 minutes.

Each of the workouts below specifies an intensity or range of intensities based on heart rate or power. Heart rate is the preferred intensity-measuring marker of aerobic endurance workouts (AE1 and AE2). Intensity measurement for muscular force, aerobic capacity, stamina, and sprint power are best done using a power meter. Few speed skills workouts require intensity measurement. See Table 3.1 for heart rate and power intensity zones.

Durations and intensities for most of the following workouts vary based on the period of the season, how you have been performing recently, your present fitness specific to the workout's demands, and your current mental and physical readiness. If unsure of your readiness to do a long or high-intensity workout, you are best advised to do less. Pushing yourself to or beyond your current limits or workout readiness is counterproductive and favors setbacks such as illness, injury, burnout, or overtraining. When in doubt, leave it out. Doing less is seldom a bad decision.

AEROBIC ENDURANCE WORKOUTS

There are two purposes for these easy and very easy workouts. The first (AE1) is to be used as a recovery ride the day after a hard ride or race, or when you don't feel up to an even slightly harder ride (or would you perhaps be better off not riding today?). It also promotes the development of aerobic capacity. The AE2 workout will also develop your aerobic endurance, which is a key determiner of your aerobic capacity (see Figure 2.1). These workouts are in many ways the most important you do. These sessions are the focus of the Preparation and Base periods, but are also continued into the Build and Peak periods to maintain early season aerobic gains.

AE1 RECOVERY

You should be doing this ride because you feel fatigued, or you simply aren't mentally up for even a slightly more demanding ride. Taking a day off is often the better choice when feeling very tired or unmotivated. This should be a relatively short workout done on a flat course. Do the entire ride in zone 1 heart rate. Pedal in the small chain ring with a comfortably high cadence. Using an indoor trainer is advised to ensure a low effort. If you use an online app when riding a trainer, do not "race" or try to keep up with other riders when doing a recovery ride.

AE2 AEROBIC THRESHOLD

The primary purpose of this workout is to improve your body's capacity for delivering oxygen to the working muscles. Over time, with many such rides, your heart's pumping volume increases, the blood's capacity for carrying oxygen to the muscles increases, and the mitochondrial capability to use the oxygen to produce energy improves. This is one of your most important workouts as it significantly boosts your aerobic capacity (VO_2 max) and positively affects your high-intensity workouts.

The aerobic threshold workout is done in zone 2 heart rate on a relatively flat course. Avoid steep hills and frequent surges in which the heart rate rises into zone 3 even if only for a minute or so. When this happens lactate production increases, which interferes with lipolysis—the use of fat for fuel, another purpose of this workout. And repeatedly going in and out of zone 3 diminishes the aerobic benefits. You should strive to ride steadily in zone 2 throughout the ride.

After finishing this workout and while briefly analyzing its data, determine your efficiency factor (EF) for the ride. EF is your power (usually "normalized power") for the ride divided by your average heart rate for the workout. Some apps, such as TrainingPeaks, do the math for you. After determining your EF, go back about eight weeks in your training diary or online app and find a previous AE2 ride with a similar duration, course, and conditions. Compare the EF data for the two rides. If your AE2 workouts are frequent and consistent, your EF should usually be higher now than it was eight weeks prior. That's a very good sign that your aerobic fitness is improving. If it is not higher, you may need more AE1 and AE2 workouts.

There is a variation of this workout that allows you to follow the aerobic threshold portion of the training ride with higher intensities, especially in the late Base and Build periods. To do this, in the first part of the ride hold steady in zone 2 heart rate, just as described above. With about 30 minutes remaining in the ride increase the intensity to zones 3, 4, or 5 in whatever manner you prefer—fartlek, intervals, repetitions, or steady state—on hills or flat terrain. After the high-intensity segment, leave at least 10 to 15 minutes for a cool-down in zone 1 heart rate. The zone 2, aerobic threshold portion of this workout must always be done prior to the higher-intensity portion. Do this easy-hard combination workout no more than twice in a week. The two combined-intensity sessions should be separated by at least two days.

Another option for boosting your aerobic endurance is to cross-train in zone 2 heart rate. This is typically done in the Preparation and early Base periods (see Table 4.1). The cross-training sport or sports should also be done at an easy intensity. This may be running, hiking, walking (with or without a weighted backpack), Nordic skiing, snowshoeing, or any other similar aerobic activity. Again, avoid hilly courses. Doing highly intense activities such as tennis, basketball, or football are not aerobically beneficial. The aerobic sport you choose should be done in heart rate zones 1 and 2, which is unlikely to be the same as your cycling zones 1 and 2. For these cross-training sports use the "talk test" (described in Chapter 3) by counting aloud from "one thousand one" to "one thousand six." The heart rate at about one thousand six is quite close to your aerobic threshold (start of zone 3) for your cross-training sport.

MUSCULAR FORCE WORKOUTS

The purpose of the muscular force workouts is to develop greater neuromuscular fitness in the legs, hips, and lower back. Essentially, it's the application of your strength workouts done in a gym to similar workouts done on the bike. This is an early-stage series of workouts in the development of power done in the Base period. You must be careful with these workouts as they come with a high risk of injury, especially to your knees. Do them conservatively—or not at all if you have especially sensitive knees, hips, or lower back. These workouts are best done in the Base period when strength training (weightlifting) starts the strength maintenance (SM) phase.

MF1 FLAT FORCE REPS

After a long warm-up, on a road that has very light traffic, such as a backstreet in a neighborhood, shift to a high gear, like 53 x 14, and slow down so that you almost come to a stop. Then accelerate by driving the cranks for only 6 or 8 strokes so that you do a total of 3 or 4 pedal strokes for each leg (of course, you are alternating legs pedaling, not just pedaling with one leg). Stay seated. Do not stand. The effort should be *extremely* high for each pedal stroke with a very low cadence of around 50 rpm or lower. The cadence will gradually rise with increasing speed. If there is uncertainty about your knees, do only one set of 6 to 8 total pedal strokes and be a bit conservative with gear selection and effort. The first time you do this workout one set is adequate. Better safe than sorry. When you eventually do a second set in a subsequent workout, recover by riding slowly in a low gear for 3 to 4 minutes after the first set before doing the second set. Experiment with gearing the first couple of times you do this workout. If you err, make it on the low-gear (easy) side at first. It's best to do only one of these workouts weekly.

MF2 HILL FORCE REPS

This Base period workout is the same as MF1, except it's done on a hill to increase the stress on the legs. Before doing this workout, you should have previously done at least three of the MF1, Flat Force Reps sessions and know that your knees do not hurt for having done them. After warming up well, go to a hill that is short (30 to 50 yards or meters) and moderately steep (about a 6 percent grade). For safety there must be little or no traffic. The hill should be a section of road you can safely make a U-turn on at the top and at the bottom. As you coast to the base of the hill to start another rep, shift to a high gear, and come to a very brief, balanced stop without unclipping from a pedal. The gear selected won't be quite as high as for the MF1, Flat Force Reps. For example, it may be 53 x 16 instead of 53 x 14. Then, *while staying seated*, alternate driving the pedals down 3 to 6 times with each leg while otherwise pedaling in a normal manner. That's 6 to 12 total pedal strokes. Do *not* stand at any time on each set. Complete up to 3 sets in a workout. After each set shift to a low (easy) gear and pedal gently for 3 to 5 minutes on flat terrain, allowing for recovery. Do *not* shorten the recovery time between sets as this will reduce the workout benefit. Also, be sure your legs are well recovered before doing the next set. This is a high-risk, high-reward workout. At the first sign of any knee tenderness stop the workout.

Do not continue even if the tenderness is only slight. Power, not heart rate, is the only gauge of intensity for this session. Strive to produce very high wattage on each pedal stroke. Do this workout no more than once per week.

MF3 HILL REPEATS

On a hill of about 6 to 8 percent grade that takes 20 to 30 seconds to climb, do 3 to 8 climbing repeats with 3 to 4 minutes of recovery between them. Maintain power zones 5a and 5b for each climb. To recover, coast while descending before starting the next rep. Climb in the saddle with minimal upper body movement. Do *not* stand. Select a gear that allows a cadence of only about 70 rpm or lower for each rep. Stop the workout if your knees become sensitive to the load. Do this workout no more than once per week. Do not do this workout at all if you are prone to knee injury.

SPEED SKILLS WORKOUTS

If you have been riding and racing for many years your speed skills are probably well honed. But if you are new to the sport, that usually means in the first three years of serious riding, developing your cycling skills will pay dividends not only in your races but also in your workouts. You will also be safer on the bike. You may notice that experienced riders keep their distance from unskilled riders. There's a reason for that. They know how common it is for novices to crash and take others out with them. One of the best indicators that you have well-developed skills is that other riders don't mind riding next to you. These workouts are best done in the Base period.

SS1 HIGH-CADENCE PEDALING

On an indoor trainer, following a brief warm-up, pedal at 95 rpm or higher for a minute or more in zone 1 heart rate. Take long breaks of 2 minutes or more with easy and comfortably low-cadence pedaling. Then raise the cadence again as before. Challenge yourself to see how high a cadence you can sustain in zone 1.

Repeat 4 to 9 times. Pedaling at high cadences with a low heart rate refines your pedaling skills. To raise your cadence, relax your entire body. Especially concentrate on the relaxation of toes and fingers. Hold the handlebars gently and try to wiggle your toes as the cadence increases.

SS2 CORNERING

In some races, especially criteriums, performance often comes down to how well you corner. If your cornering skills need improvement, a good starting point is to ride behind someone you know who has good handling skills on a course that has lots of turns. Or by yourself work on your skills in a low-traffic area with clean, dry corners. Practice several techniques: lean both the bike and your body into the turn; lean your body while keeping the bike upright; and keep your body upright while leaning the bike. Practice several speeds with different angles of approach. Heart rate and power ratings are not important for this workout. Your only concern is improving cornering skills.

SS3 DESCENDING

Descending at high speed is perhaps the most challenging skill for many riders. It can be scary, and for a good reason. The risk of having a bad crash is quite high. The best way to learn to descend skillfully is to ride with someone who has very good skills. Follow that athlete's wheel using the same braking patterns and lines on straights and corners. But realize that the first several times you do this you are unlikely to ride as fast as your model. Be patient. Skills don't happen overnight. It takes patience and persistence to master this skill. In the meantime be conservative with speed on descents.

AEROBIC CAPACITY WORKOUTS

Aerobic capacity (VO_2 max) is one of the best predictors of how fit a rider is. The best young riders have a VO_2 max that is typically in the 70s (men) and 60s (women) or even higher for extremely fit athletes. While it's interesting to know your number, it's not necessary for training. It can certainly be measured in a laboratory setting if you want to know what yours is. Under Field Tests, however, you will find a workout that puts a power number on your aerobic capacity effort and gives you a goal to gauge your progress against. As your power output improves with this test, your aerobic capacity is also improving. These workouts are best done in the Build and Peak periods.

AC1 GROUP RIDE

This is an unstructured ride with a group that simulates racing. It could also be a C-priority race. This ride should include frequent maximal efforts, as is common in fast group rides. The purpose is to achieve zones 5a and 5b power outputs for several seconds to a few minutes several times during the ride. Each high-intensity surge is a "burned match" that should closely simulate the efforts of a race. In analysis following the ride note how many matches you burned, and the total time spent in zones 5a and 5b. Be cautious with this workout not only in terms of how intense it may become, but also with regards to road safety by paying attention to traffic and other riders who may not be as skilled at riding in a group.

AC2 VO$_2$ MAX INTERVALS

After warming-up (20 to 30 minutes) do several work intervals of 30 seconds to 4 minutes duration each. The course could be flat to rolling (frequent small hills) without stop signs and with light traffic. As you progress through the Build period introduce hill climbs for this workout. Recover after each work interval with easy pedaling in zone 1 for as long as the preceding work interval lasted (for example, after a 3-minute work interval, pedal easily for 3 minutes). As fitness improves, gradually reduce the recovery time relative to the work interval durations. Start the Build period with about 5 minutes of total work interval time within a workout (for example, 10 x 30 seconds) and gradually, over several sessions, build to 15 to 20 minutes in a session (for example, 5 x 3 minutes and 5 x 4 minutes). Use your power meter to determine the intensities for each work interval. The goal intensity is power zones 5a and 5b. Cadence for these intervals should be at the high end of your comfort range. This workout is best done only once weekly.

STAMINA WORKOUTS

Stamina is another critical marker of high-performance racing. Essentially, it's a measure of how high a power output you can maintain for a long time—more than an hour. The longer your A race, the longer you should be able to maintain a certain level of power-based intensity. Under Field Tests below there is a way to measure your stamina. The purpose of the following workouts is to increase your stamina. Stamina workouts start in the late Base period and continue through the Build and Peak periods.

ST1 FARTLEK

"Fartlek" is a Swedish term first used in the 1930s as a name for an interval session in which the intensity and durations are based on how the athlete feels. This workout is commonly used in the last Base period as stamina training is initiated. After a long warm-up, include several work intervals mostly in power zones 3 (see Table 3.1). Stop the work interval when you feel you've gone long enough. That's well before fatigue sets in. Be very conservative with interval durations in this workout as you are still very early in the season. After a work interval take a long recovery break (your call for how long) before starting the next interval. Stop the workout and begin a long cool-down even though you know you could have done more. Be conservative with this workout as it will probably be your first higher-intensity effort for the season.

ST2 TEMPO INTERVALS

After a long warm-up do 3 to 5 work intervals in power zone 3 with brief recoveries. The work intervals may be 12 to 20 minutes long with recoveries that are about one-fourth as long—3 to 5 minutes. For example, following a 16-minute interval in zone 3, recover for 4 minutes. Start with about 40 minutes of total zone 3 time in a workout. Over the course of several weeks increase your total zone 3 time up to 90 minutes or even longer. Do this workout on a mostly flat course, a course with rolling hills, or an indoor trainer. Avoid roads with heavy traffic and frequent stop signs. Stay seated for each interval. Recover after each long work interval by pedaling easily in zone 1 heart rate.

ST3 CRUISE INTERVALS

This is a follow-up workout for the St2 Tempo Intervals session above. Once you have mastered that workout, increase the intensity while shortening the durations of the work intervals. The intensity of each interval is now power zone 4 and the durations are 8 to 12 minutes. Do 3 to 5 such intervals totaling about 40 to 60 minutes (for example, 5 x 8 minutes or 5 x 12 minutes). After each work interval recover in zone 1 with easy pedaling for one-fourth of the preceding interval duration. For example, after an 8-minute work interval, recover for 2 minutes with easy pedaling. The work interval intensity is very similar to that of a 40km time trial pace, making this an especially key workout for time trialists. On a time trial bike, pedal with a cadence such as you would use at such a race distance.

SPRINT POWER WORKOUTS

While "pure" sprinters need to continually hone their sprinting skills and power, *all* riders must be able to sprint in some situations. Sprinting requires not only a massive amount of power, but also highly refined skills to get the most out of one's bike and body. The following workouts are intended to do that. The skill workout below (SP1 Form Sprints) is best done in the Base period. The other workouts are intended for the Build and Peak periods.

SP1 FORM SPRINTS

Early in a ride, following a warm-up, do 4 to 6 sprints on a mostly flat terrain. Each sprint should be about 5 to 10 seconds long, followed by a 3- to 5-minute recovery. This session is done primarily for form, so limit intensity. Power should be in zone 5b (you could go higher, but don't). You should *not* be breathing hard after each of these. Alternate standing and sitting throughout this main set while focused on posture and technique. This workout is best done by yourself to avoid "competing" while refining your sprint technique. Head-to-head competition would be counterproductive this early in the season. Save it for later. Your most powerful sprints are done standing with your butt over the saddle. Your hands are in the drops with elbows bent. This lowers your torso to reduce drag. But for safety reasons in this position, you *must* have your head up and eyes looking forward.

Another key skill to be developed early in the Base period is pedaling cadence. Pure sprinters can't grind out sprint finishes in a high gear. Their cadence should be high—probably well over 100 rpm. There is room for difference here for riders for whom sprinting is not their primary ability. Time trialists and climbers when working on their sprint skills may find that using slightly higher gears and lower cadences is more effective.

SP2 COMPETITIVE SPRINTS

This is best done in the Build and Peak periods. Within a ride include several short and long, race-like sprints. These can be done with another rider or with a group to better simulate racing intensity and tactical maneuvering. Designate sprint primes such as signs. Employ all the techniques of good form sprints, only now at a high intensity. Power and effort should be maximal. Recover for several minutes between sprints. Try different distances, terrains, road conditions, wind conditions, early and late in a ride, lead outs and no lead outs. Experiment to find what works for you. Determine the tactics that work best for common distances and conditions so that when sprinting in a race you know what to do.

FIELD TESTS

To gauge cycling performance progress, it's necessary to occasionally measure how you are adapting to training. This can often be in a lab, but to limit your costs, I'd suggest using tests that are done in your normal training environment. Field tests are actually more realistic than lab testing since you are measuring progress under similar conditions as your races.

The following are field tests that measure how you are progressing. Repeat the tests every few weeks to determine improvement or where more attention is needed.

T1 FUNCTIONAL THRESHOLD POWER (FTP) AND HEART RATE (FTHR)

The purpose of this test is to determine your Functional Threshold Power (FTP) and Functional Threshold Heart Rate (FTHR) as described in Chapter 3, and to set your power and heart rate training zones. For determining FTP, you need a power meter and for FTHR, a heart rate monitor. Do this test after a few days of R&R. Warm up well before starting the test. See the introduction to this Appendix for warm-up details. Then do the following test. Ride on a road that is mostly flat to slightly uphill (3 percent grade or less). It should have a wide bike lane, light traffic, no stop signs, and few intersections or corners. It must be safe for testing at a high speed. You will need roughly 5 to 10 miles (8 to 16 kilometers) of road for the test depending on how fast you ride and the hill gradient. The test may also be done on an indoor trainer. Use the same course or indoor trainer every time you do this test. Throughout the test keep your head up so you can see ahead. Consider the test a 20-minute time trial. The bike you use should be the same one you train on. It's important to hold back slightly for the first 5 minutes (most riders start too fast). Every 5 minutes decide whether you should ride slightly harder or easier for the next 5 minutes. After the workout note your average heart rate from the 20-minute test portion. Subtract 5 percent and you have an estimate of your FTHR. Then use Table 3.1 to compute your heart rate training zones. To determine FTP from the same test, subtract 5 percent from your average power (*not* "normalized" power) and you have an estimate of FTP. Table 3.1 may then be used to set your power training zones.

T2 FUNCTIONAL AEROBIC CAPACITY TEST

The purpose of this test is to determine your Functional Aerobic Capacity (VO_2 max) power. You will need a power meter. It is best done following 3 to 5 days of R&R. The course you use for the test should be flat or slightly uphill (3 percent grade or less), have a wide bike lane, light traffic, no stop streets, and few intersections or corners. Most of all it should be safe. Use the same course every time you do this test. Look straight ahead throughout the test. Do *not* ride looking down at your power meter. The test is best done on the road, not on an indoor trainer. Following the warm-up, ride steadily at an effort you can sustain for 5 minutes. Your average power for the 5-minute test portion is a good predictor of your power at aerobic capacity. What you would like to have happen to this number over time is a steady increase. However, there may be tests in which there is no improvement or even a loss of power. That is to be expected due to the many variables on the day of the test, the most important of which is your readiness to test at a very high intensity.

T3 STAMINA TEST

This test will give you feedback on your stamina—your capability for holding a relatively high-power output for a relatively long time. The test duration is quite long, requiring a significant stretch of road, which is mostly flat. The road should also have a wide bike lane, light traffic, no stop streets, and few intersections or corners. One option is to use a repeatable loop with the above safety matters in mind. This loop may take you 15 to 30 minutes to complete one lap. Then do several laps that will give you the following test duration. The test portion of the ride is best preceded by a long warm-up, such as an AE1 and AE2 combined workout (see introduction above). The goal for the test is based on Intensity Factor (IF), which is determined by dividing your normalized power for the test ride by your FTP (see test T1 above). The test involves a 90-minute ride at a goal IF of 88 to 92 percent. If you can ride at a higher IF for that duration, you have excellent stamina. That is the ultimate goal. This test is quite stressful, usually requiring at least two days of recovery before doing the next hard ride.

T4 SPRINT POWER TEST

The purpose of this test is to gauge the progress of your sprint power and to be prepared to sprint in a race in various situations. A power meter is required. Do this test after 3 to 5 days of R&R. Following a thorough warm-up, ride to a section of road that is roughly 50 to 200 yards/meters long. The road section used for the test should have light traffic, a wide bike lane, no intersections, and no stop streets. (This test should not be done on an indoor trainer.) From a rolling start, pedal as powerfully and quickly as you can. During the test do two sprints—one that lasts 5 seconds and the other 20 seconds. Your peak and average power outputs for these two test durations are indications of your sprint power for short and long durations. Keep a record of your best sprint powers for both. At which duration are you better? Does one of them need improving? Improvement results from increased training.

GLOSSARY

Ability. In the context of this book, a category of six workout types focusing on an intended physical adaptation in preparation for racing. See *adaptation*, *aerobic endurance*, *muscular force*, *speed skills*, *stamina*, *aerobic capacity*, and *sprint power*.

Active recovery. Low-intensity exercise intended to allow for recovery. See *passive recovery*.

Adaptation. The body's physiological adjustment to a physical-training stress placed on it over a period of time. The purpose is to improve an element of fitness. Adaptation requires that the training ability be stressed repeatedly over many weeks. See *ability* and *fitness*.

Aerobic. Occurring in the presence of oxygen; aerobic metabolism uses oxygen to produce energy. See *ventilatory threshold (VT1)* and *lactate threshold (LT1)*.

Aerobic capacity (AC). The maximal volume of oxygen an athlete can process to produce energy during a maximal and prolonged exertion. Also known as VO_2 max. Aerobic capacity is determined in a graded exercise test by measuring oxygen uptake (in milliliters), dividing it by the athlete's body weight (in kilograms), then dividing the quotient by the duration of exercise (in minutes) at maximal intensity: VO_2 max = O_2 uptake (mL)/body weight (kg)/duration at maximal intensity (min). See VO_2 *max*.

Aerobic endurance. In the context of this book, a category of workouts done at or near the aerobic threshold and intended to improve an athlete's aerobic ability. See *ventilatory threshold (VT1)* and *lactate threshold (LT1)*.

Aerobic threshold. The exercise intensity at which blood lactate begins to rise above the resting level. Exercise is fully aerobic at this intensity, with fuel supplied primarily by stored body fat. In terms of heart rate, the aerobic threshold is about 20 to 40 bpm below the anaerobic or *lactate threshold*.

Agonist muscles. The primary movement muscles, which contract with the purpose of propelling the body for activities such as swimming, cycling, and running. See *antagonist muscles*.

Antagonist muscles. Muscles that oppose the contraction of agonist muscles. For example, the triceps is an antagonist muscle for the biceps because the biceps flexes the elbow and the triceps extends it. See *agonist muscles*.

Autonomic nervous system. The nervous system that regulates involuntary physiological functions such as heart rate, breathing, blood pressure, and more. The two major subsystems of the ANS are the sympathetic and parasympathetic nervous systems. See *sympathetic nervous system* and *parasympathetic nervous system.*

Base period. In seasonal periodization, the training period during which the workouts are "general," meaning not exactly like the demands of the targeted event. The purpose of training in this period is to prepare the body for the training stresses of the Build period. See *Preparation period*, *Build period*, *Peak period*, *Race period*, and *Transition period*.

Bonk. A state of extreme exhaustion during a very long endurance session related to the depletion of glycogen. See *glycogen*.

Build period. In seasonal periodization, the training period during which the workouts are "specific," meaning very much like the demands of the targeted event. The purpose of training in this period is to prepare the body for the training stresses of racing. See *Preparation period*, *Base period*, *Peak period*, *Race period*, and *Transition period*.

Cadence. Pedaling revolutions per minute.

Capillaries. Small blood vessels located between arteries and veins in which the exchange of oxygen and fuel between tissue (for example, muscle) and blood occurs. Generally, several capillaries at a given site form a capillary bed. As aerobic fitness improves in each muscle, the capillary beds for that muscle are enlarged, improving aerobic fitness.

Carbohydrate loading. A dietary procedure intended to elevate muscle and liver glycogen stores by emphasizing carbohydrate consumption for a few days prior to a race.

Cardiorespiratory system. The system comprising the heart, blood vessels, and lungs, which interact to supply fuel and oxygen to the working muscles during exercise.

Central nervous system. The brain and spinal cord.

Circuit training. Selected exercises or activities performed in a sequence. A term often used in weight training.

Compound exercise. In weightlifting, an exercise that uses multiple joints, usually in the same manner in which they are recruited during swimming, cycling, and running. For example, the squat is a compound exercise involving the hips, knees, and ankles and is somewhat similar to the lower body's movement in pedaling a bicycle.

Concentric contraction. Muscular contraction during which the muscle shortens, as when the biceps muscle is used in an arm-curling exercise. During bicycle pedaling, the quadriceps muscle is used concentrically. See *eccentric contraction*.

Cool-down. Low-intensity exercise near the end of a training session intended to return the body gradually to a resting state.

Cranks. On a bicycle, the levers to which the pedals are attached.

Cross-training. Workouts that involve activities not usually part of an athlete's primary sport. For example, weightlifting and cross-country skiing are cross-training activities for a cyclist.

Drafting. Riding closely behind another athlete to reduce drag and therefore lower effort.

Drops. The lower portion of turned-down handlebars, commonly seen on road bicycles.

Eccentric contraction. Muscular contraction during which the muscle lengthens as it contracts, as, for example, when the biceps muscle is used to slowly lower a weight that was lifted during an arm curl. See *concentric contraction*.

Economy. The physiological cost of cycling. Economy is commonly expressed as liters of oxygen consumed for a given duration or distance. As an athlete becomes more economical, the amount of oxygen that is consumed at any given power decreases. See *fitness*.

Efficiency factor (EF). In the context of this book, the normalized power divided by the average heart rate for a steady, aerobic workout or segment thereof, such as an aerobic interval. An increasing EF over time suggests improving aerobic fitness. See *normalized power (NP)*.

Ergogenic aid. A substance, device, or phenomenon that can improve athletic performance. For example, caffeine is often considered an ergogenic aid for endurance sports. Some ergogenic aids are banned from sport.

Fartlek. A Swedish term meaning speed play. An unstructured, interval-type workout in which the intensity and duration of the intervals and recovery times between them are completely subjective and spur-of-the-moment decisions.

Fast-twitch (FT) fiber. A muscle fiber characterized by a fast contraction time, high load capacity, and low aerobic capacity, all making the fiber suited for high-power activities such as sprints. See *slow-twitch fiber*.

Fitness. In endurance sport, the athlete's capacity for a unique training load. This is the result of the combined physiological functions of an athlete's aerobic capacity, stamina (as a percentage of aerobic capacity), and economy. See *aerobic capacity*, *stamina*, and *economy*.

Force. The muscular work done to overcome a resistance. For example, pushing down on a bicycle pedal exerts force. See *torque*.

Form. An athlete's readiness to race. Specifically, on race day the athlete should have a relatively high level of fitness and be fresh, without fatigue.

Free weights. Weights, such as barbells and dumbbells, that are not part of an exercise machine.

Functional threshold (FTHR, FTPo). The term *functional threshold power* (FTP) is used in cycling with a power meter, while FTHR refers to functional threshold heart rate. The term refers to an intensity level that is similar to the *lactate threshold*. The intensity level is determined through a field test. The most common test duration is 20 minutes of maximal intensity. FTPo is determined by subtracting 5 percent of the average power for the 20 minutes. FTHR is determined by subtracting 5 percent from the average heart rate for the 20-minute test. See *lactate threshold*.

Gear, high and low. On a bicycle, one crank revolution in a high gear results in the bike going a greater distance than one revolution in a low gear. During bicycle riding, greater pedal force is required to turn the cranks in a high gear than in a low gear.

Glycogen. A source of fuel for exercise derived from dietary carbohydrate. Glycogen is the body's storage form of sugar.

Hammer. A slang term used to describe a fast, sustained, nearly maximal effort.

Heart rate monitor. An electronic device that measures and displays an athlete's pulse and may be downloaded to a computer for analysis following a training session.

Heart rate variability. A measure of the time between beats of the heart which may vary considerably, either high or low, and is controlled by autonomic nervous system. See *autonomic nervous system*, *parasympathetic nervous system*, and *sympathetic nervous system*.

Hoods. On drop handlebars, the rubber covers over the brake lever mechanisms.

Individuality, principle of. The theory that any training program must consider the specific needs and abilities of the individual for whom it is designed, as individual athletes often vary considerably in their responses to training.

Intensity factor (IF). A power metric that quantifies workout intensity. IF is determined by dividing the workout's normalized power by the rider's functional threshold power (IF = NP ÷ FTP). See *intensity factor*, *normalized power*, and *functional threshold*.

Intervals. A system of generally high-intensity work marked by short but regularly repeated periods of hard exercise interspersed with periods of recovery. See *work interval* and *recovery interval*.

Isolated leg training (ILT). Pedaling a bicycle with one leg in order to focus on improving technique. Generally done on an indoor trainer.

Kilojoule (kJ). In training with a power meter, the unit used to express how much energy is expended throughout a workout or portion of a workout. The cumulative training load for a given period of time, such as a week, may also be measured in kilojoules. A kilojoule is the average power (in watts) multiplied by the number of seconds within a workout or selected portion of a workout; this product is then divided by 1,000. See *workload*.

Lactate. A chemical formed in the body that enters the bloodstream in greater amounts as intensity increases.

Lactate threshold. There are two lactate thresholds. Both are determined by the measurement of lactate accumulation in the blood. The first and lower lactate threshold (LT1) is commonly determined as 2mm of lactate accumulation in the blood. This occurs at a level of exertion which is similar to the first ventilatory threshold (VT1). The second lactate threshold (LT2) is the intensity during exercise at which blood lactate further accumulates and is usually determined by an accumulation of 4mm of lactate in the blood and is marked by labored breathing. This is similar in the second ventilatory threshold (VT2).

Long, slow distance (LSD). A form of continuous training in which an athlete performs at a relatively low intensity, usually below the aerobic threshold, for a long duration.

Macrocycle. In training periodization, a period of training that includes several mesocycles. This usually refers to an entire season but may also refer to the preparation period for a single race. See *mesocycle* and *microcycle*.

Main set. The primary portion of a workout session that is focused on a specific training ability. This typically follows the warm-up and precedes the cool-down.

Mash. To push a high gear on a bicycle at a slow cadence.

Mesocycle. In training periodization, a period of training generally two to six weeks long. See *macrocycle* and *microcycle*.

Microcycle. In training periodization, a period of training of approximately 1 week. See *macrocycle* and *mesocycle*.

Muscular force. In the context of this book, a category of workouts done as brief repeats at a maximal intensity with long recoveries between repeats for the purpose of increasing an athlete's sport-specific strength.

Normalized power (NP). A measurement of performance derived from an algorithm that computes the average power attained during cycling and assigns greater numerical significance to surges. The NP for a workout is typically somewhat higher than the workout's average power. A power meter and software are necessary to measure NP. See *power meter*.

Overload, principle of. A training load that challenges the body's current level of fitness and causes adaptation. See *adaptation* and *fitness*.

Overreaching. Training above at a workload that will produce overtraining if such a training load is continued long enough. Usually results in fatigue.

Overtraining. A physical and mental condition marked by extreme fatigue and caused by training for an excessive period of time at a workload higher than that to which the body can readily adapt. It's the result of an imbalance between training stress and rest.

Pacing. The act of carefully managing the expenditure of energy during a workout, race, or interval to produce a steady speed or power, thus leading to the best possible performance. Unsteady pacing wastes energy.

Parasympathetic nervous system. A subset of the autonomic nervous system that is activated in low-stress situations and is often described as the "rest and digest" reaction to life. See *autonomic nervous system* and *sympathetic nervous system*.

Passive recovery. A day or group of days with no workouts, the goal of which is complete rest. See *active recovery*.

Peak period. In seasonal periodization, the training period during which workouts are "specific," meaning very much like the demands of the targeted event, and workout durations are decreased while intensity remains high. The peak period typically follows the Build period and precedes the Race period. The purpose of this period is to produce form gradually by allowing the body to recover from the previous period of hard training while steadily becoming race-ready. See *form*, *Base period*, *Preparation period*, *Build period*, *Race period*, and *Transition period*.

Periodization. A seasonal planning method of structuring training into periods based on training frequency, volume, and intensity, with each period focused on a specific training objective. See *intensity*, *volume*, *macrocycle*, *mesocycle*, and *microcycle*.

Power meter. An electronic device that measures cadence and pedaling torque, thus providing a wattage reading as an indicator of intensity. The data may be downloaded to a computer for analysis following the session.

Preparation (prep) period. In seasonal periodization, the training period during which the workouts are very "general," meaning not the same as the demands of the targeted event. The purpose of training in this period is to return gradually to a structured training program following a break from focused training during the preceding Transition period. See *Base period*, *Build period*, *Peak period*, *Race period*, and *Transition period*.

Progression, principle of. The theory that an athlete's training workload must be gradually increased over time, accompanied by intermittent periods of recovery.

Quadriceps. The large muscle at the front of the thigh that extends the lower leg and flexes the hip.

Race period. In seasonal periodization, the training period during which the workouts are "specific," meaning very much like the demands of the targeted event, and workout durations are very brief while intensity remains high. This period typically follows the Peak period and culminates with the targeted race. The purpose of this period is to recover completely from the previous periods of hard training and become race-ready. See *Preparation period*, *Base period*, *Build period*, *Peak period*, and *Transition period*.

Rating of perceived exertion (RPE). A subjective assessment of how hard one is working that generally uses a scale of 0 (low) to 10 (high).

Recovery interval. The relief period between work intervals within an interval workout. The recovery interval is defined by its duration and intensity, which is usually quite low. See *work interval*.

Repetition maximum (RM). In weightlifting, the maximum load that an athlete can lift in one attempt. Also called *1-repetition maximum* (1RM).

Rest-and-recovery (R&R). In periodization, a period of moderate training that follows a block of hard training. During R&R, passive recovery and active recovery are emphasized. R&R is typically included in training after about two or three weeks of focused training in the Base and Build periods or when the athlete determines that R&R are needed.

Reversibility, principle of. The theory that if an athlete's training load is decreased for an extended period of time that fitness will gradually be lost.

Session. A single workout or race.

Slow-twitch (ST) fiber. A muscle fiber characterized by a slow contraction time, low power, and high endurance, all making the fiber suited for low-power, long-duration activities.

Specificity, principle of. The theory that training must stress the specialized systems critical for optimal performance to achieve the desired training adaptations.

Speed skills. Within the context of this book, a category of workouts focused on improving the ability to move the body efficiently to produce optimal performance—for example, the ability to pedal efficiently with a high cadence.

Sprint power. In the context of this book, a category of workouts done at a maximal effort for a very brief time and typically at a very high cadence with long recovery periods between high efforts. This workout is intended to improve sprinting ability.

Stamina. The athlete's ability to sustain a physical effort at or just below VT2 and LT2. See *ventilatory threshold* and *lactate threshold*.

Sympathetic nervous system. A subset of the autonomic nervous system that is activated under extreme situations which is often described as the "fight or flight" reaction. See *autonomic nervous system* and *parasympathetic nervous system*.

Tapering. A training method initiated a few days or weeks prior to an important race in which training volume is gradually reduced for an athlete to come into form on race day. See *form*.

Tempo. Maintaining moderately hard intensity between the ventilatory and lactate thresholds (VT1-VT2 and LT1-LT2).

Torque. In pedaling a bicycle, the rotational force applied to the pedals. See *force*.

Training. A comprehensive program or portions thereof intended to prepare an athlete for competition.

Training stress score (TSS). The numerical value assigned to a session by using an algorithm based on session duration and intensity. A power meter, heart rate monitor, or other device is required for accurately measuring intensity. Because it involves both duration and intensity, cumulative TSS may be used to create a training seasonal plan. See *power meter*, *heart rate monitor*, *periodization*, *intensity factor*, and *workload*.

Training zones. Consecutive categories of intensity based on heart rate or power that are unique to an athlete's physical capacity. Training zones are typically based on percentages of an athlete's unique physiological markers, such as max heart rate, lactate threshold, or functional threshold. Typically used to predetermine how intense a workout or portion of a workout will be. See *ventilatory threshold, lactate threshold*, and *functional threshold*.

Transition period. In seasonal periodization, the training period during which workouts are quite easy, allowing full recovery, both physical and mental, in the days immediately following a targeted race. The purpose of this period is to recover completely from the stresses of recent training and racing. See *Preparation period, Base period, Build period, Peak period,* and *Race period.*

Variability index (VI). An indicator of how steadily (or nonsteadily) paced a workout, race, or interval is when a bicycle power meter is used. It is determined by dividing normalized power by average power. A resulting quotient of 1.05 or less is, for example, an indicator of steady pacing. A VI rising above 1.05 indicates progressively nonsteady riding marked by surging. See *pacing*.

Ventilatory threshold. As with the *lactate threshold*, there are two ventilatory thresholds. The first (VT1) occurs at the moment, during steadily increasing exertion, at which breathing first becomes labored. This closely corresponds to the first *lactate threshold* (LT1). The second ventilatory threshold (VT2) is marked by an exertion level at which labored breathing makes it difficult to talk. VT2 closely corresponds to the second *lactate threshold* (LT2).

VO_2 max. An athlete's physical capacity for oxygen consumption during a maximal endurance exertion. Also known as *aerobic capacity* and maximal oxygen consumption. VO_2 max is numerically expressed as milliliters of oxygen consumed per kilogram of body weight per minute (mL/kg/min). VO_2 max is closely related to endurance performance. See *aerobic capacity* and *fitness*.

Volume. A quantitative element of training that expresses how much training is done in a given time frame, such as a week. Volume is commonly based on the cumulative training stress score (TSS), on total miles or kilometers, or on collective hours of training. Volume results from the combination of individual workout durations and their frequency. See *training stress score*.

Warm-up. The period of gradually increasing the intensity of exercise at the start of a training session or before a race, with the intent of readying the body for the physical stress of the main set or competition. See *main set*.

Work interval. High-intensity efforts within an interval workout separated by recovery intervals. Work intervals are commonly defined by their durations and intensities. See *intervals* and *recovery interval*.

Workload. The measured stress applied in training through the combination of frequency, intensity, and duration for a given period of time, such as a week. This expresses both the quantitative and qualitative aspects of training in a single number. Common measurements are cumulative training stress score (TSS) and kilojoules (kJ) for the designated time frame. See *training stress score* and *kilojoule*.

Workout. A complete training session that is focused on a specific outcome and typically includes a warm-up, main set, and cool-down. See *warm-up*, *main set*, and *cool-down*.

ACKNOWLEDGMENTS

This book is the product of having worked with hundreds of athletes throughout my four-decade coaching career. I learned a lot from them, they deserve much of the credit, and I am grateful. Without them I would never have put as much time into seeking to understand the many complex details of training for endurance sports. The nine I selected to feature in the chapters of this book are barely the tip of the iceberg. They graciously gave their permissions for me to tell their stories. They also helped me recall the details of our coach-athlete relationships from many years ago. Thank you.

Also critical to the book were the nine experts who each summarized very small portions of their vast knowledge on specific topics related to endurance cycling. Thank you to Andrew Kirkland, PhD; Paraic McGlynn; Alan Couzens; Stephen Seiler, PhD; Dirk Friel; Marco Altini, PhD; Rob Griffiths; Louise Burke, PhD; and Trevor Connor. You brought a great deal of wisdom to the book.

This book would not have come about without the encouragement of Matthew Lowing, publisher at Bloomsbury Sport. He urged me to write it and provided great support along the way. Thank you, Matt.

There were several who helped with specific topics. Bill Cofer offered insights on bodyweight management. Alan Couzens provided Figure 2.1, illustrating the contributions of low- and high-intensity training to aerobic capacity development within a season. Tim Cusick gave me Figure 2.2, showing how various types of riders compare in terms of their power-duration curves. Stephen Seiler, PhD reviewed my descriptions of polarized and pyramidal training in Chapter 5. Marco Altini, PhD provided guidance in the use of heart rate variability to manage stress, rest, and recovery. Thank you, all.

Writing this book would not have been possible without Kara Mannix, who assisted with the many time-consuming business tasks that had to be done as I devoted my time to writing. Thank you, Kara.

Thank you to the staff at Bloomsbury Sport for your editing and designs used in this book. The excellent design work was done by Sian Rance. The editing of this book made it much more readable and enjoyable. Thank you Megan Jones, Lisa Hughes and Jane Donovan.

I receive queries from athletes almost daily via social media, email, and my blog (JoeFrielTraining.com). They ask great questions which cause me to investigate focused topics I may not have otherwise considered. Their inquisitive curiosity has always played a role in my on-going growth as a coach. Thank you.

My heartfelt appreciation goes out to all who have helped me in some way who I have not mentioned here. Many little things pop up unexpectedly when writing a book that at the time seem bigger than they actually are. There were always people in my life who made the problems go away. Thank you.

And finally, I want to thank my wife, Joyce, who was always there for me to bounce weird ideas off. She put up with a huge chunk of my time spent cooped up in the office at my computer writing daily for almost a year. With her patience and support she remains the anchor and guiding light of my life. Thank you, sweetheart.

REFERENCES

Chapter 1

Iso-Ahola, S. E. "Intrapersonal and Interpersonal Factors in Athletic Performance." *Scandinavian Journal of Medicine and Science in Sports* (1995) 5 (4): 191-199.

Jones, G. "How the Best of the Best Get Better and Better." *Harvard Business Review* (2008) 86 (6): 123–127, 142.

Magean, G. and R. J. Vallerand. "The Coach-Athlete Relationship: A Motivational Model." *Journal of Sports Science* (2003) 21 (11): 883–904.

Chapter 2

Anderson, T., N. Galan-Lopez, L. Taylor, E. G. Post, J. T. Finnoff, and W. M. Adams. "Sleep Quality in Team USA Olympic and Paralympic Athletes." *International Journal of Sports Physiology and Performance* (2024) 19 (4): 383-392.

Bannister, E. W., R. H. Morton, and J. Fitz-Clarke. "Dose/Response Effects of Exercises Modeled from Training: Physical and Biochemical Measures." *Annals of Physiology and Anthropology* (1992) 11 (3): 345–356.

Bouchard, C., M. A. Sarzynski, T. K. Rice, W. E. Kraus, T. S. Church, Y. J. Sung, D. C. Rao, and T. Rankinen. "Genomic Predictors of Maximal Oxygen Uptake Response to Standardized Exercise Training Programs." *Journal of Applied Physiology* (2010) 110 (5): 1160–1170.

Busso, T., R. Candan, and J. R. Lacour. "Fatigue and Fitness Modelled from the Effects of Training on Performance." *European Journal of Applied Physiology and Occupational Physiology* (1994) 69 (1): 50–54.

Cairns, S. P. "Lactic Acid and Exercise Performance: Culprit or Friend?" *Sports Medicine* (2006) 36 (4): 279-91.

Coyle, F. F., M. E. Feltner, S. A. Kantz, M. T. Hamilton, S. J. Montain, A. M. Baylor, L. D. Abraham, and G. W. Petrek. "Physiological and Biomechanical Factors Associated with Elite Endurance Cycling Performance." *Medicine and Science in Sports and Exercise* (1991) 23 (1): 93–107.

Coyle, E. F. "Integration of the Physiological Factors Determining Endurance Performance Ability." *Exercise, Sport, and Science Review* (1995) 23: 25–63.

Ferguson B. S., M. J. Rogatzki, M. L. Goodwin, D. A. Kane, Z. Rightmire, L. B. Gladden. "Lactate Metabolism: Historical Context, Prior Misinterpretations, and Current Understanding." *European Journal of Applied Physiology* (2018) 118 (4): 691-728.

Gibson, H. and R. H. Edwards. "Muscular Exercise and Fatigue." (1985) *Sports Medicine* 2: 120-132.

Gomes, P. S. and Y. Bhambhani. "Time Course Changes and Dissociation in VO_2max at Maximum and Submaximum Exercise Levels as a Result of Training in Males." *Medicine and Science in Sports and Exercise* (1996) 28 (5): S81.

Helgerud, J., K. Hoydal, E. Wang, T. Karlsen, P. Berg, M. Bjerkaas, T. Simonsen, C. Helgesen, N. Hjorth, R. Bach, and J. Hoff. "Aerobic High-Intensity Intervals Improve VO_2max More Than Moderate Training." *Medicine and Science in Sports and Exercise* (2007) 39 (4): 665–671.

Laursen, P. B. and D. G. Jenkins. "The Scientific Basis for High-Intensity Interval Training: Optimising Training Programmes and Maximising Performance in Highly Trained Endurance Athletes." *Sports Medicine* (2002) 32 (1): 53–73.

Laursen, P. B. "Training for Intense Exercise Performance: High-Intensity or High-Volume Training?" *Scandinavian Journal of Medicine & Science in Sports* (2010) 20 (supplement 2): 1–10.

Leo, P., J. Spragg, J. Wakefield, and J. Stuart. "Predictors of Cycling Performance Success: Traditional Approaches and a Novel Method to Assess Performance Capacity in U23 Cyclists." *Journal of Science and Medicine in Sport* (2023) 26 (1): 5-57.

Lindsay, F. H., J. A. Hawley, K. H. Myburgh, H. H. Schomer, T. D. Noakes, and S. C. Dennis. "Improved Athletic Performance in Highly Trained Cyclists After Interval Training." *Medicine and Science in Sports and Exercise* (1996) 28 (11):1427–1434.

Lucia, A., J. Hoyos, M. Perez, A. Santalla, and J. L. Chicharro. "Inverse Relationship Between VO_2max and Economy/Efficiency in World-Class Cyclists." *Medicine and Science in Sports and Exercise* (2002) 34 (12): 2079–2084.

McDaniel, J., A. Subudhi, and J. C. Martin. "Torso Stabilization Reduces the Metabolic Cost of Producing Cycling Power." *Canadian Journal of Applied Physiology* (2005) 30 (4): 433–441.

Price, D. and B. Donne. "Effect of Variation in Seat Tube Angle at Different Seat Heights on Submaximal Cycling Performance in Man." *Journal of Sports Sciences* (1997) 15: 395–402.

Rogatzki, M. J., B. S. Ferguson, M. L. Goodwin, and L. B. Gladden. "Lactate Is Always the End Product of Glycolysis." *Frontiers of Neuroscience* (2015) 9: 22.

Tønnessen, E., Ø. Sylta, T. A. Haugen, E. Hem, I. S. Svendsen, and S. Seiler. (2014). "The Road to Gold: Training and Peaking Characteristics in the Year Prior to a Gold Medal Endurance Performance." *PLoS One* (2014) 9: e101796.

Tornero-Aguilera, J. F., Jiménez-Morcillo J., A. Rubio-Zarapuz, and V. J. Clemente-Suárez. "Central and Peripheral Fatigue in Physical Exercise Explained: A Narrative Review." *International Journal of Environmental Research and Public Health*. (2022) 19 (7): 3909.

Zapico, A. G., F. J. Calderon, P. J. Benito, C. B. Gonzalez, A. Parisi, F. Pigozzi, and V. Di Salvo. "Evolution of Physiological and Haematological Parameters with Training Load in Elite Male Road Cyclists: a Longitudinal Study." *Journal of Sports Medicine & Physical Fitness*. (2007) 47, 191-196.

Chapter 3

Amann, M., A. W. Subudhi, and C. Foster. "Predictive Validity of Ventilatory and Lactate Thresholds for Cycling Time Trial Performance." *Scandinavian Journal of Medicine and Science in Sports* (2006) 16 (1): 27-34.

Bendke, R., R. M. Leithauser, and Q. Ochentel. "Blood Lactate Diagnostics in Exercise Testing and Training." *International Journal of Sports Physiology and Performance* 6 (1) (2011): 8–24.

Borg, G. "Perceived Exertion as an Indicator of Somatic Stress." *Scandinavian Journal of Rehabilitation Medicine* (1970) 2 (2): 92–98.

Borszcz, F. K., A. F. Tramontin, A. H. Bossi, L. J. Carminatti, and V. P. Costa. "Functional Threshold Power in Cyclists: Validity of the Concept and Physiological Responses." *International Journal of Sports Medicine* (2018) 39 (10): 737-742.

Borszcz, F. K., A. F. Tramontin, and V. P. Costa. "Is the Functional Threshold Power Interchangeable with the Maximal Lactate Steady State in Trained Cyclists?" *International Journal of Physiology and Performance* (2019) 14 (8): 1029-1035.

Borszcz, F. K., A. F. Tramontin, and V. P. Costa. "Reliability of the Functional Threshold Power in Competitive Cyclists." *International Journal of Sports Medicine* (2020) 41 (3): 175-181.

Brooks, G. A. "Lactate as a Fulcrum of Metabolism." *Redox Biology* (2020) doi: 10.1016/j.redox.2020.101454.

Buchheit M. and P. B. Laursen. "High-Intensity Interval Training, Solutions to the Programming Puzzle. Part II: Anaerobic Energy, Neuromuscular Load and Practical Applications." *Sports Medicine* (2013) 43 (10): 927–954.

Cairns, S. P. "Lactic Acid and Exercise Performance: Culprit or Friend?" *Sports Medicine* (2006) 36 (4): 279–291.

Casado, A., C. Foster, M. Bakken, and L.I. Tjelta. "Does Lactate-Guided Threshold Interval Training Within a High-Volume Low-Intensity Approach Represent the "Next Step" in the Evolution of Distance Running Training?" *International Journal of Environmental Research and Public Health* (2023) 20 (5): 3782.

Chicharro, J. L., M. Perez, A. F. Vaquero, A. Lucia, and J. C. Legido. "Lactic Threshold vs Ventilatory Threshold During a Ramp Test on a Cycle Ergometer." *Journal of Sports Medicine and Physical Fitness* (1997) 37 (2): 117-121.

Ekblom, B. and A. N. Golobarg. "The Influence of Physical Training and Other Factors on the Subjective Rating of Perceived Exertion." *Acta Physiologica Scandinavica* (1971) 83 (3): 399–406.

Estave-Lanao, J., C. Foster, S. Seiler, and A. Lucia. "Impact of Training Intensity Distribution on Performance in Endurance Athletes." *Journal of Strength and Conditioning Research* 21 (3) (2007): 943–949.

Grossl, T., R. Dantas De Lucas, K. Mendes De Souza, and G. A. Guglielmol. "Maximal Lactate Steady-State and Anaerobic Thresholds from Different Methods in Cyclists." *European Journal of Sport Science* (2012) 12 (2): 161–167.

Harms, S. J. and R. C. Hickson. "Skeletal Muscle Mitochondria and Myoglobin, Endurance, and Intensity of Training." *Journal of Applied Physiology, Environment, and Exercise Physiology* (1983) 54 (3): 798—802.

Helgerud J., K. Høydal, E. Wang, T. Karsen, P. Berg, M. Bjerkaas, T. Simonsen, C. Helgesen, N. Hjorth, R. Bach, and J. Hoff. "Aerobic High-Intensity Intervals Improve VO_2max More Than Moderate Training." *Medicine and Science in Sports and Exercise* (2007) 39 (4): 665–671.

Impellizzeri, F., A. Sassi, M. Rodriguez-Alonso, P. Mognoni, and S. Marcora. "Exercise Intensity During Off-Road Cycling Competitions." *Medicine and Science in Sports and Exercise* (2002) 34 (11): 1808–1813.

Jacobs, I. "Blood Lactate: Implications for Training and Sports Performance." *Sports Medicine* (1986) 3 (1): 10–25. "Interval Training in Endurance-Trained Cyclists." *European Journal of Applied Physiology and Occupational Physiology* (1997) 75 (4): 298–304.

Jeanes, E. M., C. Foster, J. P. Porcari, M. Gibson, and S. Doberstein. "Translation of Exercise Testing to Exercise Prescription Using the Talk Test." *Journal of Strength and Conditioning Research* (2011) 25 (3): 590-596.

Liu, C., J. Wu, J. Zhu, et al. "Lactate Inhibits Lipolysis in Fat Cells Through Activation of an Orphan G-Protein-Coupled Receptor, GPR81." *Journal of Biology and Chemistry* (2009) 284 (5): 2811-2822.

Mahmod, S. R., L. T. Narayanan, R. A. Hasan, and E. Supriyauto. "Regulated Mono-Syllabic Talk Test vs. Counting Talk Test During Incremental Cardiorespiratory Exercise: Determining the Implications of the Utterance Rate on Exercise Intensity Estimation." *Frontiers in Physiology* (2022) doi: 10.3389.

McGehee, J. C., C. J. Tanner, and J. A. Houmard. "A Comparison of Methods for Estimating the Lactate Threshold." *Journal of Strength and Conditioning Research* (2005) 19 (3): 553–558.

Myers, J. and E. Ashley. "Dangerous Curves. A Perspective on Exercise, Lactate, and the Anaerobic Threshold." *Chest* (1997) 111 (3): 787–795.

Nicholls, J. F., S. L. Phares, and M.J. Buono. "Relationship Between Blood Lactate Response to Exercise and Endurance Performance in Competitive Female Master Cyclists." *International Journal of Sports Medicine* (1997) 18 (6): 458–463.

Norman, J. F., E. Hopkins, and E. Crapo. "Validity of the Counting Talk Test in Comparison with Standard Methods of Estimating Exercise Intensity in Young Healthy Adults." *Journal of Cardiopulminary Rehabilitation Preview* (2008) 28 (3): 199-202.

Owen, J., R. Simmons, S. D. Patterson, and M. Waldron. "Functional Threshold Power Is Not Equivalent to Lactate Parameters in Trained Cyclists." *Journal of Strength and Conditioning Research* (2021) 35 (10): 2790-2794.

Persinger, R., C. Foster, M. Gibson, D. C. W. Fater, and J. P. Porcari. "Consistency of the Talk Test for Exercise Prescription." *Medicine & Science in Sports and Exercise* (2004) 36 (9): 1632–1639.

Plato, P. A., M. McNulty, S. M. Crunk, and A. Tugergun. "Predicting Lactate Threshold Using Ventilatory Threshold." *International Journal of Sports Medicine* (2008) 29 (9): 732-737.

Quinn, T. J. and B. A. Coons. "The Talk Test and Its Relationship with the Ventilatory and Lactate Thresholds." *Journal of Sports Science* (2011) 29 (11) 1175-1182.

Rodriguez-Marroyo, J. A., J. G. Villa, J. Garcia-Lopez, and C. Foster. "Relationship Between the Talk Test and Ventilatory Thresholds in Well-Trained Cyclists." *Journal of Strength and Conditioning Research* (2013) 27 (7): 1942-1949.

Seiler, S. and E. Tønnessen. "Intervals, Thresholds, and Long Slow Distance: The Role of Intensity and Duration in Endurance Training." *SportScience* (2009) sportsci.org. 13. 32 – 53.

Sitko, S., R. Cirer-Sastre, F. Corbi, and I. Lopez-Laval. "Functional Threshold Power as an Alternative to Lactate Thresholds in Road Cycling." *Journal of Strength and Conditioning Research* (2022) 36 (11): 3129-3183.

Skinner, J. and T. McLellan. "The Transition from Aerobic to Anaerobic Metabolism." *Research Quarterly for Exercise and Sport* (1980) 51 (1): 234–248.

Stöggl, T. and B. Sperlich. "Polarized Training Has Greater Impact on Key Endurance Variables than Threshold, High Intensity, or High-Volume Training." *Frontiers in Physiology* (2014) 5: 33.

Swensen, T. C., C. R. Harnish, L. Beltman, and B. A. Keller. "Noninvasive Estimation of the Maximal Lactate Steady State in Trained Cyclists." *Medicine and Science in Sports and Exercise* (1999) 31 (5): 742–746.

Tramontin, A. F., F. K. Borszcz, and V. Costa. "Functional Threshold Power Estimates From a 20-Minute Time-Trial Test Is Warm-up Dependent." *International Journal of Sports Medicine* (2022) 43 (5): 411-417.

Westgarth-Taylor, C., J. A. Hawley, S. Rickard, K.H. Myburgh, T. D. Noakes, and S. C. Dennis. "Metabolic and Performance Adaptations" to Loftin, M. and B. Warren. "Comparison of a Simulated 16.1-km Time Trial, VO_2max and Related Factors in Cyclists with Different Ventilatory Thresholds." *International Journal of Sports Medicine* (1994) 15 (8): 498–503.

Woltmann, M. L., C. Foster, J. P. Porcari, C. L. Camic, C. Dodge, S. Haible, and R. P. Mikat. "Evidence That the Talk Test Can be Used to Regulate Exercise Intensity." *Journal of Strength and Conditioning Research* (2015) 29 (5): 1248-1254.

Chapter 4

Aceto, M., J. Cassinat, Y. S. Ghattas, and V. Wright. "Lower Body Weightlifting Injuries Treated in United States Emergency Departments from 2012–2021." *International Journal of Sports Medicine* (2024) doi: 10.1055/a-2335-4304.

Bosquet, L., J. Montpetit, D. Arvisais, and I. Mujika. "Effects of Tapering on Performance: A Meta-Analysis." *Medicine and Science in Sports and Exercise* (2007) 39 (8): 1358–1365.

Casado, A., F. Gonzalez-Mohino, J. M. Gonzalez-Rave, and C. Foster. "Training Periodization, Methods, Intensity Distribution, and Volume in Highly Trained and Elite Distance Runners: A Systematic Review." *International Journal of Sports, Physiology, and Performance* (2022) 17 (6): 820-833.

Filipas, L., M. Bonato, G. Gallo, and R. Codella. "Effects of 16 Weeks of Pyramidal and Polarized Training Intensity Distributions in Well-Trained Endurance Runners." *Scandinavian Journal of Medicine and Science in Sports* (2011) 32 (3): 498-511.

Fitz-Clarke J. R., R. H. Morton, and E. W. Banister. "Optimizing Athletic Performance by Influence Curves." *Journal of Applied Physiology* (1991) 71 (3): 1151–1158.

Houmard, J. A. "Impact of Reduced Training on Performance in Endurance Athletes." *Sports Medicine* (1991) 12 (6): 380–393.

Kiely, J. "Periodization Theory: Confronting an Inconvenient Truth." *Sports Medicine* (2017) 48: 753-764.

Muñoz, I., R. Cejuela, S. Seiler, E. Larumbe, and J. Esteve-Lanao. "Training-Intensity Distribution During an Ironman Season: Relationship with Competition Performance." *International Journal of Sports Physiology and Performance* (2014) 9 (2): 332–339.

Neal, C. M., A. M. Hunter, L. Brennan, A. O'Sullivan, D. L. Hamilton, G. DeVito, and S. D. Galloway. "Six Weeks of a Polarized Training Intensity Distribution Leads to Greater Physiological and Performance Adaptations Than a Threshold Model in Trained Cyclists." *Journal of Applied Physiology* (2013) 114 (4): 461–471.

Seiler, S. and G. Kjerland. "Quantifying Training Intensity Distribution in Elite Endurance Athletes: Is There Evidence for an 'Optimal' Distribution?" *Scandinavian Journal of Medicine & Science in Sports* (2006) 16 (1): 49–56.

Seiler, S. and E. Tonnessen. "Intervals, Thresholds, and Long Slow Distance: The Role of Intensity and Duration in Endurance Training." *Sportscience* (2009) 13: 32–53.

Seiler, S. "What Is Best Practice for Training Intensity and Duration Distribution in Endurance Athletes?" *International Journal of Sports Physiology and Performance* (2010) 5 (3): 276–291.

Seiler, S. and E. Tonnessen. "Intervals, Thresholds, and Long Slow Distance: The Role of Intensity and Duration in Endurance Training." *Sportscience* (2009) 13: 32–53.

Stoggl, T. and B. Sperlich. "Polarized Training Has Greater Impact on Key Endurance Variables Than Threshold, High Intensity, or High Volume Training." *Frontiers in Physiology* (2014) 4 (5): 33.

Taha, T. and S. G. Thomas. "Systems Modelling of the Relationship Between Training and Performance." *Sports Medicine* (2003) 33 (14): 1061–1073.

Chapter 5

Almquist, N. W., I. Loullen, P. T. Byrkjedal, and M. Spencer. "Effects of Sprints in One Weekly Low-Intensity Training Session During the Transition Period of Elite Cyclists." *Frontiers in Physiology* (2020) 11: 1000.

Asplund, C. and M. Ross. "Core Stability and Bicycling." *Current Sports Medicine Reports* (2010) 9 (3): 155–160.

Banister, E. W., R. H. Morton, and J. Fitz-Clarke. "Dose/Response Effects of Exercise Modeled from Training: Physical and Biochemical Measures." *Annals of Physiology and Anthropology* (1992) 11 (3): 345–356.

Beattie, K., I. C. Kenny, M. Lyons, and B. P. Carson. "The Effect of Strength Training on Performance in Endurance Athletes." *Sports Medicine* (2014) 44 (6): 845-865.

Beatty, T., D. Webner, and S. J. Collina. "Bone Density in Competitive Cyclists." *Current Sports Medicine Report* (2010) 9 (6): 352–355.

Bosquet, L., J. Montpetit, D. Arvisais, and I. Mujika. "Effects of Tapering on Performance: A Meta-Analysis." *Medicine and Science in Sports and Exercise* (2007) 39 (8): 1358–1365.

Bouchard, C., T. Rankinen, Y. C. Chagnon, T. Rice, L. Perusse, J. Gagnon, I. Borecki, P. An, A. S. Leon, J. S. Skinner, J. H. Wilmore, M. Province, and D. C. Rao. "Genomic Scan for Maximal Oxygen Uptake and Its Response to Training in the HERITAGE Family Study." *Journal of Applied Physiology* (2000) 88 (2): 551–559.

Busso, T. "Variable Dose-Response Relationship Between Exercise Training and Performance." *Medicine and Science in Sports and Exercise* (2003) 35 (7): 1188-1195.

Campion F., A. M. Nevill, M. K. Karlsson, J. Lounana, M. Shabani, P. Fardellone, and J. Medell. "Bone Status in Professional Cyclists." *International Journal of Sports Medicine* (2010) 31(7): 511–515.

Cormie, P., M. R. McGuigan, and R. U. Newton. "Developing Maximal Neuromuscular Power: Part 1—Biological Basis of Maximal Power Production." *Sports Medicine* (2011) 41 (1): 17–38.

Cormie, P., M. R. McGuigan, and R. U. Newton. "Developing Maximal Neuromuscular Power: Part 2—Training Considerations for Improving Maximal Power Production." *Sports Medicine* (2011) 41 (2): 125–146.

Davies, T., R. Orr, M. Halaki, and D. Hackett. "Effect of Training Leading to Repetition Failure on Muscular Strength: A Systematic Review and Meta-Analysis." *Sports Medicine* (2016) 46 (4): 487–502.

Ebben, W. P., A. G. Kindler, K. A. Chirdon, N. C. Jenkins, A. J. Polichnowski, and A. V. Ng. "The Effect of High-Load vs. High-Repetition Training on Endurance Performance." *Journal of Strength and Conditioning Research* (2004) 18 (3): 513–517.

Goto, K., M. Nagasawa, O. Yanagisawa, T. Kizuka, N. Ishii, and K. Takamatsu. "Muscular Adaptations to Combinations of High- and Low-Intensity Resistance Exercises." *Journal of Strength and Conditioning Research* (2004) 18 (4): 730–737.

Hautala A. J., A. M. Kiviniemi, T. H. Makikallio, H. Kinnunen, S. Nissila, H. V. Huikuri, and M. P. Tulppc. "Individual Differences in the Responses to Endurance and Resistance Training." *European Journal of Applied Physiology* (2006) 96 (5): 535–542.

James, C. A., A. J. Richardson, P. W. Watt, A. G. B. Willmott, O. R. Gibson, and N. S. Maxwell. "Short-Term Heat Acclimation Improves the Determinants of Endurance Performance and 5-KM Running Performance in the Heat." *Applied Physiology, Nutrition, and Metabolism* (2017) 42 (3): 285–294.

Kubukeli, Z. N., T. D. Noakes, and S. C. Dennis. "Training Techniques to Improve Endurance Exercise Performances." *Sports Medicine* (2002) 32 (8): 489–509.

Laursen, P. B. and D. G. Jenkins. "The Scientific Basis for High-Intensity Interval Training: Optimising Training Programmes and Maximising Performance in Highly Trained Endurance Athletes." *Sports Medicine* (2002) 32 (1): 53–73.

Lindner, R., I. S. Raj, A. W. H. Yang, S. Zamen, J. Larsen, and J. Denham. "Moderate to Vigorous-Intensity Continuous Training Versus High Intensity Training for Improving VO_2 max in Women: A Systematic Review and Meta-Analysis." *International Journal of Sports Medicine* (2023) 44 (7): 484–495.

Lorenzo, S., J. R. Halliwell, M. N. Sawka, and C. T. Munson. "Heat Acclimation Improves Exercise Performance." *Journal of Applied Physiology* (2010) 109 (4): 1140–1147.

Louis, J. C., Hausswirth, C. Easthope, and J. Brisswalter. "Strength Training Improves Cycling Efficiency in Master Endurance Athletes." *European Journal of Applied Physiology* (2012) 112 (2): 631–640.

Martinez-Noguera, F. J., P. E. Alcaraz, R. Ortolano-Ríos, S. Dufour, C. Marin-Pagán. "Professional Cyclists Have Lower Levels of Bone Markers Than Amateurs. Is There a Risk of Osteoporosis in Cyclists?" *Bone* (2021) 153: 116102.

Maun, T., R. P. Lamberts, and M. I. Lambert. "Methods of Prescribing Relative Exercise Intensity: Physiological and Practical Considerations." *Sport Medicine* (2013) 43 (7): 613–625.

Millet, G. P., B. Jaouen, F. Borrani, and R. Candau. "Effects of Concurrent Endurance and Strength Training on Running Economy and VO_2 Kinetics." *Medicine and Science in Sports and Exercise* (2002) 34 (8): 1351–1359.

Mitchell, C. J., T. A. Churchward-Venne, D. W. West, N. A. Burd, L. Breen, S. K. Baker, and S. M. Phillips. "Resistance Exercise Load Does Not Determine Training-Mediated Hypertrophic Gains in Young Men." *Journal of Applied Physiology* (2012) 113 (1): 71–77.

Mojock, C. D., M. J. Ormsbee, J. S. Kim, B. H. Arjmandi, G. A. Louw, R. J. Contreras, and L. B. Panton. "Comparisons of Bone Mineral Density Between Recreational and Trained Male Road Cyclists." *Clinical Sport Medicine* (2016) 26 (2): 152–156.

Mujik, I. and S. Padilla. "Scientific Bases for Precompetition Tapering Strategies." *Medicine and Science in Sports and Exercise* (2003) 35 (7): 1182-1187.

Mujika, I., B. R. Ronnestad, and D. T. Martin. "Effects of Increased Muscle Strength and Muscle Mass on Endurance-Cycling Performance." *International Journal of Sports, Physiology, and Performance* (2016) 11 (3): 283–289.

Neary, J. P., T. P. Martin, D. C. Reid, R. Burnham, and H. A. Quinney. "The Effects of a Reduced Exercise Duration Taper Programme On Performance and Muscle Enzymes on Endurance Cyclists." *European Journal of Applied Physiology and Occupational Physiology* (1992) 65 (1): 30–36.

Oystein, S., E. Tonnessen, O. Sandbakk, D. Hammarstrom, J. Danielsen, K. Skovereng, B. R. Ronnestad, and S. Seiler. "Effects of High-Intensity Training on Physiological and Hormonal Adaptations in Well-Trained Cyclists." *Medicine and Science in Sports and Exercise* (2017) 49 (6): 1137–1146.

Pate, R. R. and J. D. Branch. "Training for Endurance Sport." *Medicine and Science in Sports and Exercise* (1992) 24 (9): S340–S343.

Paton, C. D. and W. G. Hopkins. "Seasonal Changes in Power of Competitive Cyclists: Implications for Monitoring Performance." *Journal of Science and Medicine in Sport* (2005) 8 (4): 375–381.

Phillips, S. M. "A Brief Review of Critical Processes in Exercise-Induced Muscular Hypertrophy." *Sports Medicine* (2014) 44 (S1): S71–S77.

Rønnestad, B. R., E. A. Hansen, and T. Raastad. "Effect of Heavy Strength Training on Thigh Muscle Cross-Sectional Area, Performance Determinants, and Performance in Well-Trained Cyclists." *European Journal of Applied Physiology* (2010) 108 (5): 965–975.

Rønnestad, B. R., E. A. Hansen, and T. Raastad. "In-Season Strength Maintenance Training Increases Well-Trained Cyclists' Performance." *European Journal of Applied Physiology* (2010) 110 (6): 1269–1282.

Rønnestad, B. R., E. A. Hansen, and T. Raastad. "Strength Training Improves 5-Min All-Out Performance Following 185 Min of Cycling." *Scandinavian Journal of Medicine and Science in Sports* (2011) 21 (2): 250–259.

Rønnestad, B. R., J. Hansen, I. Hollan, and S. Ellefsen. "Strength Training Improves Performance and Pedaling Characteristics in Elite Cyclists." *Scandinavian Journal of Medicine and Science in Sports* (2014) 25 (1): e89–98.

Rønnestad, B. R. and I. Mujika. "Optimizing Strength Training for Running and Cycling Endurance Performance." *Scandinavian Journal of Medicine and Science in Sports* (2014) 24 (4): 603–612.

Rønnestad, B. R., E. A. Hansen, I. Hollan, M. Spencer, and S. Ellefsen. "In-Season Strength Training Cessation Impairs Performance Variables in Elite Cyclists." *International Journal of Sports, Physiology, and Performance* (2015) 11 (6): 727–735.

Rumpf, M. C., R. G. Lockie, J. B. Cronin, and F. Jalilvand. "The Effect of Different Sprint Training Methods on Sprint Performance Over Various Distances: A Brief Review." *Journal of Strength and Conditioning Research* (2016) 30 (6):1767–1785.

Sekiguchiy, Y., C. L. Benjamin, C. N. Manning, J. F. Struder, L. E. Armstrong, E. C. Lee, R. A. Huggins, R. L. Stearns, L. J. Distefano, and D. J. Casa. "Effects of Heat Acclimatization, Heat Acclimation, and Intermittent Exercise Heat Training on Time-Trial performance." *Sports Health* (2022) 14 (5): 694–701.

Shepley, B., J. D. MacDougall, N. Cipriano, J. R. Sutton, M. A. Tarnopolsky, and G. Coates. "Physiological Effects of Tapering in Highly Trained Athletes." *Journal of Applied Physiology* (1992) 72 (2): 706–711.

Simão, R., B. F. de Salles, T. Figueiredo, I. Dias, and J. M. Willardson. "Exercise Order in Resistance Training." *Sports Medicine* (2012) 42 (3): 251–265.

Smoliga, J. "Relationship Between Cycling Mechanics and Core Stability." *The Journal of Strength and Conditioning Research* (2021) 21 (4): 1300–1304.

Sunde, A., O. Støren, M. Bjerkaas, M. H. Larsen, J. Hoff, and J. Helgerud. "Maximal Strength Training Improves Cycling Economy in Competitive Cyclists.*" Journal of Strength and Conditioning Research* (2010) 24 (8): 2157–2165.

Taha, T. and S. G. Thomas. "Systems Modelling of the Relationship Between Training and Performance." *Sports Medicine* (2003) 33 (14): 1061–1073.

Thomas, L., I. Mujika, and T. Busso. "Computer Simulations Assessing the Potential Performance Benefit of a Final Increase in Training During Pre-Event Taper.*" Journal of Strength and Conditioning Researc*h (2009) 23 (6): 1729–1736.

Tønnessen, E., Ø. Sylta, T. A. Haugen, E. Hem, I. S. Svendsen, and S. Seiler. "The Road to Gold: Training and Peaking Characteristics in the Year Prior to a Gold Medal Endurance Performance." *PLoS One* (2014) 9 (7): e101796.

Chapter 6

Antunes, B. M., E. Z. Campos, S. S. Parmezzani, R. V. Santos, E. Franchini, and F. S. Lira. "Sleep Quality and Duration Are Associated With Performance in Maximal Incremental Test." *Physiology and Behavior* (2017) 1 (177): 252–256.

Aubry, A., C. Hausswirth, J. Louis, A. J. Coutts, and Y. Le Meur. "Functional Overreaching: The Key to Peak Performance During the Taper?" *Medicine and Science in Sports and Exercise* (2014) 46 (9): 1769–1777.

Billman, G. E. "Heart Rate Variability–A Historical Perspective." *Frontiers in Physiology* (2011) 2: 86.

Bosquet, L., S. Merkari, D. Arvisais, and A. E. Aubert. "Is Heart Rate a Convenient Tool to Monitor Over-Reaching? A Systematic Review of the Literature." *British Journal of Sports Medicine* (2008) 42 (9): 709–714.

Bourdillon, N. S., S. Bellenoue, L. Schmitt, and G. P. Millet. "Daily Cardiac Autonomic Responses During the Tour de France in a Male Professional Cyclist." *Frontiers in Neuroscience* (2023) doi: 103389/fnins.2023.1221957.

Busso, T., R. Candau, and J. R. Lacour. "Fatigue and Fitness Modelled from the Effects of Training on Performance." *European Journal of Applied Physiology and Occupational Physiology* (1994) 69 (1): 50–54.

Cadegiani, F. A. and C. E. Kater. "Novel Insights of Overtraining Syndrome Discovered from the EROS Study." *BMJ Open Sport & Exercise Medicine* (2019) 5 (1): e000542.

Chung, J., M. Choi, and K. Lee. "Effects of Short-Term Intake of Montmorenoy Tart Cherry Juice on Sleep Quality After Intermittent Exercise in Elite Female Hockey Players: A Randomized Controlled Trial." *International Journal of Environmental Research and Public Health* (2022) 19 (16): 10272.

Crispim, C. A., I. Z. Zimberg, B. G. dos Reis, R. M. Diniz, S. Tufik, and M. T. de Mello. "Relationship Between Food Intake and Sleep Pattern in Healthy Individuals." *Journal of Clinical Sleep and Medicine* (2011) 7 (6): 659–664.

DaSilva, D. F., Z. M. Ferro, K. B. Adamo, and F. A. Machado. "Endurance Running Training Individually Guided by HRV in Untrained Women." *Journal of Strength and Conditioning Research* (2019) 33 (3): 736–746.

Davies, D. J., K. S. Graham, and C. M. Chow. "The Effect of Prior Endurance Training on Nap Sleep Patterns." *International Journal of Sports Physiology and Performance* (2010) 5 (1): 87–97.

De Pauw, K., B. De Geus, B. Roelands, F. Lauwens, J. Verschueren, E. Heyman, and R.R. Meeusen. "Effect of Five Different Recovery Methods on Repeated Cycle Performance." *Medicine and Science in Sports and Exercise* (2011) 43 (5): 890–897.

Ebrahim, I. O., C.M. Shapiro, A. J. Williams, and P. B. Fenwick. "Alcohol and Sleep I: Effects on Normal Sleep." *Alcoholism, Clinical and Experimental Research* (2013) 37 (4): 539–549.

Eliakim, M., E. Bodner, Y. Meckel, D. Nemet, and A. Eliakim. "Effect of Rhythm on the Recovery from Intense Exercise." *Journal of Strength and Conditioning Research* (2012) 27 (4): 1019–1024.

Flatt, A. A., M. R. Esco, and F. Y. Nakamura. "Individual Heart Rate Variability Responses to Preseason Training in High Level Female Soccer Players." *Journal of Strength and Conditioning Research* (2017) 31 (2): 531–538.

Foster, C., K. M. Heimann, P. L. Esten, G. Brice, and J. P. Porcari. "Differences in Perceptions of Training by Coaches and Athletes." *South African Journal of Sports Medicine* (2001) 8 (2): 3-7.

Fry, R. W., A. R. Morton, and D. Keast. "Periodisation of Training Stress—A Review." *Canadian Journal of Sport Sciences* (1992) 17 (3): 234–240.

Garrido, M., D. González-Gómez, M. Lozano, C. Barriga, S. D. Paredes, and A. B. Rodríguez. "A Jerte Valley Cherry Product Provides Beneficial Effects on Sleep Quality. Influence on Aging." *Journal of Nutrition, Health & Aging* (2013) 17 (6): 553–560.

Hagberg, J. M., R. C. Hickson, A. A. Ehsani, and J. O. Holloszy. "Faster Adjustment to and Recovery from Submaximal Exercise in the Trained State." *Journal of Applied Physiology* (1980) 48 (2): 218–224.

Hausswirth, C., J. Louis, A. Aubry, G. Bonnet, R. Duffield, and Y. Le Meur. "Evidence of Disturbed Sleep and Increased Illness in Overreached Endurance Athletes." *Medicine and Science in Sports and Exercise* (2014) 46 (5): 1036–1045.

Hautala, A. J., A. M. Kiviniemi, and M. P. Tulppo. "Individual Responses to Aerobic Exercise: The Role of the Autonomic Nervous System." *Neuroscience, Biology, and Behavior Review* (2009) 33 (2): 107–115.

Hedelin, R., G. Kentta, U. Wiklund, P. Bjerle, and K. Henriksson-Larsen. "Short-Term Overtraining: Effects on Performance, Circulatory Responses, and Heart Rate Variability." *Medicine and Science in Sports and Exercise* (2000) 32 (8): 1480–1484.

Hemmings, B., M. Smith, J. Graydon, and R. Dyson. "Effects of Massage on Physiological Restoration, Perceived Recovery, and Repeated Sports Performance." *British Journal of Sports Medicine* (2000) 34 (2): 109–114.

Hill, D. W., D. O. Borden, K. M. Darnaby, and D. N. Hendricks. "Aerobic and Anaerobic Contributions to Exhaustive High-Intensity Exercise After Sleep Deprivation." *Journal of Sports Sciences* (1994) 12 (5): 455–461.

Hooper, S. L., L. T. MacKinnen, A. Howard, R. D. Gordon, and A. W. Bachmaan. "Markers for Monitoring Overtraining and Recovery." *Medicine and Science in Sports and Exercise* (1995) 27 (1): 106–112.

Howatson, G., P. G. Bell, J. Tallent, B. Middleton. M. P. McHugh, and J. Ellis. "Effect of Tart Cherry Juice (Prunuscerasus) on Melatonin Levels and Enhanced Sleep Quality." *European Journal of Nutrition* (2012) 51 (8): 909–916.

Impey, S. G., M. A. Hearris, K. M. Hammond, J. D. Bartlett, J. Louis, G. L. Close, and J. P. Morton. "Fuel for the Work Required: A Theoretical Framework for Carbohydrate Periodization and the Glycogen Threshold Hypothesis." *Sports Medicine* (2018) 48 (5): 1031–1048.

Kaikkonen, P., E. Hynynen, T. Mann, H. Rusko, and A. Nummela. "Heart Rate Variability Is Related to Training Load Variables in Interval Running Exercises." *European Journal of Applied Physiology* (2012) 112 (3): 829–838.

Killer, S. C., I. S. Svendsen, A. E. Jeukendrup, and M. Gleeson. "Evidence of Disturbed Sleep and Mood State in Well-Trained Athletes During Short-Term Intensified Training With and Without a High Carbohydrate Nutritional Intervention." *Journal of Sports Sciences* (2015): 1–9.

Kivinemi, A. M., A. J. Hautala, H. Kinnunen, and M. P. Tulppo. "Endurance Training Guided Individually by Daily Heart Rate Variability Measurements." *European Journal of Applied Physiology* (2007) 101 (6): 743–751.

Lamberts, R. P., J. Swart, B. Capostagno, T. D. Noakes, and M. I. Lambert. "Heart Rate Recovery as a Guide to Monitor Fatigue and Predict Changes in Performance Parameters." *Scandinavian Journal of Medicine & Science in Sports* (2010) 20 (3): 449–457.

Le Meur, Y., A. Pichon, K. Schaal, L. Schmitt, J. Louis, J. Gueneron, P. P. Vidal, and C. Hausswirth. "Evidence of Parasympathetic Hyperactivity in Functionally Overreached Athletes." *Medicine and Science in Sports and Exercise* (2013) 45 (11): 2061–2071.

Lehmann, M. J., W. Lormes, A. Opitz-Gress, J. M. Steinacker, N. Netzer, C. Foster, and U. Gastman. "Training and Overtraining: An Overview and Experimental Results in Endurance Sports." *Journal of Sports Medicine and Physical Fitness* (1997) 37 (1): 7–17.

Levy, W. C., M. D. Cerqueira, G. D. Hood, K. A. Johannessen, I. B. Abraiss, R. S. Schwartz, and J. R. Stratton. "Effect of Endurance Exercise Training on Heart Rate Variability at Rest in Healthy Young and Older Men." *American Journal of Cardiology* (1990) 82: 1236–1241.

Li, J., M. V. Vitello, and N. S. Gooneratne. "Sleep in Normal Aging." *Sleep Medicines Clinic* (2018) 13 (1): 1–11.

Lindseth, G., P. Lindseth, and M. Thompson. "Nutritional Effects on Sleep." *Western Journal of Nursing Research* (2013) 35 (4): 497–513.

Lundstrom, C. J., N. A. Foreman, and G. Biltz. "Practices and Applications of Heart Rate Variability Monitoring in Endurance Athletes." *International Journal of Sports Medicine* (2023) 44 (01): 9–19.

McAinch, A. J., M. A. Febbraio, J. M. Parkin, S. Zhao, K. Tangalakis, L. Stojanovska, and M. F. Carey. "Effect of Active Versus Passive Recovery on Metabolism and Performance During Subsequent Exercise." *International Journal of Sport Nutrition and Exercise Metabolism* (2004) 14 (2): 185–196.

Meeusen, R., D. Martine, C. Foster, A. Fry, M. Gleeson, D. Nieman, J. Raglin, G. Rietjens, J. Steinacker and A. Urhausen, European College of Sport Science, and American College of Sports Medicine. "Prevention, Diagnosis and Treatment of the Overtraining Syndrome: Joint Consensus Statement of the European College of Sport Science (ECSS) and the American College of Sports Medicine (ACSM)." *European Journal of Sport Science* (2013) 13 (1): 1–24.

Meth, E. M. S., L. E. M. Braudao, L. T. van Egmond, P. Xue, A. Grip, J. Wu, A. Adan, F. Andersson, A. P. Pacheco, K. Uvnas-Moberg, J. Cedernaes, and J. Cedernaes. "A Weighted Blanket Increases Pre-Sleep Salivary Concentrations of Melatonin in Young, Healthy Adults." *Journal of Sleep Research* (2013) 32 (2): e13743.

Mika, A., P. Mika, B. Fernhall, and V. B. Unnithan. "Comparison of Recovery Strategies on Muscle Performance After Fatiguing Exercise." *American Journal of Physical Medicine & Rehabilitation* (2007) 86 (6): 474–481.

Millet, G. P., A. Lambert, B. Barbier, J. D. Rouillon, and R. B. Candan. "Modelling the Relationships Between Training, Anxiety, and Fatigue in Elite Athletes." *International Journal of Sports Medicine* (2005) 26 (6): 492–498.

Mishica, C., H. Kyrolainene, E. Hynynen, H. C. Holmberg, and V. Linnamo. "Relationships Between Heart Rate Variability, Sleep Duration, Cortisol and Physical Training in Young Athletes." *Journal of Sports Science and Medicine* (2021) 20 (4): 778–788.

Morton, R. H. "Modeling Training and Overtraining." *Journal of Sports Sciences* (1997) 15 (3): 335–340.

Mujika, I. and S. Padilla. "Detraining: Loss of Training-Induced Physiological and Performance Adaptations. Part I: Short Term Insufficient Training Stimulus." *Sports Medicine* (2000) 30 (2): 79–87.

Mujika, I. and S. Padilla. "Detraining: Loss of Training-Induced Physiological and Performance Adaptations. Part II: Long Term Insufficient Training Stimulus." *Sports Medicine* (2000) 30 (3): 145–54.

Neufer, P. D. "The Effect of Detraining and Reduced Training on the Physiological Adaptations to Aerobic Exercise Training." *Sports Medicine* (1989) 8 (5): 302–320.

Penev, P. D. "Association Between Sleep and Morning Testosterone Levels in Older Men." *Sleep* (2007) 30 (4): 427–432.

Pigeon, W. R., M. Carr, C. Gorman, and M. L. Perlis. "Effects of a Tart Cherry Juice Beverage on the Sleep of Older Adults with Insomnia: A Pilot Study." *Journal of Medicine and Food* (2010) 13 (3): 579–583.

Plews, D. J., P. B. Laursen, A. E. Kilding, and M. Buchheit. "Evaluating Training Adaptation with Heart Rate Measures: A Methodological Comparison." *International Journal of Sports Physiology and Performance* (20113) 8 (6): 688–691.

Reichel, T., S. Hacker, J. Palmowski, T. K. Bosslau, T. Frech, P. Tirekoglou, E. Bothur, S. Samel, R. Walscheid, and K. Kruger. "Neurophysiolgical Markers for Monitoring Exercise and Recovery Cycles in Endurance Sports." *Journal of Sports Science and Medicine* (2022) 21 (3): 446–457.

Reynolds, A. C., J. Dorrian, P. Y. Liu, H. P. Van Dongen, G. A. Wittert, L. J. Harmer, and S. Banks. "Impact of Five Nights of Sleep Restriction on Glucose Metabolism, Leptin and Testosterone in Young Adult Men." *PLoS One* (2012) 7 (7): e41218.

Roberts, L. A., T. Raastad, J. F. Markworth, V. C. Figueiredo, I. M. Egner, A. Shield, D. Cameron-Smith, J. S. Coombes, and J. M. Peake. "Post-Exercise Cold Water Immersion Attenuates Acute Anabolic Signalling and Long-Term Adaptations in Muscle to Strength Training." *The Journal of Physiology* (2015) 593 (18): 4285-4301.

Seiler, S., O. Haugen, and E. Kuffel. "Autonomic Recovery After Exercise in Trained Athletes: Intensity and Duration Effects." *Medicine and Science in Sports and Exercise* (2007) 39 (8): 1366–1373.

Tomlin, D. L. and H. A. Wenger. "The Relationship Between Fitness and Recovery from High Intensity Intermittent Exercise." *Sports Medicine* (2001) 31 (1): 1–11.

Tseng, C. Y., J. P. Lee, Y. S. Tsai, S. D. Lee, C. L. Kao, T. C. Liu, C. Lai, M. B. Harris, and C. H. Kuo. "Topical Cooling (Icing) Delays Recovery from Eccentric Exercise-Induced Muscle Damage." *Journal of Strength and Conditioning Research* (2013) 27 (5): 1354–1361.

Urhausen, A. and W. Kindermann. "Diagnosis of Overtraining: What Tools Do We Have?" *Sports Medicine* (2002) 32 (2): 95–102.

Van Cauter, E., R. Leproult, and L. Plat. "Age-Related Changes in Slow-Wave Sleep and REM Sleep and Relationship with Growth Hormone and Cortisol Levels in Healthy Men." *Journal of the American Medical Association* (2000) 284 (7): 861–868.

VanHelder, T. and M. W. Radomski. "Sleep Deprivation and the Effect on Exercise Performance." *Sports Medicine* (1989) 7 (4): 235–247.

Vesterinen, V., K. Hakkinen, E. Hynynen J. Mikkola, L. Hokka, and A Nummela. "Heart Rate Variability in Prediction of Individual Adaptation to Endurance Training in Recreational Endurance Runners." *Scandinavian Journal of Medicine and Science in Sports* (2013) 23 (2): 171–180.

Vesterinen, V., A. Nummela, I. Heikura, T. Laine, E. Hynynen, J. Botella, and K. Hakkinen. "Individual Endurance Training Prescription with Heart Rate Variability." *Medicine and Science in Sports and Exercise* (2016) 48 (7): 1347–1354.

Zulfiqar, V., D. A. Jurivich, W. Gao, and D. H. Singer. "Relation of High Heart Rate Variability to Healthy Longevity." *American Journal of Cardiology* (2010) 105 (8): 1181–1185.

Chapter 7

Blanchfield, A. W., J. Hardy, H. M. De Morree, W. Staiano, and S. M. Marcora. "Talking Yourself Out of Exhaustion: The Effects of Self-Talk on Endurance Performance." *Medicine and Science in Sports and Exercise* (2014) 46 (5): 998–1007.

Brick, N. E. and M. J. McElhinney. "The Effects of Facial Expression and Relaxation Cues on Movement Economy, Physiological, and Perceptual Responses During Running." *Psychology of Sport and Exercise* (2017) 34: 20–28.

Damisch, L., B. Stoberock, and T. Mussweiler. "Keep Your Fingers Crossed!: How Superstition Improves Performance." *Psychological Science* (2010) 21 (7): 1014–1020.

Giles, G. E., J. A. Cantelon, M. D. Eddy, T. T. Brunye, H. L. Urry, H. A. Taylor, C. R. Mahoney, and R. B. Kavarek. "Cognitive Reappraisal Reduces Perceived Exertion During Endurance Exercise." *Motivation and Emotion* (2018) 42: 482-496.

Gould, D., K. Dieffenbach, and A. Moffett. "Psychological Talent and Its Development in Olympic Champions." Unpublished Final Grant Report, Coaching and Sports Sciences Division, IS. S. Olympic Olympic Committee, Colorado Springs, Colorado.

Hamilton, R. A., D. Scott, and M. P. MacDougal. "Assessing the Effectiveness of Self-Talk Interventions on Endurance Performance." *Journal of Applied Sport Psychology* (2007) 19 (2): 226–239.

Jones, G. "How the Best of the Best Get Better and Better." *Harvard Business Review* (2008) 86 (6): 123–127, 142.

Machida, M., R. M. Ward, and R. S. Vealey. "Predictors of Sources of Self-Confidence in Collegiate Athletes." *International Journal of Sport, Exercise, and Psychology* (2012) 10 (3): 172–185.

Mahoney, M. J. and M. Avener. "Psychology of the Elite Athlete: An Exploratory Study." *Cognitive Therapy and Research* (1977) 1: 135–141.

Moore, L. J., S. J. Vine, M. R. Wilson, and P. Freeman. "Reappraising Threat: How to Optimize Performance Under Pressure." *Journal of Sport & Exercise* (2015) 37: 339-343.

Ofori, P. K., D. Tod, and D. LaVallee. "An Exploratory Investigation of Superstitious Behaviors, Coping, Control Strategies, and Personal Control in Ghanian and British Student-Athletes." *International Journal of Sport, Exercise, and Psychology* (2015) 16 (1): 3–19.

Vealey, R. S., S. W. Hayashi, M. Garner-Holman, and P. Giacobbi. "Sources of Sport-Confidence: Conceptualization and Instrument Development." *Journal of Sport, Exercise, and Psychology* (1998) 20: 54–80.

Williams, S. and J. Cumming. "Challenge vs. Threat: Investigating the Effect of Using Appraisal of a Dart Throwing Task." *Sport and Exercise Psychology Review* (2012) 8 (1): 4–21.

Wilson, R. C., P. J. Sullivan, N. D. Myers, and D. L. Feltz. "Sources of Sport Confidence of Masters Athletes." *Journal of Sport, Exercise, and Psychology* (2004) 26: 369–384.

Chapter 8

Allison, K. C., C. M. Hopkins, M. Ruggiers, A. M. Spaeth, R. S. Ahuma, Z. Zhang, D. M. Taylor, and N. Goel. "Prolonged Controlled Versus Delayed Eating Impacts Weight and Metabolism." *Current Biology* (2020) 31 (3): 650–657.

Antonio, J., C. A. Peacock, A. Ellerbroek, B. Fromhoff, and T. Silver. "The Effects of Consuming a High Protein Diet (4.4g/kg/d) on Body Composition in Resistance-Trained Individuals." *Journal of the International Society of Sports Nutrition* (2014) 11: 19 doi: 101186/1550-2783-11-19.

Antonio, J. "High-Protein Diets in Trained Individuals." *Research in Sports and Medicine* (2019) 27 (2): 195–203.

Berardi, J. M., T. B. Price, E. E. Noreen, and P. W. Lemon. "Postexercise Muscle Glycogen Recovery Enhanced with a Carbohydrate-Protein Supplement." *Medicine and Science in Sports and Exercise* (2006) 38 (6): 1106–1113.

Bossingham, M. J., N. S. Carnell, and W. W. Campbell. "Water Balance, Hydration Status, and Fat-Free Mass Hydration in Younger and Older Adults." *American Journal of Clinical Nutrition* (2005) 81 (6): 1342–1350.

Breen, L., A. Philip, O. C. Witard, S. R. Jackman, A. Selby, K. Smith, K. Barr, and K. D. Tipton. "The Influence of Carbohydrate-Protein Co-ingestion Following Endurance Exercise on Myofibrillar and Mitochondrial Protein Synthesis." *Journal of Physiology* (2011) 589 (16): 4011–4025.

Burke, L. M., J. A. Hawley, S. H. S. Wong, and A E. Jeukendrup. "Carbohydrates for Training and Competition." *Journal of Sports Science and Supplements* (2011) S17—27.

Cirius, C., H. M. Lynch, C. Wharton, and C. S. Johnston. "A Comparison of Dietary Protein Digestibility, Based on DIAAS Scoring, in Vegetarian and Non-vegetarian Athletes." *Nutrients* (2019) 11 (12): 3016.

Correia, J. M., P. Pezarat-Correia, C. Minderico, J. Infante, and G. V. Mendonca. "Effects of Time-Restricted Eating on Aerobic Capacity, Body Composition and Markers of Metabolic Health in Healthy-Male Recreational Runners: A Randomized Crossover Trial." *Journal of Academics, Nutrition*, and Diet (2024) doi: 10.1016/j.jand.2024.01.005.

Craddock, J. C., Y. C. Probst, and G. E. Peoples. "Vegetarian and Omnivorous Nutrition—Comparing Physical Performance." *International Journal of Sports Nutrition and Exercise Metabolism* (2016) 26 (3): 212–220.

Currell, K. and A. E. Jeukendrup. "Superior Endurance Performance with Ingestion of Multiple Transportable Carbohydrates." *Medicine and Science in Sports and Exercise* (2008) 40 (2): 275–281.

Deuries, M. C. and S. M. Phillips. "Supplemental Protein in Support of Muscle Mass and Health: Advantage Whey." *Journal of Food Science* (2015) 80 Supplement 1: A8—A15.

Fowles, J. R., M. W. O'Brien, K. G. Comeau, B. Thurston, and H. J. Petrie. "Flattened Cola Improves High-Intensity Interval Performance in Competitive Cyclists." *European Journal of Applied Physiology* (2021) 121 (10): 2859–2867.

REFERENCES

Halson, S. L., G. I. Lancaster, J. Achten, M. Gleeson, and A. E. Jeukendrup. "Effects of Carbohydrate Supplementation on Performance and Carbohydrate Oxidation After Intensified Cycling Training." *Journal of Applied Physiology* (2004) 97 (4): 1245–1253.

Hearris, M. A., J. N. Pugh, C. Langan-Evans, S. J. Mann, L. Burke, T. Stellingwerff, J. T. Gonzalez, and J. P. Morton. "C-Glucose/Fructose Labelling Reveals Comparable Exogenous CHO Oxidation During Exercise When Consuming 120g/h in Fluid, Gel, Jelly Chew, or Coingestion." *Journal of Applied Physiology* (2022) 132 (6): 1327–1591.

Impey, S. G., M. A. Hearris, K. M. Hammond, J. D. Bartlett, J. Louis, G. L. Close, and J. P. Morton. "Fuel the Work Required: A Theoretical Framework for Carbohydrate Periodization and the Glycogen Threshold Hypothesis." *Sports Medicine* (2018) 48 (5): 1031–1048.

Ivy, J. L. "Dietary Strategies to Promote Glycogen Synthesis After Exercise." *Canadian Journal of Applied Physiology* (2001) 26 (Supplement): S236–S245.

Ivy, J. L., H. W. Goforth Jr., B. M. Damon, T. R. McCauley, E. C. Parsons, and T. B. Price. "Early Postexercise Muscle Glycogen Recovery Is Enhanced with a Carbohydrate-Protein Supplement." *Journal of Applied Physiology* (2002) 3 (4): 1337–1344.

James, L. J., E. J. Stevenson, P. L. S. Rumbold and C. J. Hulston. "Cow's Milk as a Post-Exercise Recovery Drink: Implications for Performance and Health." *European Journal of Sport Science* (2019) 19 (1): 40–48.

Jensen, K., L. Johansen, and N. H. Secher. "Influence of Body Mass on Maximal Oxygen Uptake: Effect of Sample Size." *European Journal of Applied Physiology* (2001) 84 (3): 201–205.

Jentjens, R. and A. Jeukendrup. "Determinants of Post-Exercise Glycogen Synthesis During Short-Term Recovery." *Sports Medicine* (2003) 33 (2): 117–144.

Jeukendrup, A. E., M. K. Hesselink, A. C. Snyder, H. Kuipers, and H. A. Keizer. "Physiological Changes in Male Competitive Cyclists After Two Weeks of Intensified Training." *International Journal of Sports Medicine* (1992) 13 (7): 534–541.

Jeukendrup, A. E., L. Moseley, G. I. Mainwaring, S. Samuels, S. Perry, and C. H. Mann. "Exogenous Carbohydrate Oxidation During Ultra Endurance Exercise." *Journal of Applied Physiology* (2006) 100 (4): 1134–1141.

Jeukendrup, A. E. "Carbohydrate and Exercise Performance: The Role of Multiple Transportable Carbohydrates." *Current Opinion in Clinical Nutrition and Metabolic Care* (2010) 13 (4): 452–457.

Jeukendrup, A. E. "Periodized Nutrition for Athletes." *Sports Medicine* (2017) 47: 51–63.

Kenney, W. L., C. G. Tankersley, D. L. Newswanger, D. E. Hyde, S. M. Puhl, and N. L. Turner. "Age and Hypohydration Independently Influence the Peripheral Vascular Response to Heat Stress." *Journal of Applied Physiology* (1990) 68 (5): 1902–1908.

Kenney, W. L. and Chiu P. "Influence of Age on Thirst and Fluid Intake." *Medicine and Science in Sports and Exercise* (2001) 33 (9): 1524–1532.

Kovacs, E. M., J. M. Senden, and F. Brouns. "Urine Color, Osmolality and Specific Electrical Conductance Are Not Accurate Measures of Hydration Status During Postexercise Rehydration." *Journal of Sports Medicine and Physical Fitness* (1999) 39 (1): 47–53.

Lane, S. C., D. M. Camera, D. G. Lassiter, J. L. Areta, S. R. Bird, W. K. Yeo, N. A. Jeacocke, A. Krook, J. R. Zierath, L. M. Burke, and J. A. Hawley. "Effects of Sleeping with Reduced Carbohydrate Availability on Acute Training Responses." *Journal of Applied Physiology* (2015) 119 (6): 643–655.

Levenhagen, D. K., J. D. Gresham, M. G. Carlson, D. J. Maron, M. J. Borel, and P. J. Flakoll. "Postexercise Nutrient Intake Timing in Humans Is Critical to Recovery of Leg Glucose and Protein Homeostasis." *American Journal of Physiology. Endocrinology and Metabolism* (2001) 280 (6): E982–E993.

Levenhagen, D. K., C. Carr, M. G. Carlson, D. J. Maron, M. J. Borel, and P. J. Flakoll. "Postexercise Protein Intake Enhances Whole-Body and Leg Protein Accretion in Humans." *Medicine and Science in Sports and Exercise* (2002) 34 (5): 828–837.

Maffetone, P. B. and P. B. Laursen. "Athletes: Fit But Unhealthy?" *Sports Medicine Open* (2016) doi: 10.1186/s40798-016-0048-x.

Marquet, L-A., J. Brisswalter, J. Louis, E. Tiollier, L. M. Burke, J. A. Hawley, and C. Hausswirth. "Enhanced Endurance Performance by Periodization of Carbohydrate Intake: 'Sleep Low' Strategy." *Medicine and Science in Sports and Exercise* (2016) 48 (4): 663–672.

Montain, S. J. and E. F. Coyle. "Influence of Graded Dehydration on Hyperthermia and Cardiovascular Drift During Exercise." *Journal of Applied Physiology* (1992) 73 (4): 1340–1350.

Moon, J. and G. Koh. "Clinical Evidence and Mechanisms of High-Protein Diet-Induced Weight Loss." *Journal of Obesity and Metabolic Syndrome* (2020) 29 (3): 166–173.

Nielsen, L. L. K., M. N. T. Lambert, and P. B. Jeppesen. "The Effect of Ingesting Carbohydrate and Proteins on Athletic Performance: A Systematic Review and Meta-Analysis of Randomized Controlled Trials." *Nutrients* (2020) 12 (5): 1483.

Noakes, T. D. "Drinking Guidelines for Exercise: What Evidence Is There That Athletes Should Drink 'as Much as Tolerable', 'to Replace the Weight Lost During Exercise' or 'Ad Libitum'?" *Journal of Sports Sciences* (2007) 25 (7): 781–796.

Pakosz, O., M. Konieczny, P. Domaszewski, T. Dybek, O. García-García, M. Gnoiński, and E. Skorupska. "Muscle Contraction Time After Caffeine Intake Is Faster After 30 Minutes Than After 60 Minutes." *Journal of the International Society of Sports Nutrition* (2024) doi: 101080/15502783.2024.2306295.

Parkin, J. A., M. F. Carey, I. K. Martin, L. Stojanovska, and M. A. Febbraio. "Muscle Glycogen Storage Following Prolonged Exercise: Effect of Timing of Ingestion of High Glycemic Index Food." *Medicine and Science in Sports and Exercise* (1997) 29 (2): 220–224.

Peeling, P., M. J. Binnie, P. S. R. Goods, M. Sim, and L. M. Burke. "Evidence-Based Supplements for the Enhancement of Athletic Performance." *International Journal of Sports Nutrition and Exercise Metabolism* (2018) 28 (2): 178–187.

Pennings, B., R. Koopman, M. Beelen, J. M. G. Senden, W. H. M. Saris, and L. J. C. van Loon. "Exercising Before Protein Intake Allows for Greater Use of Dietary Protein-Derived Amino Acids for De Novo Muscle Protein Synthesis in Both Young and Elderly Men." *American Journal of Clinical Nutrition* (2011) 93 (2): 322–331.

Perez-Schindler, J., D. L. Hamilton, D. R. Moore, K. Baar, and A. Philp. "Nutritional Strategies to Support Concurrent Training." *European Journal of Sport Science* (2015) 15 (1): 41–52.

Phillips, S. M., J. E. Tang, and D. R. Moore. "The Role of Milk- and Soy-Based Protein in Support of Muscle Protein Synthesis and Muscle Protein Accretion in Young and Elderly Persons." *Journal of the American College of Nutrition* (2009) 28 (4): 343–354.

Phillips, S. M. and L. J. C. Van Loon. "Dietary Protein for Athletes: From Requirements to Optimum Adaptation." *Journal of Sports Sciences* (2011) 29 S1: 529–538.

Phillips, S. M., S. Chevalier, and H. J. Leidy. "Protein 'Requirements' Beyond the RDA: Implications for Optimizing Health." *Applied Physiology, Nutrition, and Metabolism* (2016) 41 (5): 565–572.

Prieto-Beliver, G., J. Diaz-Lara, D. J. Bishop, J. Fernandez-Saez, J. Abian-Vicen, I. San-Millan, and J. Santos-Concejero. "A Five-Week Periodized Carbohydrate Diet Does Not Improve Maximal Lactate Steady-State Exercise Capacity and Substrate Oxidation in Well-Trained Cyclists Compared to a High-Carbohydrate Diet." *Nutrients* (2024) 16 (2): 318–324.

Res, P. T., B. Groen, B. Pennings, M. Beelen, G. A. Wallis, A. P. Gijsen, J. M. Senden, and L. J. Van Loon. "Protein Ingestion Before Sleep Improves Postexercise Overnight Recovery." *Medicine and Science in Sports and Exercise* (2012) 44 (8): 1560–1569.

Rowe, J. T., R. F. G. J. King, A. J. King, D. J. Morrison, T. Preston, O. J. Wilson, and J. P. O'Hara. "Glucose and Fructose Hydrogel Enhances Running Performance, Exogenous Carbohydrate Oxidation, and Gastrointestinal Tolerance." *Medicine and Science in Sports and Exercise* (2022) 54 (1): 129–140.

Rustad, P. I., M. Sailer, K. T. Cumming, P. B. Jeppesen, K.J. Kolnes, O. Sollie, J. French, J. L. Ivy, H. Daniel, and J. Jensen. "Intake of Protein Plus Carbohydrate During the First Two Hours After Exhaustive Cycling Improves Performance the Following Day." *PLoS One* (2016) 11 (4): e0153229.

Speedy, D. B., J. M. D. Thompson, I. Rodgers, M. Collins, K. Sharwood, and T. D. Noakes. "Oral Salt Supplementation During Ultradistance Exercise." *Clinical Journal of Sports Medicine* (2002) 12 (5): 279–284.

Suzuki, M. "Glycemic Carbohydrates Consumed with Amino Acids or Protein Right After Exercise Enhance Muscle Formation." *Nutrition Review* (2003) 61 (5 Pt 2): S88–S94.

Symons, T. B., M. S. Moore, and R. R. Wolfe. "A Moderate Serving of High-Quality Protein Maximally Stimulates Muscle Protein Synthesis in Young and Elderly Subjects." *Journal of the American Dietetic Association* (2009) 109 (9): 1582–1586.

Tipton, K. D., A. A. Ferrando, S. M. Phillips, D. Doyle Jr, and R. R. Wolfe. "Postexercise Net Protein Synthesis in Human Muscle from Orally Administered Amino Acids." *American Journal of Physiology* (1999) 276 (4 Pt 1): E628–E634.

Tipton, K. D., B. B. Rasmussen, S. L. Miller, S. E. Wolf, S. K. Owens-Stovall, B. E. Petrini, and R. R. Wolfe. "Timing of Amino Acid-Carbohydrate Ingestion Alters Anabolic Response of Muscle to Resistance Exercise." *American Journal of Physiology. Endocrinology and Metabolism* (2001) 281 (2): E197–E206.

Tøien, T., J. L. Nielsen, and O. K. Berg. "The Impact of Life-Long Strength Versus Endurance Training on Muscle Fiber Morphology and Phenotype Composition in Older Men." *Journal of Applied Physiology* (2023) doi.org/10.1152/japplphysiol.00208.2023.

Trommelen, J., G. A. A. vanLieshout, J. Nyakayiru, A. M. Holiwerda, J. S. J. Smeets, F. K. Hendriks, J. X. M. vanKranenburg, A. H. Zorence, J. M. Senden, J. P. B. Goessens, A. P. Gigsen, and L. J. C. VanLoon. "The Anabolic Response to Protein Ingestion During Recovery from Exercise Has No Upper Limit in Magnitude and Duration in Vivo in Humans." *Cell Reports Medicine* (2023) 4 (12): 101324.

Valenzuela, P. L., N. A. Maffiuletti, M. J. Joyner, A. Lucia, and R. Lepers. "Lifelong Endurance Exercise as a Countermeasure Against Age-Related [Formula: see text]

REFERENCES

Decline: Physiological Overview and Insights from Masters Athletes." *Sports Medicine* (2020) 50 (4): 703–716.

Valtin, H. "'Drink at Least Eight Glasses of Water a Day.' Really? Is There Scientific Evidence for '8 x 8'?" *American Journal of Physiology. Regulatory, Integrative and Comparative Physiology* (2002) 283 (5): R993–R1004.

Van Loon, L. J., M. Kruijshoop, H. Verhagen, W. H. Saris, and A. J. Wagenmakers. "Ingestion of Protein Hydrolysate and Amino Acid-Carbohydrate Mixtures Increases Postexercise Plasma Insulin Responses in Men." *Journal of Nutrition* (2000) 130 (10): 2508–2513.

Venderly, A. M, and W. W. Campbell. "Vegetarian Diets: Nutritional Considerations for Athletes." *Sport Medicine* (2006) 36 (4): 293–305.

Williamson, E., H. J. W. Fung, C. Adams, D. W. D. West, and D. R. Moore. "Protein Requirements Are Increased in Endurance-Trained Athletes but Similar between Females and Males during Postexercise Recovery." *Medicine and Science in Sports and Exercise* (2012) 55 (10): 1866–1875.

Zhou, H.-H., Y. Liao, X. Zhou, Z. Peng, S. Xu, S. Shi, L. Liu, L. Hao, and W. Yang. "Mass, Strength and Physical Performance in Adults Undergoing Resistance Training: A Network Meta-Analysis." *International Journal of Sport Nutrition and Exercise Metabolism* (2023) doi.org/10.1123/ijsnem. 2023–0118.

Chapter 9

Afonso, J., J. Brito, E. Abade, G. Rendeiro-Pinho, I. Baptista, P. Figueiredo, and F. Y. Nakamura. "Revisiting the 'Whys' and 'Hows' of the Warm-Up: Are We Asking the Right Questions?" *Sports Medicine* (2024) 54 (1): 23–30.

Armstrong, L. E., R. W. Hubbard, E. W. Askew, J. P. DeLuca, C. O'Brien, A. Pasqualicchio, and R. P. Francesconi. "Responses to Moderate and Low Sodium Diets During Exercise-Heat Acclimation." *International Journal of Sport Nutrition* (1993) 3 (2): 207–221.

Azevedo, R. de A., R. Cruz, P. Couto, M. D. Silva-Cavalcante, D. Boari, N. Okuno, and R. Bertuzzi. "Effects of Prior High-Intensity Endurance Exercise in Subsequent 4-km Cycling Time Trial Performance and Fatigue Development." *Science & Sports* (2022) 37 (1): 70.e1-70.e11.

Barranco-Gil, D., L. B. Alejo, P. L. Valenzuela, J. Gil-Cabrera, A. Montalvo-Pérez, E. Talavera, and A. Lucia. "Warming Up Before a 20-Minute Endurance Effort: Is It Really Worth It?" *International Journal of Sports Physiology and Performance* (2020) 15 (7): 964–970.

Bishop, D. "Warmup II: Performance Changes Following Active Warmup and How to Structure the Warmup." *Sports Medicine* (2003) 33 (7): 483–498.

Burke, L. M. "Nutritional Needs for Exercise in Heat." *Comparative Biochemistry and Physiology. Part A, Molecular & Integrative Physiology* (2001) 128 (4): 735–748.

Carr, A., L. Garvican-Lewis, B. Vallance, A. Drake, P. Saunders, C. Humberstone, and C. Gore. "Training to Compete at Altitude: Natural Altitude or Simulated Live High: Train Low?" *International Journal of Sports Physiology and Performance* (2019) 14 (4): 509–517.

Chapman, R. F., J. L. Stickford, and B. D. Levine. "Altitude Training Considerations for the Winter Sport Athlete." *Experimental Physiology* (2010) 95 (3): 411–421.

Christensen, P. M. and J. Bangsbo. "Warm-Up Strategy and High-Intensity Endurance Performance in Trained Cyclists." *International Journal of Sports Physiology and Performance* (2015) 10 (3): 353–360.

Corbett, J., R. A. Neal, H. C. Lunt, and M. J. Tipton. "Adaptation to Heat and Exercise Performance Under Cooler Conditions: A New Hot Topic." *Sports Medicine* (2014) 44 (10): 1323–1331.

Dugas, J. "Ice Slurry Ingestion Increases Running Time in the Heat." *Clinical Journal of Sport Medicine* (2011) 21 (6): 541–542.

Esh, C. J., S. Carter, N. Galan-Lopez, F Garrandes, S. Bermon, P. E. Adamia, S. Racinais, L. James, T. Stellingwerff, W. M. Adams, B. Chrismas, C. J. Stevens, J. D. Periard, C. Brade, M. J. Henderson, and L. Taylor. "A Review of Elite Athlete Evidence-Based Knowledge and Preparation for Competing in the Heat." *Journal of Science in Sport and Exercise* (2024) doi.org/10.1007/s42973-024-00283-y

Foss, J., K. Constantini, T. Mickleborough, and R. Chapman. "Short-Term Arrival Strategies for Endurance Exercise at Moderate Altitude." *Journal of Applied Physiology* (2017) 123 (5): 1258–1265.

Foster, C., A. C. Snyder, N. N. Thompson, M. A. Green, M. Foley, and M. Schrager. "Effect of Pacing Strategy on Cycle Time Trial Performance." *Medicine and Science in Sports and Exercise* (1993) 25 (3): 383–388.

Fraakin, A. J., T. R. Zazryn, and J. M. Smogla. "Effects of Warming-Up on Physical Performance: A Systematic Review with Meta-Analysis." *Journal of Strength and Conditioning Research* (2010) 24 (1): 140–148.

González-Alonso, J., C. Teller, S. L. Andersen, F. B. Jensen, T. Hyldig, and B. Nielsen. "Influence of Body Temperature on the Development of Fatigue During Prolonged Exercise in the Heat." *Journal of Applied Physiology* (1999) 86 (3): 1032–1039.

Goulet, E. D. "Effect of Exercise-Induced Dehydration on Time-Trial Exercise Performance: A Meta-Analysis." *British Journal of Sports Medicine* (2011) 45 (14): 1149–1156.

Hajoglou, A., C. Foster, J. J. DeKoning, A. Lucia, T. W. Kernozek, and J. P. Porcari. "Effect of Warm-Up on Cycle Time Trial Performance." *Medicine and Science in Sports and Exercise* (2005) 37 (9): 1608–1614.

Jentjens, R. L. P. G., A. J. M. Wagenmakers, and A. E. Jeukendrup. "Heat Stress Increases Muscle Glycogen Use But Reduces the Oxidation of Ingested Carbohydrates During Exercise." *Journal of Applied Physiology* (2001) 92 (4): 1562–1572.

McGowan, C. J., D. B. Pyne, K. G. Thompson, and B. Rattray. "Warm-Up Strategies for Sport and Exercise: Mechanisms and Applications." *Sports Medicine* (2015) 45 (11): 1523–1546.

McIntyre, J. P. R. and A. E. Kilding. "Effects of High-Intensity Intermittent Priming on Physiology and Cycling Performance." *Journal of Sports Sciences* (2015) 33 (6) 561–567.

Mitchell, J. B. and J. S. Huston. "The Effect of High- and Low-Intensity Warm-up on the Physiological Responses to a Standardized Swim and Tethered Swimming Performance." *Journal of Sports Science* (1993) 11 (2): 159–163.

Morris, C. J., J. N. Yang, J. I. Garcia, S. Myers, I. Bozzi, W. Wang, O. M. Buxton, S. A. Shea, and F. A. J. L. Scheer. "Endogenous Circadian System and Circadian Misalignment Impact Glucose Tolerance Via Separate Mechanisms in Humans." *Proceedings of the National Academy of Sciences* (2015) doi: 10.1073/pnas. 1418955112.

Morris, N. B. and J. Ollie. "To Drink or to Pour: How Should Athletes Use Water to Cool Themselves?" *Taylor, Francis Online* (2016) 3 (2): 191–194.

Mujika, I., R. Gonzalez de Txabarri, S. Maldonado-Martin, and D. B. Pyne. "Warm-Up Intensity and Duration's Effect on Traditional Rowing Time-Trial Performance." *International Journal of Sports Physiology and Performance* (2012) 7: 186–188.

Ronnestad, B. R., T. Urianstad, H. Hamarsland, J. Hansen, H. Nygaard, S. Ellefsen, D. Hammarstrom, and C. Lundby. "Heat Training Efficiently Increases and Maintains Hemoglobin Mass and Temperate Endurance Performance in Elite Cyclists." *Medicine and Science in Sports and Exercise* (2022) 54 (9): 1515–1526.

Sawka, M. N., S. J. Montain, and W. A. Latzka. "Hydration Effects on Thermoregulation and Performance in the Heat." Comparative Biochemistry and Physiology Part A, *Molecular & Integrative Physiology* (2001) 128 (4): 679–690.

Terrados, N. and R. J. Maughan. "Exercise in the Heat: Strategies to Minimize the Adverse Effects on Performance." *Journal of Sports Science* (1995) 13: 555–462.

Tomaras, E. K. and B. R. MacIntosh. "Less Is More: Standard Warm-Up Causes Fatigue and Less Warm-Up Permits Greater Cycling Power Output." *Journal of Applied Physiology* (2011) 111 (1), 228–235.

Tyler, C. J., T. Reeve, G. J. Hodges, and S. S. Cheung. "The Effects of Heat Adaptation on Physiology, Perception and Exercise Performance in the Heat: A Meta-Analysis." *Sports Medicine* (2016) 46 (11): 1699–1724.

Wei, C., L. Yu, B. Duncan, and A. Renfree. "A Plyometric Warm-Up Protocol Improves Running Economy in Recreational Endurance Athletes." *Frontiers in Physiology* (2020) 11, 197.

Zourdos, M. C., C. D. Bazyler, E. Jo, A. V. Khamoui, B.-S. Park, S.-R. Lee, J.-S. Kim. "Impact of a Submaximal Warm-Up on Endurance Performance in Highly Trained and Competitive Male Runners." *Research Quarterly for Exercise and Sport* (2017) 88 (1), 114–119.

Appendix

Hawley, J. A. and T. D. Noakes. "Peak Power Output Predicts Maximal Oxygen Uptake and Performance Time in Trained Cyclists." *European Journal of Applied Physiology and Occupational Physiology* (1992) 65 (1): 79–83.

ABOUT THE AUTHOR

Joe Friel has a Master's degree in Exercise Science. His training methods are grounded in the principles of science and have been further shaped by more than 40 years of personal coaching experience. The athletes he has coached range from novice to elite amateur to professional to Olympian. He is a frequent presenter at athletic seminars and coaching conferences. Sports federations from various countries have had him update their national coaches on current best practices in training. Joe occasionally leads camps for athletes around the world, and advises top endurance athletes and coaches in several sports. He also consults with companies in the sports equipment industry.

Joe has written numerous books on training for endurance sports, including his best-selling *Cyclist's Training Bible*, and various other books for triathletes, cyclists, and mountain bikers. He is also a frequent contributor to such magazines as *VeloNews*, *Bicycling*, *Triathlete* and *220 Triathlon*.

In 1999, Joe cofounded TrainingPeaks.com along with his son Dirk and close friend Gear Fisher. TrainingPeaks is widely considered the world's leading provider of training software for endurance athletes and is used by grand tour teams, leading coaches in many sports, and some of the world's best athletes.

Joe lives and trains in Sedona, Arizona.

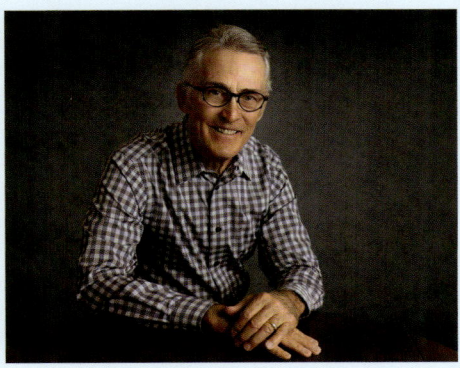

INDEX

A
adaptation, training 9, 162–3
aerobic endurance (AE) training 65–6, 75, 101–2, 103, 119, 131, 138, 140, 142, 154–5, 234, 241–2
aerobic fitness/capacity 44–5, 48–9, 52, 65–6, 75, 78, 131–3, 137, 138, 140, 198–9, 206, 209, 236, 244–5
    testing 76–7, 78, 118, 248
affirmations, using 182
age factors 46, 156, 157, 193, 206–9
    older riders 206–7
    young riders — starting out 208, 209
anaerobic fitness 44–5
apps, training 165–6

B
Base period 66, 75, 90, 94, 101–2, 108, 115, 119, 121, 129, 130, 131, 135, 137, 138, 140, 142, 155, 156, 157, 234
bike checks, pre-race 226
bike fitting 31, 36–7
bike-handling skills 66, 130, 137
blood pressure levels 173
bone density 120, 207
Build period 66, 75, 90, 102, 108, 118, 131–2, 135–6, 137, 138–9, 140, 142, 156, 157, 234

C
carbohydrates 45–6, 132, 137, 164–5, 194–5, 207, 209, 218–19
cardiac capacity 60, 61
celebrating successes 176–7, 230
climbing and descending 66, 130
clothing 215, 217
coach-athlete relationships 16–17, 41, 173
cold-water immersion 163
competition/competitors 23–4
compression boots 163
confidence building 177–80
consistency, training 39–40, 234–5
cool-downs 230
core strength exercises 121, 125–6
cornering 66, 130, 244
cortisol 199
cross-training 92, 100, 101, 115, 120, 132, 137, 154

D
data analysis, training 116–17
decoupling metric 117
diet/fuel 45–7, 132, 137, 164–5, 192–3, 198, 207, 209
    daily requirements 193–4
    nutrition periodization 196
    race week and race day 226
    during races 218–19, 228–9
    snacks 200–1
    sports drinks 197, 198
    supplements 190–1, 220–1
    workout fuel 194–5
    see also weight, body
doping 50
duration, training 62, 94, 104–6

E
efficiency factor (EF) 45–6, 60, 79, 117, 141, 142, 159, 236–7
erythropoietin (EPO) 50
exertion
    see intensity, training
experience, rider 25
experts/professionals 18–19

F
family and friends, support from 18, 178
fat 45–6, 60, 61, 165, 194–5
fatigue 103, 151, 152–4, 155, 158–9, 166
fitness loss 103, 154, 155
fitness testing *see* testing fitness; zones, setting intensity
frequency, training 62, 94, 115
fuel/refueling *see* diet/fuel
functional threshold power (FTP) 53, 69, 72, 74, 77, 137, 141, 142, 166, 206, 247–8

G
goals 20–4, 98, 99, 179
    see also plans, linear periodized training; races, B and C
group rides 91, 92, 102, 103, 117–18, 132, 135, 136, 140, 185, 225
gym workouts 100, 101, 102, 115, 117, 120–9, 140

H
health, general 40–1, 120, 153, 155, 199
    see also rest and recovery (R&R); stress
heart rate 173
    average 116
    functional threshold (FTHR) 69, 70, 71, 72, 74, 141, 142, 247–8
    lactate (LHR) 70, 71
    maximal (MHR) 68–9, 71, 72
    monitors 27–8, 79
    variability (HRV) 150–1, 159–60

heart size 60, 61
heat/hot rides 132–3, 137, 216–19
heated clothing 215
high-altitude races 219–21
hip mobility exercises 121, 126–8
hobbies and other activities 177
hormones 152–3, 155, 172, 199
hunger and stress 199
hydration 132, 136, 137, 164, 197, 218

I

imposter syndrome 172
individuality and training 9, 97
injuries 41, 120, 124
intensity factor (IF) 77
intensity, training
    high-intensity 60–1, 62, 74, 92, 93, 132, 137, 140, 154, 164, 234, 235–6
    low-intensity 60–1, 62, 74, 76, 92, 93–4, 164, 235–6
    obsessive behaviour 235
    power meters and heart rate monitors 27–8, 79
    training balance 235–6
    see also Base zone; Build zone; Peak zone; plans, linear periodized training; Preparation zone; Race zone; zones, setting intensity
international travel 222, 225, 227
iron supplements 220–1

L

lactate 46, 51–2
lactate threshold power (LTP) 74, 77
lactate thresholds 70, 71, 154
lifestyle 25, 38, 152
limiters 98–9, 102, 103, 108, 136–7, 138, 140
listening to your body 40–1, 166
losing weight 199–201

M

massage 164
measuring performance 27–8, 76–9
mental health *see* mindset, rider
metrics, making sense of 116
mindset, rider 40, 170–3, 185, 199, 226–7
    building self-confidence 177–80
    enjoyment factor 236–7
    focus 180–1, 227
    impact on physiology 172–3
    motivation 176–7
    patience 184
    self-assessment 174–5
    self-efficacy 173
    self-talk 182–3
mitochondria 50, 60, 61
motivation 159, 176–7
multiple races *see* race categories, B and C

muscle fatigue and soreness 51–2
muscle function 45–6
muscle glycogen stores 218–19
muscle mass 22, 199, 207
muscles, fast- and slow-twitch fibers 54, 60–1
muscular force (MF) training 65–6, 75, 93, 94, 102, 119–25, 137, 138, 207, 209, 234, 242–3

N

National Time Trial Championship, US 14–15
neurotransmitters 173
normalized power (NP) 116
nutrition periodization 196

O

obsessive behaviour 235
osteoporosis 120, 207, 209
overtraining 151, 153–4, 155, 235

P

Peak period 66, 75, 90, 103, 108, 139–40, 234
pedaling 66, 244
physical therapists/physiotherapists 30
plans, linear periodized training 10, 26, 47, 83, 181
    Preparation period 100–1, 108, 115, 121, 129, 137, 155, 156, 234
    Base period 101–2, 108, 115, 117–18, 119, 121, 129, 130, 131, 135, 137, 138, 140, 142, 155, 156, 157, 234
    Build period 102, 108, 118, 131–2, 135–6, 137, 138–9, 140, 142, 156, 157, 234, 234
    Peak period 103, 108, 139–40, 234
    Race period 104, 139–40, 223–31
    Transition period 104, 108
    goal setting 20–4, 98, 99
    limiters 98–9, 102, 103, 108, 136–7, 138, 140
    periods chronologically
        Preparation period 100–1, 108, 115, 121, 129, 137, 155, 156, 234
        Base period 101–2, 108, 115, 117–18, 119, 121, 129, 130, 131, 135, 137, 138, 140, 142, 155, 156, 157, 234
        Build period 102, 108, 118, 131–2, 135–6, 137, 138–9, 140, 142, 156, 157, 234, 234
        Peak period 103, 108, 139–40, 234
        Race period 104, 139–40, 223–31
    scheduling weekly hours 104–8
    seasonal progression transitions 91–4, 115–18
    seasonal plan table 142
    time limitations and missed workouts 202–5
    training balance - moderation 235–6
    training schedule flexibility 97
    see also aerobic endurance (AE) training; aerobic fitness/capacity; muscular force (MF) training; speed skills (SS) training; sprint power; stamina

polarized training approach 86–7, 88, 89, 94, 102, 166
power meters 27–8, 79
Preparation period 66, 90, 100–1, 108, 115, 121, 129, 137, 155, 156, 234
protein 194–5, 207, 209
psychology, sports 11
pyramidal training 88–9, 94, 101

R

race categories, B and C 21, 108, 109, 131, 135, 140, 162, 185, 225
Race period and race days 66, 90, 104, 108, 139–40, 234
    challenging conditions 215–22
    day-before preparation 226
    mental preparation 228, 229
    post-race analysis 230, 231
    preparing for a high-altitude race 219–21
    preparing for a hot race 216–19
    race strategy and tactics 223–4, 226, 227
    race-week form 223
    race week sleep 225–6
    refueling 226, 228–9
    warm-up and VO_2 priming 214–15, 228
rate of perceived exertion (RPE) 26, 67, 218, 236
real-life stories
    Dirk — training for lifetime passion 34–5, 40, 55
    Elizabeth — self-perception 170–2, 185
    Johnny — race day preparation 212–13, 231
    Laurie — the Leadville Trail 100 112–13, 143
    Lynda — low- vs high-intensity training 58–9, 81
    Ralph — asking questions 188–9, 209
    Steve — goal accomplishment 21–2, 31
    Tom — improving stamina 84–5, 109
    Wes — R&R 146–8, 167, 235
resistance work 93
rest and recovery (R&R) 11, 41–2, 102, 103, 104, 118, 146–8, 149, 151–3, 155, 156, 160, 166, 236
    adaption and recovery tools 162–4
    day-to-day — hard and easy days 161–2
    planned 156–8
    recovery on demand 158–60
reversibility and training 9, 20
role models 238

S

sarcopenia 207, 209
self-confidence 177–80
self-talk, positive 182–3, 226
sleep 42–3, 149, 152–3, 155, 164, 225–6
SMART goals 21–2, 98, 99
specificity and training 9, 90
speed skills (SS) 65–6, 75, 102, 129–30, 138, 243–4
sprint power/sprinting 53–5, 65–6, 75, 103, 130, 136–7, 138, 140, 246–7
    testing 77–8, 248

stamina/durability 51–2, 65–6, 75, 78, 104, 133, 135, 137, 138, 140, 245–6
    testing 77, 78, 141, 248
strategy and tactics, race 223–4, 226, 227
stress, positive and negative 11, 41–2, 148-151, 155, 199
Stress Scores, Training 116
stretching and recovery 163
'success savings account' 178–9
superstitions 179–80
supplements, diet/food 190–1, 220–1
support from others 18–19, 178, 179

T

talk tests/ventilatory threshold tests 71
tapering 20–1, 103, 139, 227
teams/team work, high-performance 18–19, 223–4, 226, 227, 230
testing fitness 141, 142, 150–1, 247–8
    see also zones, setting intensity
time limitations and missed workouts 202–5
time to exhaustion 67–8
training principles overview 9–10
TrainingPeaks app 165–6
Transition period 90, 104, 108
travel, international 222, 225, 227

U

undertraining 154–5

V

VO_2 max 48–51, 76, 131, 133, 198, 206–7, 209
VO_2 priming 214–15

W

warm-ups 214–15, 228
weight, body 22, 198–201
weightlifting/strength training see muscular force (MF) training

Z

zones, setting intensity 62–3, 75, 141
    functional threshold heart rate (FTHR) tests 69, 70, 71, 72, 74, 141, 142, 247–8
    functional threshold power (FTP) 69, 72, 74, 141, 247–8
    lactate heart rate tests 70, 71, 74
    lactate power tests (LTP) 74
    lactate threshold 70, 71
    matching intensities and workouts 62–4, 74
    maximal heart rate (MHR) tests 68–9, 71, 72
    rating of perceived exertion (RPE) 67, 75
    talk tests 71, 75
    time to exhaustion 67–8, 75
    Training Triad Abilities 65–6